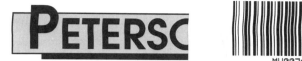

JOB OPPORTUNITIES IN HEALTH CARE
1995

Peterson's
Princeton, New Jersey

To order additional copies of these books, call Peterson's
Customer Service at 800-338-3282.

Editorial inquiries concerning this book should be addressed to the editor at
Peterson's Guides, P.O. Box 2123, Princeton, New Jersey 08543-2123.

ISSN 1071-0671
ISBN 1-56079-370-8
Printed in the United States of America

10 9 8 7 6 5 4 3 2 1

CONTENTS

HOW TO USE THIS BOOK

*P*eterson's *Job Opportunities in Health Care 1995* provides job hunters with vital information on over 1,500 employers in the health-care field. With this information, readers can identify and research companies that are seeking their skills and, by surveying the opportunities presented, build a picture of the various career alternatives in health care.

About Employer Profiles

This guide is not a definitive listing of health-care organizations. If you do not find a particular organization within the pages of this guide, it doesn't necessarily mean that the company has no employment opportunities. Similarly, a listing in the guide does not mean that the organization has immediate openings in the field of expertise mentioned; it simply means that the organization, by virtue of its business, typically seeks employees with the background cited.

Companies and other organizations profiled in this guide were selected based on recent growth in number of employees and sales stability and were then contacted for specific information on the type of employees sought, and appropriate contacts for employment inquiries. Employers were also asked to provide a contact for recent college graduates, if college recruiting is handled separately from overall employment recruiting within the organization. In addition to the above, profiles contain a business description; annual sales and number of employees (last reported publicly available figures as of January 1994); and in most instances, a founding date. Founding dates generally refer to the year in which the organization was first established; however, they may in some cases indicate when the organization underwent the last major change resulting in its current corporate structure. Profiles also contain the number of professional and managerial hires, if the company surveyed was able to provide this information.

About Employer Descriptions

Some organizations have chosen to augment their profile with narrative information about their activities and job opportunities. Short descriptions follow the organizational profile; longer descriptions, in which organizations provide detailed information about their businesses, future employment opportunities, and quality of work life, appear in a separate section following the organizational profiles.

In addition to the information about specific organizations, this book also includes the following valuable features:

Diagnosing Your Health-Care Options
Today's health-care job landscape has its peaks and valleys. But, as the author of this article shows, if you are vigilant about examining each sector of the industry, you can find companies within industry sectors that have strong records of financial stability and growth and job opportunities that fit your expertise.

Search Strategies for Today's Challenging Job Market
Simply keeping your résumé neat and updated isn't enough in today's competitive job market. Here are some insightful tips to help you stand above the crowd.

Finding Jobs With Smaller, Rapid-Growth Companies
It's probably not news to you that smaller companies create a large portion of today's jobs. Learn how to track trends that will help you find these rising stars and how to position yourself for potential employment in a smaller, fast-moving organization.

DIAGNOSING YOUR HEALTH-CARE OPTIONS

By Carter A. Prescott

The health-care industry isn't waiting for Congress to pass reform legislation. It's busy doing what industries across America have been doing for the past five years—reinventing itself.

And a good thing, too. Not even the experts can predict the final shape of the extensive reforms contained in President Clinton's 1,342-page Health Security Act. Congressional deliberations have focused on three major alternatives: a single-payer system, in which the federal government would provide health insurance to all Americans; an employer mandate, under which employers would have to pay most of the bills; and an individual mandate, under which people would have to buy their own insurance, with subsidies or tax credits for those of modest incomes.

Regardless of the final outcome, however, one thing is certain: there will be stepped-up reliance on managed care, where health-care providers team up to share expenses and reduce costs. The goal is to guarantee health insurance to everyone—including the 39 million Americans now without it—and to reduce the cost of health care in the bargain.

What does this mean for job seekers? That health-care reform is likely to force a slowdown in future hiring—at least for the near term. But make no mistake about it: Health-care jobs will continue to grow, as the U.S. Labor Department points out, just more slowly than in the 1980s.

Good News/ Bad News

There's plenty of good news here—and some bad news, too. But if you're vigilant about examining each sector of the health-care industry then you can find a company within a sector that has a strong record of financial stability and innovation and maybe a berth for you as well.

But that's not to say that rose petals will litter your path. Montgomery Securities analyst Leonard Yaffe predicts a "phenomenal consolidation" in the health-care industry—with resulting job cuts. Already, health-care cost increases have slowed. Nonetheless, overall spending in 1993 was up 10.2 percent, to an estimated $903.3 billion. Medical price increases are estimated to lift health care's share of the nation's economy from one-seventh to one-fifth by the year 2000.

That means the health services industry will continue to be a major driver of job growth. After all, this sector has added 1.4 million jobs since 1990. But the widespread downsizing and restructuring that has hit other industries has affected health care, too. Expect to hunt hard for your first job, and when you get it, expect to work harder and do more with less.

How to Make Your Search Successful

The key to a successful job search, Yaffe advises, is to survey the scene with a cold analytical eye, then ferret out those companies that are scoring at the expense of other companies. For example, health maintenance organizations (HMOs) look like winners in an era of "managed competition," where large groups negotiate steep discounts on the price of doctors' care, hospital services, and prescription drugs. But not all HMOs are created equal, and smaller ones are likely to be gobbled up by bigger fish. Ergo, aim for the whales, not the minnows.

Companies whose market is health-care providers—but whose products or services aren't in health care at all—are other potential winners. For example, check out companies that market billing software for managed-care providers. If your skills are in computers and their clients are rock-solid HMOs, you may have yourself a job.

Carter A. Prescott is a business writer and corporate communications consultant based in New York City.

Another sector that stands to gain is managed-care drug companies, which could control 80 percent of this $60-billion-a-year market in the next five years. Also called pharmacy benefit managers, these firms sprang up in the last few years to buy prescription drugs for HMOs—and to wring out substantial discounts from drug manufacturers, who risked losing millions of potential customers otherwise. Led by PCS Health Systems, a unit of McKesson Corporation, as well as Medco Containment Services, Diversified Pharmaceutical Services, Caremark International, Value Health, and Express Scripts, managed-care drug companies already have taken charge of more than half the nation's drug business. As a result, drug companies are laying off many of their salespeople, or "detailers," as they're known in the trade.

In response, several major pharmaceutical firms have moved into this sector, hoping to increase sales to managed-care customers. Merck & Company started the stampede in 1993, paying $6.6 billion for Medco. In the spring of 1994, SmithKline Beecham bought Diversified, and Pfizer announced alliances with Value Health and Caremark. Analysts say the British drug maker Glaxo Holdings might acquire PCS, while Value Health and Express Scripts are promising candidates for a takeover by Glaxo or Sandoz, Ltd., a major Swiss-based drug company.

Elsewhere on the pharmaceutical horizon, Kodak decided to get out of the drug business altogether, putting its Sterling Winthrop subsidiary up for sale. Roche Holding, another big Swiss drug maker, took the opposite tack. Aiming to expand its U.S. presence, it acquired Syntex of California, whose aging product line made it highly vulnerable. Industry executives believe that more mergers and acquisitions lie ahead as drug makers, hospitals and HMOs struggle with growing competition and demands for lower prices for drugs and health-care services.

The moral here is to pick your targets wisely. Many pharmaceutical companies will continue to do very well in coming years. As the population ages—and if millions of previously uninsured people can finally afford prescriptions—many drug makers' fortunes should not sag precariously. Also, the savvy ones are deadly serious about maintaining market share. They're expanding overseas sales and making cheaper generic equivalents of their own products as they come off patent.

Star Biotech Firms

If you want to work for a pharmaceutical company, take a close look at sizzling hot biotech firms—especially those engaged in genetic

HOW TO TRACK AN INDUSTRY

Once you have used this book to identify employers you may be interested in, take the time to investigate their industry group. The current financial performance and future prospects of an industry, as a whole, in which you take a job will directly affect your job security, along with your chance for raises and promotions. It is easy to become better informed. Consult with general business magazines such as *Business Week*, *Forbes*, or *Fortune*. They do most of the work for you.

For instance, each year these magazines publish industry-by-industry analyses of the top corporations in the United States. Use the industry-by-industry figures provided to judge the overall prospects of a company you are interested in, regardless of whether it is actually listed. Look for industries that are rated above average in sales growth, profits as a percentage of sales, and growth in the number of employees. Keep in mind that one or two years of bad results for an industry does not necessarily mean the industry is in permanent decline; some industries are more sensitive to short-term economic conditions than others.

The point is that tracking an industry takes many different forms. You should study the raw data— the numbers—but look at the intangibles and, especially, at the future.

research. Decoding the fundamental secrets of life is expected to produce novel and uniquely effective medicines that attack the causes of disease, not just the symptoms. Analysts see a $7-billion-a-year industry taking shape in the next few years.

Human Genome Sciences (HGS) in Rockville, Maryland, is the largest and most lavishly financed of about a dozen new companies racing to crack the human genetic code. Some analysts think HGS is so far ahead of the field that it may be the Microsoft of genetics in the making. Even better, it has the backing of drug giant SmithKline Beecham. Hoffman-La Roche has invested in Millennium Pharmaceuticals of Cambridge, Massachusetts, and Eli Lilly has joined forces with Myriad Genetics of Salt Lake City. Other comers: Sequana Therapeutics of La Jolla, California; Genica Pharmaceuticals of Worcester, Massachusetts; Darwin Molecular of Bothwell, Washington; and GenVec of Rockville, Maryland. "This is biotech's

OCCUPATIONS FOR THE FUTURE

How does the job scene shape up for the years ahead? Here's a look at projected percentage growth for 1990–2005 for selected health-services occupations:

1. Physical therapists (87%)
2. Medical scientists (87%)
3. Medical assistants (77%)
4. Radiologic technicians (72%)
5. Occupational therapists (65%)
6. Human services workers (64%)
7. Speech-language pathologists (62%)

8. Medical records technicians (58%)
9. Surgical technicians (55%)
10. Respiratory therapists (53%)
11. Recreation workers (50%)
12. Registered nurses (49%)
13. Physicians (44%)
14. Pharmacists (35%)

From the U.S. Department of Labor Bureau of Labor Statistics Occupational Outlook: 1990–2005.

---

counterpart of the Oklahoma land rush," says Kevin Kinsella, a veteran venture capitalist and founder and CEO of Sequana Therapeutics.

Challenges for Hospital Hiring

In those areas of health care that deal directly with patients, the immediate hiring picture is murky. Many hospitals, for example, have empty beds and huge overheads ever since Medicare began reimbursing on fixed rates rather than a percentage of full costs. Accounting firm Kenneth Leventhal & Co. predicts that hospitals will eliminate 5 percent to 10 percent of their 920,000 beds to cut overhead in each of the next several years.

On the other hand, many hospitals may get a financial windfall under the Clinton plan if all Americans are assured of some type of health insurance, because hospitals would be paid to provide care to people who now pay little or nothing. Most hospital administrators reject this scenario, however, arguing that hospitals would reduce their charges under managed competition.

Four Million New Health-Care Jobs by 2005

Despite rising costs and other job deflating factors, the demand for health-care services will ultimately fuel growth in job opportunities. The U.S. Bureau of Labor Statistics predicts that the health services industry will add 3.9 million jobs by 2005—17 percent of total employment growth, the most of any single field. Some 1.3 million of these jobs will be in hospitals, 900,000 in physician's offices and 700,000 in nursing and personal-care facilities. Even if you're only qualified or interested in a minute percentage of those four million jobs, that still means thousands of open-

ings. In fact, half of the 30 fastest-growing occupations the Bureau projected to the year 2005 are professional and technical health-care jobs. Some require significant postsecondary education, like psychologists; others don't require college degrees at all, like home health aides and medical secretaries.

Key Trends Fuel Growth

What's fueling all this growth? Four trends stand out, according to the Bureau of Labor Statistics and industry analysts:

■ **An aging population.** Those people age 75 and older, who require the most health care, will increase by 35 percent, much faster than the total population. Baby-boomers are aging, too, and their health-care needs also will rise.

■ **New medical technology.** It creates higher demand for more services and more intensive care.

■ **Increased public and private financing of health-care services.** Even if Congress waters down President Clinton's reform proposals, employers will increasingly seek out HMOs and PPOs (preferred provider organizations, which allow patients to see doctors outside the network) or set up their own health networks to hold the line on costs.

■ **Phenomenal growth in home health care.** This $22 billion industry benefits as insurers force hospitals to restrict lengthy stays. And as more and more sophisticated treatment becomes available on an outpatient basis, patients can conclude their recuperation in the comfort of their own homes.

HOW TO TRACK A COMPANY

Once you have checked the overall performance of a company's industry, you can use the library or your computer to gather more information about the company itself. Perform database searches to look for mention in the press of new products or new contracts, along with comments from industry analysts. You invariably will impress the people who are conducting an interview by informing yourself about their company before you get there. An hour's worth of research time will make you look sharp and prepared and put you in a position to interview them while they are interviewing you.

If a company is publicly traded on a stock exchange, you can also take advantage of a good indicator of a company's future performance. Look at the P/E (price-to-earnings) ratio of companies you are interested in over the last year or so. Compare this ratio to other companies in the same industry. You can find up-to-date figures for most publicly traded companies in the *Wall Street Journal* or *Barron's*. If the P/E of a company in a healthy industry is significantly higher than other, similar companies, the stock market's judgment is that the near- to mid-term prospects for profitability of that company are good.

Companies that are achieving profitability through sales growth and high profit margins typically will be hiring. The stock market is full of smart people doing their best to judge the prospects of companies year in and year out. They are not always right, of course, but they have more sources of information at their disposal than the average job seeker. Take advantage of them.

National health-care reform notwithstanding, the Bureau of Labor Statistics has indicated that occupations concentrating in the health services industry will be among the most rapidly growing occupations, with very favorable employment prospects.

The big questions are, Which jobs and where? Generally speaking, the Bureau of Labor Statistics sees relatively rapid job growth for physical therapists (87 percent) and registered nurses (40 percent), for example. But even with strong job growth predicted, surpluses in certain occupations still can occur. Here's a closer look.

Nurses: Surplus or Shortage?

It depends on where you live. Rose Houston, in nurse recruitment since 1967 and now president of a Chicago temporary-nurse agency called HealthStaffers, Inc., says there is "no across-the-board shortage now, but there are always shortages in rural areas and in expensive places to live, like Hawaii." California, she adds, "no longer feels like it has a severe shortage."

One of her competitors agrees—and disagrees. "There is minimum demand for medical-surgical nurses, except in rural areas," says Bruce Male, president of TravCorps in Malden, Massachusetts, a company that provides temporary health-care professionals around the country. "But there is still a shortage of critical care and labor and delivery nurses."

Adds Houston: "Opportunities have been more limited for nurses, but we're on the verge of an upturn because the economy is better. A lot of health care is elective, and people now have more money to pay for it." Economic fluxes notwithstanding, however, she says overall there are "still more opportunities for nurses than in most any other field."

Indeed, for the first time, the highest-paid 1993 graduates of the University of Delaware were nurses. They started at an average of $32,858, displacing engineers, who started at $32,298.

WORK IN A HOSPITAL, THEN GO HOME—TO SOMEONE ELSE'S HOME, THAT IS

No doubt about it: Home health care is the hottest segment of the industry now and into the foreseeable future, as the population ages and hospital stays shorten.

But it's not the best area for new nursing graduates, cautions Karen S. Peters, RN, former director of nursing at Alpha Home Health Care in Green Bay, Wisconsin. "Too many independent decisions are needed that they don't have the experience to handle," she observes.

"When you're catheterizing a patient in the home, for example, you're on your own with no one to help you. Solidify your skills first in a hospital for a year or two."

"DON'T BECOME A DOCTOR"

That's the strongly worded advice of Leonard Yaffe, an analyst for Montgomery Securities in San Francisco. "They have too much debt at graduation, and they enter a practice that is not as lucrative or enjoyable as it was in the past," he says. "Managed care is placing greater restrictions on what they can and can't do in their practices, but if they don't work in a managed-care environment, the paperwork is unbelievable."

On the other hand, physicians working in HMOs, for example, are generally assured of steady hours. Yes, salaries can be lower (how much lower depends on the specialty) and tend not to increase much over the years, but the steadier hours mean fewer on-call, sleepless nights.

If you want to be a doctor, rural America desperately needs you, especially if you want to set up a family practice. Think about it: Overjoyed patients, clean air, a great place to raise a family . . . and maybe even a hit TV show if you move to Alaska.

A good way to "call your own shots and go anywhere" is to "get the additional training and become a nurse practitioner," advises Karen S. Peters, RN, former assistant director of nursing at the University of Illinois Medical Center. "Many people believe that successful health-care reform will involve reducing the number of medical specialists and increasing the number of generalists and nurse practitioners."

Allied Health Care Personnel—The More, The Better

"Severe shortages of allied health personnel "have gone virtually unnoticed by the general public," says TravCorps president Bruce Male.

For example, there's always a shortage of physical therapists. "It's one of the hottest fields," he notes. With the rise of PT-owned orthopedic and sports rehabilitation centers, newly minted physical therapists have a wide choice of employers, along with flexible hours and continuing education opportunities. In May 1994, a New York City rehabilitation center was offering physical therapists annual salaries of up to $50,000 plus $3,000 sign-on bonuses. Nor should PTs—and speech and language pathologists—overlook early-childhood intervention programs in schools, where toddlers from three years and up can receive therapy through Head Start initiatives.

Ads in mid-1994 issues of *The New York Times* offered occupational therapists their choice of full-time, part-time, or contract jobs—and specifically targeted new grads. OTs are in demand because rehabilitation services increase the survival rate of accident victims. And an aging population increases the need for long-term care.

The ranks of respiratory therapists are expected to swell by an additional 31,000 jobs by 2005. A significant percentage of the coming bulge of middle-aged and elderly people will suffer from cardiopulmonary diseases. Employment will grow fastest in home health-care services, though hospitals will continue to be primary employers.

The relatively new field of "portable" X-ray technology—as in, Have X-Ray Machine, Will Travel—offers applicants their choice of full-time or part-time positions. In New York City, some candidates with "previous portable experience" have garnered a $3,000 sign-on bonus, full benefits, and a brand-new car.

For medical technologists and technicians, a host of federal regulations have raised the bar for credentials for lab personnel. As a result, lab staffing structures are changing faster, and fewer—but more highly educated and higher paid—technologists and technicians will be used. Depending on the region, lab technologists (who typically have bachelor's degrees) may earn an additional $3 to $6 an hour over the hourly wages of lab technicians. In the meantime, while hospitals and clinics determine the impact of the new regulations, it's a seller's market for highly credentialed technologists and technicians.

Jobs for pharmacists also are expected to increase by 35 percent by the year 2005, according to the Bureau of Labor Statistics. In addition to drug stores, pharmacists are finding jobs in HMOs, drug companies, and even grocery store chains.

Health-Care Managers: A Rosy Forecast for MBAs

If you can cut costs the way Paul Bunyan cut trees, there's a secure job in your future. Positions for health-care administrators will increase by more than 50 percent by 2005, according to Labor Department figures. HMOs and long-term care facilities will be eager employers, as will those hospitals striving to stay competitive. While an M.A. in public health or hospital administration has been the usual ticket to success, the more generalist M.B.A. degree is growing in favor.

WANT FLEXIBLE HOURS AND HIGH PAY?

"Temp" nursing is a good field for returning nurses, assuming you've taken refresher courses. You can choose your own hours and make about twice the hourly pay that full-time staff nurses earn—with full benefits to boot. If you'd rather, some agencies will let you decline the benefits in exchange for more pay.

Temporary nursing is not a good bet for brand-new nurses, however. Most reputable agencies won't take new graduates. "Wait until you feel comfortable with your skills," counsels Rose Houston, president of HealthStaffers, Inc., in Chicago. "We require one to five years' experience in a specialty, not just experience in a medical-surgical unit."

Temporary nurses work on a per-diem (day-rate) basis. In contrast, traveling nurses usually work three months at a time—often in such locations as Hawaii, Australia, or Saudi Arabia—with their travel and living expenses fully paid.

Temp agencies' biggest competitors are hospitals, which often set up their own part-timer pools to save money and standardize training and the quality of care provided. Most hospital pool nurses work a few days a week in addition to holding full-time jobs.

And Let's Not Forget . . .

Bless those aging teeth . . . and eyes . . . and feet. As baby boomers age, dentists, optometrists, opticians, and podiatrists will be overwhelmed with business, as will their assistants.

And opportunities for nutritionists and dieticians extend beyond the hospital kitchen. Food companies, public relations agencies that have food clients, and restaurant chains—all of whom must meet the needs of an increasingly health-conscious public and stringent new federal food labeling requirements—are welcoming applicants with nutrition and dietetics backgrounds. Employment will increase by more than 25 percent by the year 2005, government data shows.

Stay the Course

As you work your way through this maze of options, take heart in knowing that you're still on the right track: By some measures, the explosion in health-care spending accounted for all of the nation's job growth since 1989. And it still appears that health-care spending will continue to account for a significant chunk of new jobs for the rest of the century. You just may have to print up a few more résumés to get the job that's right for you.

LIKE YOUR GRANDMA? YOU'LL LOVE THIS JOB

Geriatric medicine will be a booming business as Americans live longer. Doctors, nurses, and physical therapists specializing in the needs of the elderly will find plenty of jobs in hospitals, nursing homes, patients' homes, hospices, and continuing-care facilities.

SEARCH STRATEGIES FOR TODAY'S CHALLENGING JOB MARKET

Finding a job is never a cakewalk, but if you follow these guidelines, you'll be a stand-out in your first job—and for the rest of your career.

■ ***Do your homework: Carefully research prospective employers.*** "I have to beat people up about this," says Belinda Plutz, who worked 15 years in hospitals before founding Career Mentors, a New York–based career development consulting firm. "Employers like to know that you really want to work for them. The best way to prove that is to research their products and markets so you can show how your skills can contribute to their growth potential."

■ ***Get the right training.*** That's especially important if you're switching careers, Plutz notes. She tells the story of a woman who got a certificate in counseling from New York University, only to discover she couldn't get a job because she needed a Masters of Social Work degree instead. Plutz's advice: "Research what credentials you need from the employer's—not the school's—end. Talk to physical therapists if you want to be a PT, to registered nurses if you want to be an RN."

■ ***Read and write English well.*** Whether you're born in America or overseas, you can stand out by communicating well, especially if you have a science background (where it's expected that your math skills will far outweigh your verbal abilities).

■ ***Know a foreign language.*** Better yet, spend time living or working abroad. Health care is an increasingly global business as American companies go overseas for fresh markets and European and Japanese firms establish footholds in the United States. French, Japanese, and Spanish are the most useful languages.

■ ***Be results-oriented.*** Show what you can do for employers, not how wonderful you are (that goes for both the interview and any introductory or thank you letters). Employers look for problem-solvers who can be productive quickly.

■ ***Get as much practical experience as possible.*** "Everyone comes out of school looking and smelling like each other," complains Bob Jacobs, president of Health Resources Optimization, Inc., in Metuchen, New Jersey. "You need practical skills, not just theoretical discussions." While still in school, work part-time in health care, get internships, volunteer—do projects that take you out of the classroom and into the field. Not only will you get valuable experience, you'll find out what areas you like and don't like.

■ ***Don't try to change the system to fit you; adapt yourself to the system.*** "When people lose their jobs, eighty percent of the time it's due to personality conflicts, not performance," says Wendy Alfus Rothman, an organizational psychologist and president of Wenroth, Inc., a management consulting firm in New York. "Understand the corporate or departmental culture to be sure you can—and want to—fit in. Then do so."

■ ***Network, network, network.*** This is especially true for minorities, Plutz says. "Professional groups composed of minorities make a big effort to help newcomers," she notes. "Take advantage of that help. You can never know too many people."

■ ***Have your own career goals.*** Remember, only you control your destiny, Rothman notes. So research your options and determine the fit. "Hiring managers like to know that you have thought through what you want in life—even if that changes over time. People want to hire those who are clear about their direction rather than those they'll have to baby-sit or who might change their minds two weeks into the job."

■ ***Pay attention to the details.*** Spell people's names right (is it "John" or "Jon"? "Karen," "Karin," or "Karyn"?). Check the gender of androgynous names (don't assume, for example, that the author of this article is a man). Always address elders as "Mr." "Ms." or "Dr." on first meeting. And if you go to work in a hospital, never ask patients, "How are we feeling today?" Patients figure that if you don't know how you're feeling, how can you help them.

FINDING JOBS WITH SMALLER, RAPID-GROWTH COMPANIES

Emerging companies may be small, but they're sizzling with employment prospects for people who have the right technical abilities and are nimble enough to keep pace in fast-moving environments.

In fact, small business continues to drive most job creation. Small businesses showed a 45 percent increase in hiring in 1993 according to a survey conducted by Olsten Corporation, a temporary placement firm. These job gains occurred at twice the rate of major corporations, a trend expected to continue throughout 1994. The Olsen survey also indicated that small companies experience fewer layoffs—25 percent in 1993, compared with 52 percent in big businesses. Even better, small business provides two of every three workers with their first jobs, according to Arthur Andersen's Enterprise Group. And with 20 million companies employing fewer than 500 people, that's a lot of opportunity.

"Young, emerging growth companies have the flexibility and energy to respond to market needs," notes Robert C. Czepiel, manager of the Robertson Stephens Emerging Growth Fund. In contrast, many big companies are continuing to focus on downsizing and cost containment instead of product development.

The examples that follow highlight the qualities that aggressive, young firms are looking for in new employees. You'll find plenty of other examples of small, dynamic companies throughout the Employer Profiles section of this book—many looking for similar attributes in future employees.

Flexibility and Energy Wanted

Generic drug maker Geneva Pharmaceuticals is a good example of a dynamic, young firm. In the last two years alone, its workforce has doubled, to 814 employees. This Ciba Pharmaceuticals subsidiary manufactures and distributes more than 1,000 generic drugs.

Geneva hires *a lot* of temporary summer help, mostly the sons and daughters of people already working there. "One guy started sweeping floors in high school and he's now a marketing analyst," reports Joni Cuevas, human resources manager. "We're very much a family company."

But you don't have to be related to a Geneva employee to get hired. Just make sure you're customer-focused and a good team player, she advises. And be flexible. Cuevas landed her current position with no experience in human resources. However, her six years as a field sales rep meant that she knew the customers well and "had the respect of my peers," as she puts it. "They figured you can teach someone human resources, but you can't teach them to have a good feel for the company and its customers."

Team Orientation a Prerequisite

Healthsource, Inc., is another fast-growing firm. Just since its inception in 1985, Healthsource has grown from a start-up HMO plan in New Hampshire to become the operator or manager of health plans in 12 states, providing managed care services to more than 750,000 people. It was recently ranked 26th in *Business Week*'s 250 Companies on the Move and 106th in *Forbes*' listing of "best small companies."

From its base in Concord, Healthsource continues to import jobs into the state. In mid-1994, the company employed 600 workers in three different New Hampshire locations and more than 1,300 nationwide. Its New Hampshire base doubled in size from mid-1992 to mid-1993, as the company acquired many of the managed care plans it now operates throughout the Northeast, Southeast and Midwest. "We're still growing significantly," says Tim Dean, public relations manager.

Dean joined Healthsource in 1989 after being laid off from Digital Equipment Corporation, a worldwide company with more than 100,000 employees. "When I first arrived, there were only

75 to 80 people working here," he recalls. "Our corporate culture has been formed by the personality and contributions of those original employees, many of whom now direct major functional areas of the company."

Comparing his experience working for a giant employer, Dean says, It's much more personal working for a small company that's growing quickly, more like a family. You can form close relationships with people." Nor is the environment "rigidly structured," he notes. Communication and decision making are "spontaneous," with problem solving occurring in teams of workers cooperating across departments.

A Commitment to Customers—
Internal and External

As with Geneva Pharmaceuticals, a commitment to serving customers—both internal and external—is central to employees' mission. He cites "Super Saturdays" as a case in point. Hundreds of employees from all departments rally together, volunteering their time on Saturdays to help departments reduce the backlog of work created by the company's unprecedented growth. And a new Job Exchange program—in which department managers, the CEO and other senior executives spend one day a month working in a different department—helps company leadership better understand and appreciate the kind and quality of work done. As for pay and benefits, they're "very competitive" with large corporations, Dean says.

For People Who Want to Make a Difference

If tons of intensity and excitement set your blood pumping, then check out Chiron Corporation, one of the "powerhouses of biotechnology," according to analyst Andre Garnet at A. G. Edwards & Sons. Says Larry Kurtz, vice president of corporate communications, "The atmosphere here is very intense, like it is with most biotech and smaller, entrepreneurial companies. We're very lean. Every possible dollar is spent on research."

Despite the intensity, it's "a fun place to work," Kurtz reports. "We're very informal. Even though we have 2,300 employees worldwide, it still feels like a small company. People wear jeans, shorts and T-shirts in the labs, and Friday is a formal dress-down day."

Founded in 1981 by three university scientists, Chiron "draws from the strengths of a university environment," he explains. Work groups interact frequently, and seminars are held weekly with outside speakers discussing their work.

Chiron has partnered with leading drug makers to develop the first treatment available for multiple sclerosis and the first genetically engineered vaccine for hepatitis B. Other key products improve vision, fight cancer, and treat infectious diseases.

"Young people get opportunities faster here than they would in large companies, and they can move up quickly," Kurtz notes. "There's a strong demand for talent here." Workforce growth mushroomed 320 percent between 1989 and 1993, from 680 to 2,179 employees.

Chiron attracts people "with a sense of purpose, who want to make a difference," he says. Indeed, the company's mission statement says its products "transform the practice of medicine," and Chiron employees believe they "change people's lives."

But you won't succeed at Chiron—or any other biotech company—if you want to do routine work from 9 to 5. "Safe people wouldn't enjoy it here," Kurtz says. "We try not to penalize people for taking risks and reward them for their successes instead. You have to be confident of your skills, because we push responsibility to the lowest possible level."

EMPLOYER PROFILES

A listing of U.S. health-care and related companies and select government organizations, organized alphabetically

ABBOTT LABORATORIES
1 ABBOTT PARK ROAD
ABBOTT PARK, ILLINOIS 60064-3500

Description: Manufactures pharmaceutical, nutritional, hospital, and laboratory products
Founded: 1888
Annual Sales: $8.4 billion
Number of Employees: 50,000
Number of Managerial and Professional Employees Hired 1993: 497
Expertise Needed: Biochemistry, chemical engineering, chemistry, biomedical engineering, marketing, finance, molecular biology, laboratory technology
Contact: Ms Jean Jackson-Swopes, PhD
Manager of College Relations
(708) 937-9016

ABBOTT-NORTHWESTERN HOSPITAL
800 EAST 28TH STREET
MINNEAPOLIS, MINNESOTA 55407-3723

Description: General medical and surgical hospital
Parent Company: Lifespan, Inc.
Annual Sales: $310.0 million
Number of Employees: 5,167
Expertise Needed: Nursing, occupational therapy
Contact: Ms Nancy Paine
Employment Manager
(612) 863-4842

ABINGTON MEMORIAL HOSPITAL
1200 OLD YORK ROAD
ABINGTON, PENNSYLVANIA 19001-3720

Description: General medical and surgical hospital
Founded: 1913
Annual Sales: $185.4 million
Number of Employees: 2,889
Expertise Needed: Physical therapy, occupational therapy, laboratory technology, medical technology
Contact: Ms Meghan Patton
Employment Manager
(215) 576-2000

ABRASIVE TECHNOLOGY, INC.
8400 GREEN MEADOWS DRIVE
WESTERVILLE, OHIO 43081

Description: Manufactures dental equipment and supplies
Founded: 1971
Number of Employees: 100
Expertise Needed: Mechanical engineering, industrial engineering
Contact: Ms Dotti Riggs
Human Resources Department
(614) 548-4100

ACCESS HEALTH MARKETING
11020 WHITE ROCK ROAD
RANCHO CORDOVA, CALIFORNIA 95670

Description: Provides medical education and training services and markets medical data processing software
Annual Sales: $124.0 million
Number of Employees: 165
Expertise Needed: Nursing, marketing
Contact: Ms Joanne Paglucia
Human Resources Representative
(416) 851-4000

ACOUSTIC IMAGING TECHNOLOGY, INC.
10027 SOUTH 51ST STREET
PHOENIX, ARIZONA 85044-5204

Description: Manufactures diagnostic ultrasound imaging equipment and transducers
Parent Company: Dornier Medical Systems, Inc.
Annual Sales: $26.0 million
Number of Employees: 230
Expertise Needed: Electrical engineering, computer science, mechanical engineering
Contact: Ms Patty Fenger
Human Resources Administrator
(602) 496-6681

ACUFEX MICROSURGICAL, INC.
130 FORBES BOULEVARD
MANSFIELD, MASSACHUSETTS 02048-1145

Description: Manufactures microsurgical instruments
Parent Company: American Cyanamid Company
Annual Sales: $42.0 million
Number of Employees: 250
Expertise Needed: Accounting, marketing, finance, management information systems, sales
Contact: Director of Human Resources
(508) 339-9700

ACUSON CORPORATION
1220 CHARLESTON ROAD
MOUNTAIN VIEW, CALIFORNIA 94043-1330

Description: Manufactures medical diagnostic ultrasound imaging systems
Founded: 1979
Annual Sales: $342.8 million
Number of Employees: 1,722
Number of Managerial and Professional Employees Hired 1993: 100
Expertise Needed: Hardware engineering, marketing, sales, finance, software engineering/development, mechanical engineering, accounting, management information systems
Contact: Department of Employment
(415) 969-9112

ADAMS LABORATORIES, INC.
14801 SOVEREIGN ROAD
FORT WORTH, TEXAS 76155-2645

Description: Pharmaceuticals laboratory
Annual Sales: $22.5 million
Number of Employees: 250
Expertise Needed: Chemistry, biochemistry, microbiology
Contact: Ms Joni Walpole
        Assistant Director of Human Resources
        (817) 545-7791

ADDICTION RESEARCH & TREATMENT
22 CHAPEL STREET
BROOKLYN, NEW YORK 11201-1903

Description: Drug rehabilitation center
Founded: 1969
Annual Sales: $18.6 million
Number of Employees: 350
Expertise Needed: Registered nursing, licensed practical nursing, physical therapy, social work, occupational therapy
Contact: Mr Mario Hoyle
        Personnel Recruiter
        (718) 260-2900

ADVACARE, INC.
9696 SKILLMAN
DALLAS, TEXAS 75243-2219

Description: Provides third-party claims management and medical practice management consulting services
Annual Sales: $54.8 million
Number of Employees: 1,600
Expertise Needed: Data processing, management information systems, business management
Contact: Ms. Donna Elwell
        Director of Human Resources
        (214) 226-0348

ADVANCED TECHNOLOGY LABORATORIES
221 BOTHELL HIGHWAY
SEATTLE, WASHINGTON 98021-8431

Description: Manufactures ultrasound devices
Founded: 1958
Annual Sales: $504.7 million
Number of Employees: 2,100
Expertise Needed: Mechanical engineering, design engineering, electrical engineering, manufacturing engineering, acoustic engineering, customer service and support, sales, engineering technology, software engineering/development, accounting
Contact: Ms Pam Kovarik
        Personnel Recruiter
        (206) 487-7418

ADVANTAGE HEALTH CORPORATION
304 CAMBRIDGE ROAD
WOBURN, MASSACHUSETTS 01801-6040

Description: Operates medical rehabilitation facilities and provides home health-care services
Founded: 1982
Annual Sales: $80.8 million
Number of Employees: 2,500
Expertise Needed: Physical therapy, occupational therapy, accounting, medical technology, registered nursing, licensed practical nursing
Contact: Ms Lynne Aston
        Human Resources
        (617) 935-2500

ADVENTIST HEALTH SYSTEMS SUNBELT
2400 BEDFORD ROAD
ORLANDO, FLORIDA 32803-1418

Description: Church-operated, multi-hospital health-care system
Founded: 1973
Annual Sales: $21.5 million
Number of Employees: 8,000
Expertise Needed: Physicians, pharmacy, radiology
Contact: Ms Debbie Bishop
        Manager of Recruiting
        (407) 897-1919

ADVENTIST HEALTH SYSTEMS/SUNBELT
2400 BEDFORD ROAD
ORLANDO, FLORIDA 32803-1418

Description: Owns and operates hospitals and medical centers
Founded: 1973
Annual Sales: $805.7 million
Number of Employees: 9,500
Expertise Needed: Accounting, finance, data processing, marketing, health insurance, law
Contact: Mr James Thompson
        Senior Vice President of Human Resources
        (407) 897-1919

ADVENTIST HEALTH SYSTEMS/WEST
2100 DOUGLAS BOULEVARD
ROSEVILLE, CALIFORNIA 95661-3808

Description: Church-operated, multi-hospital health-care system
Founded: 1973
Annual Sales: $1.4 billion
Number of Employees: 13,500
Expertise Needed: Accounting, finance, data processing, nursing, computer programming
Contact: Mr Roger Ashley
        Director of Human Resources
        (916) 781-4740

ADVENTIST HEALTHCARE/MIDDLE ATLANTIC
10800 LOCKWOOD DRIVE
ROCKVILLE, MARYLAND 20850-1554

Description: Owns and operates hospitals and medical centers
Parent Company: Columbia Union Conference
Annual Sales: $961.2 million
Number of Employees: 20,359
Expertise Needed: Accounting, data processing
Contact: Mr Daryl Milam
　　　Director of Human Resources
　　　(301) 279-6256

AETNA HEALTH PLANS OF SOUTHERN CALIFORNIA
303 EAST VANDERBILT WAY
SAN BERNARDINO, CALIFORNIA 92408-3519

Description: Health maintenance organization
Parent Company: Partners National Health Plans
Annual Sales: $561.2 million
Number of Employees: 283
Expertise Needed: Finance, business, case management
Contact: Human Resources Department
　　　(909) 888-2060

AFFILIATED MEDICAL CENTERS OF PENNSYLVANIA, WILLMAR CLINIC
101 WILLMAR AVENUE SOUTHWEST
WILLMAR, MINNESOTA 56201-3556

Description: Multi-specialty clinic
Founded: 1971
Annual Sales: $36.4 million
Number of Employees: 530
Expertise Needed: Licensed practical nursing, data processing
Contact: Ms Pat Phrolson
　　　Manager of Nursing/Patient Relations
　　　(612) 231-5000

AKRON GENERAL MEDICAL CENTER
400 WABASH AVENUE
AKRON, OHIO 44307-2433

Description: General medical and surgical hospital
Parent Company: Health Network of Ohio, Inc.
Founded: 1914
Annual Sales: $193.9 million
Number of Employees: 2,400
Expertise Needed: Radiation technology, physical therapy, occupational therapy, registered nursing
Contact: Ms B. J. Aberlinger
　　　Coordinator of Human Resources
　　　(216) 384-6090

AL LABORATORIES, INC.
1 EXECUTIVE DRIVE
FORT LEE, NEW JERSEY 07024-3303

Description: Develops and manufactures pharmaceuticals and animal health products
Founded: 1975
Annual Sales: $295.1 million
Number of Employees: 2,000
Expertise Needed: Veterinary, agricultural science
Contact: Ms Patricia Lewis
　　　Recruiter
　　　(201) 947-7774

ALACARE HOME HEALTH SERVICE
1945 HOOVER COURT
BIRMINGHAM, ALABAMA 35226-3606

Description: Home health-care agency
Founded: 1970
Annual Sales: $20.0 million
Number of Employees: 550
Expertise Needed: Registered nursing, licensed practical nursing, physical therapy, occupational therapy, social work
Contact: Ms Kay Sykes
　　　Human Resources Manager
　　　(205) 823-7081

ALADAN CORPORATION
630 COLUMBIA HIGHWAY
DOTHAN, ALABAMA 36303-5412

Description: Manufactures latex gloves and condoms
Annual Sales: $60.7 million
Number of Employees: 438
Expertise Needed: Engineering, accounting
Contact: Ms Belinda Bracewell
　　　Director of Personnel
　　　(205) 793-4509

ALBERT EINSTEIN MEDICAL CENTER
5501 OLD YORK ROAD
PHILADELPHIA, PENNSYLVANIA 19141-3001

Description: Private hospital
Founded: 1952
Annual Sales: $257.8 million
Number of Employees: 4,450
Expertise Needed: Administration, registered nursing
Contact: Ms Nancy Glassburg
　　　Director of Human Resources
　　　(215) 456-8035

ALCO HEALTH SERVICES CORPORATION
300 CHESTER FIELD PARKWAY
MALVERN, PENNSYLVANIA 19355-9726

Description: Distributes pharmaceuticals and health-care products
Founded: 1933
Annual Sales: $3.3 billion

Alco Health Services Corporation (continued)
Number of Employees: 2,269
Expertise Needed: Accounting, finance, management
Contact: Mr Robert Gregory
Vice President of Human Resources
(610) 296-4480

ALCON LABORATORIES, INC.
6201 SOUTH FREEWAY
FORT WORTH, TEXAS 76134-2001

Description: Manufactures ophthalmic pharmaceuticals, surgical instruments and kits, and diagnostic instruments
Founded: 1947
Annual Sales: $872.7 million
Number of Employees: 4,600
Expertise Needed: Microbiology, research and development, chemistry, pharmaceutical, toxicology, computer programming, data processing, accounting, customer service and support
Contact: Mr Mike Farell
Recruiter
(817) 293-0450

ALCON SURGICAL, INC.
6201 SOUTH FREEWAY
FORT WORTH, TEXAS 76134-2001

Description: Manufactures ophthalmic instruments and pharmaceuticals for eye surgery
Parent Company: Alcon Laboratories, Inc.
Annual Sales: $117.8 million
Number of Employees: 1,400
Expertise Needed: Manufacturing engineering, mechanical engineering, ophthalmological engineering
Contact: Mr Ken Stevens
Director of Recruiting
(817) 293-0450

ALDRICH CHEMICAL COMPANY, INC.
1001 WEST SAINT PAUL AVENUE
MILWAUKEE, WISCONSIN 53233-2625

Description: Commercial physical research company specializing in industrial inorganic and organic chemicals, medicinals, and botanicals
Founded: 1951
Number of Employees: 920
Expertise Needed: Chemistry, laboratory technology
Contact: Ms Laura Backe
Administrator
(414) 273-3850

ALEXIAN BROTHERS MEDICAL CENTER
800 BIESTERFIELD ROAD
ELK GROVE VILLAGE, ILLINOIS 60007-3311

Description: General medical and surgical hospital
Founded: 1966

Annual Sales: $112.5 million
Number of Employees: 2,250
Expertise Needed: Physical therapy, nursing
Contact: Mr Don Giancaterino
Employment Manager
(708) 981-3586

ALL CHILDREN'S HOSPITAL, INC.
P.O. BOX 31020
ST. PETERSBURG, FLORIDA 33701-4816

Description: Public hospital specializing in pediatric care
Founded: 1928
Annual Sales: $93.8 million
Number of Employees: 1,530
Expertise Needed: Nursing, physical therapy
Contact: Ms Wendy Smith
Nursing Recruiter
(813) 898-7451

ALL SAINTS EPISCOPAL HOSPITAL
1400 8TH AVENUE
FORT WORTH, TEXAS 76104-4110

Description: General medical and surgical hospital and nursing home
Parent Company: All Saints Health Care, Inc.
Founded: 1900
Annual Sales: $112.8 million
Number of Employees: 1,600
Expertise Needed: Nursing
Contact: Ms Brenda Riddle
Nurse Recruitment and Employment Manager
(817) 927-6285

ALLEGHENY HEALTH SERVICES
320 EAST NORTH AVENUE
PITTSBURGH, PENNSYLVANIA 15212-4772

Description: Public hospital specializing in acute care and trauma
Annual Sales: $578.7 million
Number of Employees: 9,200
Expertise Needed: Registered nursing
Contact: Mr Keith Allen
Manager of Employment
(412) 359-3131

ALLEN HEALTHCARE SERVICES, INC.
175-20 HILLSIDE AVENUE
JAMAICA, NEW YORK 11432

Description: Provides home health-care services
Number of Employees: 450
Expertise Needed: Registered nursing
Contact: Ms Caroline Weinstein
Director of Human Resources
(718) 657-2966

ALLERGAN, INC.
2525 DUPONT DRIVE
IRVINE, CALIFORNIA 92715-1531

Description: Manufactures ophthalmic, optical, and pharmaceutical products
Founded: 1948
Annual Sales: $859.0 million
Number of Employees: 4,750
Expertise Needed: Sales, pharmaceutical, research and development, science
Contact: Ms Chris Montagua
Manager of Human Resources
(714) 752-4500

ALLERGAN MEDICAL OPTICS, INC.
9701 JERONIMO ROAD
IRVINE, CALIFORNIA 92718-2020

Description: Manufactures optical lenses and cleansers
Parent Company: Allergan, Inc.
Founded: 1986
Annual Sales: $100.0 million
Number of Employees: 900
Expertise Needed: Accounting, marketing, optics
Contact: Ms Sarah Cardona
Recruiter
(714) 951-0455

ALLIANCE HEALTH, INC.
4250 PERIMETER PARK SOUTH
ATLANTA, GEORGIA 30341

Description: Provides hospital management, chemical dependency, surgical, and physical therapy services
Number of Employees: 270
Expertise Needed: Accounting, finance, health care, nursing management and administration, data processing
Contact: Human Resources Department
(404) 452-1221

ALLIANCE IMAGING, INC.
3111 NORTH TUSTIN STREET
ORANGE, CALIFORNIA 92665-1752

Description: Provides MRI services to hospitals and other health-care providers
Annual Sales: $63.7 million
Number of Employees: 315
Expertise Needed: CAT/MRI technology
Contact: Personnel Department
(714) 921-5656

ALLIED CLINICAL LABORATORIES, INC.
4225 EXECUTIVE SQUARE
SAN DIEGO, CALIFORNIA 92037

Description: Clinical testing laboratory
Parent Company: National Health Labs
Annual Sales: $114.0 million
Number of Employees: 2,400

Expertise Needed: Laboratory technology, laboratory assistance
Contact: Human Resources
(619) 550-0600

ALLIED HEALTHCARE PRODUCTS
1720 SUBLETTE AVENUE
SAINT LOUIS, MISSOURI 63110-1927

Description: Manufactures and markets medical gas and respiratory therapy equipment
Parent Company: Harbour Group, Ltd.
Founded: 1933
Annual Sales: $61.2 million
Number of Employees: 500
Number of Managerial and Professional Employees Hired 1993: 15
Expertise Needed: Accounting, finance, data processing, mechanical engineering, computer programming
Contact: Mr Jim MacNee
Director of Human Resources
(314) 771-2400

ALLIED PHARMACY MANAGEMENT
8615 FREEPORT PARKWAY SOUTH
IRVING, TEXAS 75063-2551

Description: Owns drug stores
Annual Sales: $35.5 million
Number of Employees: 300
Expertise Needed: Pharmaceutical technology, pharmacology, pharmacy, business management, administration, accounting, finance, data processing, human resources
Contact: Ms Christine Poen
Director of Human Resources
(214) 929-5000

ALPHA MICROSYSTEMS
3511 WEST SUNFLOWER AVENUE
SANTA ANA, CALIFORNIA 92704

Description: Manufactures and markets computer hardware and software products
Founded: 1977
Expertise Needed: Hardware engineering, software engineering/development, computer programming
Contact: Mr William Mitchell
Director of Human Resources
(714) 957-8500

THE ALTOONA HOSPITAL
620 HOWARD AVENUE
ALTOONA, PENNSYLVANIA 16601-4804

Description: General hospital specializing in open-heart surgery
Annual Sales: $107.2 million
Number of Employees: 1,700

The Altoona Hospital (continued)

Expertise Needed: Medical technology, occupational therapy, physical therapy, accounting, management information systems

Contact: Ms Patricia Geesey
Employment Coordinator
(814) 946-2011

ALZA CORPORATION
950 PAGE MILL ROAD
PALO ALTO, CALIFORNIA 94304-0802

Description: Develops and tests pharmaceutical products
Founded: 1968
Annual Sales: $250.2 million
Number of Employees: 850
Expertise Needed: Chemistry, biology

Contact: Ms Susan Halsted
In-house Recruiter
(415) 494-5000

AMALGAMATED LIFE INSURANCE COMPANY, INC.
730 BROADWAY
NEW YORK, NEW YORK 10003-9522

Description: Provides life and health-care insurance services
Founded: 1943
Annual Sales: $26.0 million
Number of Employees: 425
Expertise Needed: Health insurance, allied health, accounting, data processing, disability insurance, actuarial

Contact: Ms Nancy Wood
Recruitment & Placement Specialist
(212) 473-5700

AMARILLO HOSPITAL DISTRICT
1501 COULTER DRIVE
AMARILLO, TEXAS 79106-1770

Description: General medical and surgical hospital
Founded: 1959
Annual Sales: $124.4 million
Number of Employees: 2,163
Expertise Needed: Physical therapy, occupational therapy, dietetics, pharmacy

Contact: Ms Tammy Horton
Professional Recruiter
(806) 354-1000

AMERICA'S BEST CONTACTS & EYEGLASSES
7255 NORTH CRESCENT BOULEVARD
PENNSAUKEN, NEW JERSEY 08110-1516

Description: Owns and operates eyeglass and contact lens retail stores
Founded: 1978
Annual Sales: $45.0 million
Number of Employees: 560

Expertise Needed: Accounting, data processing, optics, optometry, ophthalmological engineering

Contact: Ms Patty Price
Manager of Personnel
(609) 486-4300

AMERICAN BAPTIST HOMES OF THE WEST
400 ROLAND WAY
OAKLAND, CALIFORNIA 94621-2012

Description: Owns and operates nursing homes
Founded: 1955
Annual Sales: $50.0 million
Number of Employees: 1,600
Expertise Needed: Accounting, management, management information systems

Contact: Mr William Nelson
Associate Vice President of Personnel
(510) 635-7600

AMERICAN BRANDS, INC.
1700 EAST PUTMAN AVENUE
OLD GREENWICH, CONNECTICUT 06870-1321

Description: Diversified company producing tobacco products, alcoholic beverages, hardware, optical goods, and office supplies
Founded: 1904
Annual Sales: $14.6 billion
Number of Employees: 47,000
Expertise Needed: Accounting, finance

Contact: Mr Robert M Garber
Manager of Human Resources
(203) 698-5000

AMERICAN CYANAMID COMPANY
1 CYANAMID PLAZA
WAYNE, NEW JERSEY 07470-2012

Description: Produces agricultural, animal health and nutrition, and medical products
Founded: 1907
Annual Sales: $43.0 billion
Number of Employees: 26,500
Expertise Needed: Sales, marketing, finance, chemistry, biochemistry, manufacturing engineering

Contact: Mr Robert Koegel
Director of Personnel Resources
(201) 831-2000

AMERICAN DRUG STORES, INC.
1818 SWIFT DRIVE
OAKBROOK, ILLINOIS 60521-1576

Description: Drug store chain
Parent Company: American Stores Company
Founded: 1930
Annual Sales: $3.7 billion
Number of Employees: 25,000

Expertise Needed: Management, pharmacy
Contact: Ms Elizabeth Cardello
  Director of Recruitment
  (708) 572-5000

AMERICAN FAMILY ASSURANCE COLLECTIVE
1932 WYNNTON ROAD
COLUMBUS, GEORGIA 31999-0001

Description: Provides health-care insurance services
Founded: 1973
Annual Sales: $3.2 billion
Number of Employees: 3,314
Number of Managerial and Professional Employees Hired 1993: 225
Expertise Needed: Customer service and support, telecommunications, computer engineering, actuarial, computer programming, finance, law, marketing, underwriting, accounting
Contact: Ms Beverly Alexander
  Assistant Vice President of Human Resources
  (706) 323-3431

AMERICAN HEALTH SERVICES CORPORATION
4440 VON KARMAN AVENUE
NEWPORT BEACH, CALIFORNIA 92660-2011

Description: Operates outpatient, diagnostic imaging centers
Annual Sales: $38.3 million
Number of Employees: 210
Expertise Needed: Marketing, accounting, magnetic resonance imaging
Contact: Ms Cecelia Guastaferro
  Director of Personnel
  (714) 476-0733

AMERICAN HOME PRODUCTS
5 GIRALDA FARMS
MADISON, NEW JERSEY 07940

Description: Manufactures and markets pharmaceuticals, medical supplies, food products, and household products
Founded: 1909
Annual Sales: $7.9 billion
Number of Employees: 50,653
Expertise Needed: Biochemistry, marketing, public relations, nursing, sales
Contact: Mr Shawn Powell
  Director of Human Resources
  (201) 660-5000

AMERICAN MEDICAL ELECTRONICS
250 EAST ARAPAHO ROAD
RICHARDSON, TEXAS 75081-2768

Description: Manufactures medical devices for orthopedic and surgical use

Annual Sales: $32.7 million
Number of Employees: 240
Expertise Needed: Electronics/electronics engineering, electrical engineering, manufacturing engineering, biomedical technology, medical technology, accounting, marketing, product design and development, mechanical engineering
Contact: Ms Kay Hughes
  Employee Relations Specialist
  (214) 918-8300

AMERICAN MEDICAL INTERNATIONAL
14001 DALLAS PARKWAY
DALLAS, TEXAS 75240

Description: Owns and operates general and specialty hospitals
Founded: 1957
Annual Sales: $2.2 billion
Number of Employees: 27,500
Expertise Needed: Accounting, marketing, law, finance, auditing, treasury management, human resources
Contact: Mr Ed French
  Senior Vice President of Human Resources
  (214) 360-6300

AMERICAN MEDICAL SYSTEMS, INC.
11001 EAST BREN ROAD
MINNETONKA, MINNESOTA 55343-9605

Description: Manufactures medical devices for treating impotence and incontinence
Parent Company: Pfizer Pharmaceuticals
Annual Sales: $81.6 million
Number of Employees: 673
Expertise Needed: Biomedical engineering, physicians, research and development, engineering, public administration
Contact: Mr Ned Vandellen
  Human Resources Administrator
  (612) 930-6181

AMERICAN ONCOLOGIC HOSPITAL
7701 BURHOME AVENUE
PHILADELPHIA, PENNSYLVANIA 19111

Description: Hospital specializing in cancer treatment
Founded: 1904
Annual Sales: $56.7 million
Number of Employees: 1,400
Expertise Needed: Research, oncology
Contact: Ms Mary Ann Michini
  Employment Manager
  (215) 728-6900

AMERICAN PHYSICIANS SERVICES GROUP
1301 CAPITAL OF TEXAS HIGHWAY
AUSTIN, TEXAS 78746-6548

Description: Provides diverse financial services for the health-care industry
Founded: 1974

American Physicians Services Group (continued)

Annual Sales: $18.0 million
Number of Employees: 139
Expertise Needed: Credit/credit analysis, law
Contact: Mr Bill Hayes
      Chief Financial Officer
      (512) 328-0888

AMERICAN SHARED-CURE CARE

444 MARKET STREET
SAN FRANCISCO, CALIFORNIA 94117

Description: Provides diagnostic imaging services
Founded: 1971
Expertise Needed: Sales, accounting
Contact: Ms Shirley Tunick
      Director of Human Resources
      (415) 788-5300

AMERICAN SHARED HOSPITAL SERVICES

444 MARKET STREET
SAN FRANCISCO, CALIFORNIA 94111

Description: Provides diagnostic imaging, radiosurgery, and respiratory therapy services
Founded: 1980
Annual Sales: $49.3 million
Number of Employees: 720
Expertise Needed: Medical technology, respiratory therapy, radiology
Contact: Human Resources Director
      (415) 788-5300

AMERICAN SPECIALTIES, INC.

441 SAW MILL RIVER ROAD
YONKERS, NEW YORK 10701

Description: Manufactures hospital furniture and patient aids
Founded: 1961
Number of Employees: 220
Expertise Needed: Sales
Contact: Ms Bernice Fern
      Personnel Manager
      (914) 476-9000

AMERICAN STERILIZER COMPANY

2424 WEST 23RD STREET
ERIE, PENNSYLVANIA 16506-2921

Description: Manufactures sterilizers for hospitals and laboratories
Parent Company: Amsco International, Inc.
Annual Sales: $498.0 million
Number of Employees: 3,300
Expertise Needed: Medical technology, laboratory technology, mechanical engineering, engineering
Contact: Mr Sid Booker
      Director of Employee Relations
      (814) 452-3100

AMERICAN WHITE CROSS LABORATORIES, INC.

349 LAKE ROAD
DAYVILLE, CONNECTICUT 06241

Description: Manufactures surgical appliances and supplies
Founded: 1915
Annual Sales: $40.0 million
Number of Employees: 360
Expertise Needed: Manufacturing engineering, design engineering, mechanical engineering
Contact: Ms Roxanne Peckham
      Human Resources Manager
      (203) 774-8541

AMERIHEALTH, INC.

100 GALLERIA PARKWAY
ATLANTA, GEORGIA 30339

Description: Owns and operates hospitals
Annual Sales: $64.2 million
Number of Employees: 775
Expertise Needed: Marketing, finance, accounting
Contact: Mr William Gerry White
      President
      (404) 953-9600

AMERSHAM MEDI-PHYSICS, INC.

2636 SOUTH CLEARBROOK DRIVE
ARLINGTON HEIGHTS, ILLINOIS 60005-4626

Description: Manufactures medicines and botanical products
Annual Sales: $77.4 million
Number of Employees: 500
Expertise Needed: Accounting, sales, marketing
Contact: Mr John Moses
      Director of Organizational Development
      (708) 593-6300

AMGEN, INC.

1840 DEHAVILLAND DRIVE
THOUSAND OAKS, CALIFORNIA 91320-1701

Description: Develops biotechnology products used in medical research and disease treatment
Founded: 1980
Annual Sales: $1.4 billion
Number of Employees: 3,500
Expertise Needed: Pharmaceutical, biology, chemistry
Contact: Sally Fox
      Staffing Department
      (805) 447-1000

AMITY CARE CORPORATION

4415 HIGHLINE BOULEVARD
OKLAHOMA CITY, OKLAHOMA 73108-1866

Description: Operates nursing homes
Founded: 1976
Annual Sales: $35.4 million

Number of Employees: 1,550
Expertise Needed: Registered nursing, licensed practical nursing, accounting, finance, data processing
Contact: Mr Gene Clark
        Regional Manager
        (405) 943-1144

AMRESCO, INC.
30175 SOLON INDUSTRIAL PARK
SOLON, OHIO 44139-4321

Description: Manufactures and markets biochemicals, chemicals, diagnostic reagents, and test kits
Number of Employees: 120
Expertise Needed: Laboratory technology, chemistry, marketing
Contact: Human Resources Department
        (216) 349-1199

AMSCO INTERNATIONAL, INC.
2424 WEST 23RD STREET
ERIE, PENNSYLVANIA 16506-2502

Description: Manufactures operating room tables, sterilization equipment, and lights
Annual Sales: $231.2 million
Number of Employees: 4,161
Expertise Needed: Management information systems, accounting, finance, computer programming, mechanical engineering, medical technology, product design engineering, electrical engineering, design engineering, manufacturing engineering
Contact: Mr Sid Booker
        Director of Employee Relations
        (814) 870-8192

ANDERSEN GROUP, INC.
NEY INDUSTRIAL PARK
BLOOMFIELD, CONNECTICUT 06002

Description: Manufactures electronic parts for dentistry and ultrasound cleaners
Founded: 1950
Annual Sales: $45.5 million
Number of Employees: 348
Expertise Needed: Electrical engineering, mechanical engineering, design engineering
Contact: Mr Franklin R Stoner
        Director of Human Resources
        (203) 242-0761

ANGELICA CORPORATION
424 SOUTH WOODSMILL ROAD
CHESTERFIELD, MISSOURI 63017

Description: Manufactures, sells, and rents textiles and uniforms for hospitals
Founded: 1878
Annual Sales: $434.5 million
Number of Employees: 9,100

Expertise Needed: Manufacturing engineering, mechanical engineering, textiles, accounting, marketing, sales
Contact: Human Resources
        (314) 854-3800

APOTHECARE PRODUCTS, INC.
11531 RUPP DRIVE
BURNSVILLE, MINNESOTA 55337

Description: Manufactures and sells pharmaceutical supply equipment and patient aids
Founded: 1943
Number of Employees: 185
Number of Managerial and Professional Employees Hired 1993: 6
Expertise Needed: Pharmacy, sales, marketing
Contact: Ms Lori Peterson
        Personnel Administrator
        (612) 890-1940

APPLIED BIOSCIENCE INTERNATIONAL, INC.
4350 NORTH FAIRFAX DRIVE
ARLINGTON, VIRGINIA 22203-1619

Description: Tests chemicals and drugs for public health and environmental safety
Founded: 1986
Annual Sales: $181.0 million
Number of Employees: 1,800
Expertise Needed: Laboratory technology, medical technology, environmental engineering, life sciences, research and development
Contact: Ms Penny Williams
        Director of Human Resources
        (703) 516-2490

ARA ENVIRONMENTAL SERVICES, INC.
1101 MARKET STREET
PHILADELPHIA, PENNSYLVANIA 19107

Description: Provides cleaning services for hospitals and businesses
Founded: 1968
Number of Employees: 5,000
Expertise Needed: Food services, accounting, marketing, sales
Contact: Ms Bonnie Duckworth
        Human Resources Department
        (215) 238-3485

ARBOR HEALTH CARE COMPANY
1100 SHAWNEE ROAD
LIMA, OHIO 45805

Description: Owns and operates medical and nursing care centers
Founded: 1985
Annual Sales: $90.0 million
Number of Employees: 2,700

Expertise Needed: Registered nursing, accounting
Contact: Ms Cindy Moller
Human Resources Assistant
(419) 227-3000

JOHN D. ARCHBOLD MEMORIAL HOSPITAL
GORDON AT MIMOSA
THOMASVILLE, GEORGIA 31792

Description: Nonprofit hospital with rehabilitation and psychiatric units
Founded: 1925
Annual Sales: $61.3 million
Number of Employees: 2,200
Expertise Needed: Nursing, physical therapy, occupational therapy
Contact: Mr Jeff English
Recruiter/Human Resources
(912) 228-2747

ARIZONA PHYSICIANS IPA, INC.
4041 NORTH CENTRAL AVENUE
PHOENIX, ARIZONA 85012-1949

Description: Provides health-care and accident insurance services
Founded: 1985
Annual Sales: $195.3 million
Number of Employees: 250
Expertise Needed: Claims adjustment/examination, registered nursing, health care
Contact: Ms Jeanne Norton
Director of Human Resources
(602) 274-6102

ARKANSAS CHILDREN'S HOSPITAL
800 MARSHALL STREET
LITTLE ROCK, ARKANSAS 72202-3591

Description: General children's hospital
Founded: 1912
Annual Sales: $131.7 million
Number of Employees: 2,600
Expertise Needed: Laboratory technology, child therapy, physical therapy, registered nursing, licensed practical nursing, occupational therapy, purchasing, activity therapy, behavioral health
Contact: Department of Human Resources
(501) 320-1100

ARLINGTON HOSPITAL ASSOCIATION
1701 NORTH GEORGE MASON DRIVE
ARLINGTON, VIRGINIA 22205-3671

Description: General medical and surgical hospital
Annual Sales: $102.6 million
Number of Employees: 1,700
Expertise Needed: Nursing, administration
Contact: Department of Human Resources
(703) 558-5000

ARLINGTON MEMORIAL HOSPITAL
800 WEST RANDOL MILL ROAD
ARLINGTON, TEXAS 76012-2504

Description: Nonprofit hospital
Founded: 1958
Annual Sales: $103.9 million
Number of Employees: 1,783
Expertise Needed: Nursing
Contact: Ms Louise Harris
Nursing Recruiter
(817) 548-6100

ARROW INTERNATIONAL, INC.
3000 BUNVILLE ROAD
READING, PENNSYLVANIA 19612-2888

Description: Manufactures disposable medical products
Founded: 1975
Annual Sales: $133.4 million
Number of Employees: 1,127
Expertise Needed: Mechanical engineering, biomedical engineering
Contact: Ms Linda Silva
Staffing Manager
(215) 378-0131

ARTROMICK INTERNATIONAL, INC.
4800 HILTON CORPORATE DRIVE
COLUMBUS, OHIO 43232

Description: Manufactures drug administration equipment
Founded: 1973
Number of Employees: 150
Expertise Needed: Manufacturing engineering, mechanical engineering
Contact: Ms Carolyn Anderson
Manager of Human Resources
(614) 864-9966

ANNE ARUNDEL MEDICAL CENTER
FRANKLIN & CATHEDRAL STREETS
ANNAPOLIS, MARYLAND 21401

Description: Private hospital
Annual Sales: $107.9 million
Number of Employees: 1,800
Expertise Needed: Registered nursing
Contact: Ms Cathy Sulzer
Nursing Recruitment
(410) 267-1000

ASKLEPIOS HOSPITAL CORPORATION
249 EAST OCEAN BOULEVARD
LONG BEACH, CALIFORNIA 90802-4806

Description: Owns and operates hospitals
Annual Sales: $80.6 million
Number of Employees: 1,000

Expertise Needed: Accounting, finance, management

Contact: Mr Don Scheliga
Director of Human Resources
(310) 437-2117

ASPEN LABORATORIES, INC.
14603 EAST FREEMONT AVENUE
ENGLEWOOD, CALIFORNIA 80112

Description: Manufactures electrosurgical equipment
Founded: 1975
Number of Employees: 120
Number of Managerial and Professional Employees Hired 1993: 3
Expertise Needed: Electrical engineering, mechanical engineering
Contact: Ms Taffy Dean
Human Resources Manager
(303) 699-7600

ASSOCIATED GROUP
120 MONUMENT CIRCLE
INDIANAPOLIS, INDIANA 46204-4902

Description: Provides medical and health-care insurance services
Founded: 1944
Annual Sales: $2.2 billion
Number of Employees: 6,779
Expertise Needed: Auditing, real estate, actuarial, accounting, human resources
Contact for College Students and Recent Graduates:
Mr Matt Kennedy
Manager of Corporate Human Resources
(317) 488-6213
Contact for All Other Candidates:
Ms Renee Eberhardt
Staffing Assistant
(317) 488-6262

ASSOCIATED REGIONAL UNIVERSITY PATHOLOGISTS
500 CHIPETA WAY
SALT LAKE CITY, UTAH 84108-1221

Description: Medical and veterinary pathology laboratory
Parent Company: Associated University Pathologists
Annual Sales: $44.7 million
Number of Employees: 625
Expertise Needed: Veterinary, pathology, chemistry, biology
Contact: Mr Joel Deaton
Manager of Recruitment
(801) 583-2787

ASTRA USA, INC.
50 OTIS STREET
WESTBORO, MASSACHUSETTS 01581-3323

Description: Develops and manufactures anesthetics, antivirals, and cardiac critical care drugs
Founded: 1947
Annual Sales: $143.3 million
Number of Employees: 780
Expertise Needed: Sales, pharmacology, research and development
Contact: Personnel Department
(508) 366-1100

ASTRO-MED, INC.
600 EAST GREENWICH AVENUE
WEST WARWICK, RHODE ISLAND 02893

Description: Designs and develops specialty high-speed printers for use in medical electronics and other fields
Founded: 1969
Annual Sales: $29.8 million
Number of Employees: 240
Expertise Needed: Research and development, manufacturing engineering, mechanical engineering, sales
Contact: Ms Jackie Verduzco
Personnel Assistant
(401) 828-4000

ATHENS REGIONAL MEDICAL CENTER
1199 PRINCE AVENUE
ATHENS, GEORGIA 30606-2767

Description: Nonprofit medical center
Founded: 1918
Annual Sales: $109.7 million
Number of Employees: 1,864
Expertise Needed: Registered nursing, occupational therapy, physical therapy, general nursing, health care, radiology, licensed practical nursing
Contact: Ms Barbara Keesler
Employment Coordinator
(706) 549-9977

ATI/ORION
529 MAIN STREET
BOSTON, MASSACHUSETTS 02129-1101

Description: Manufactures analytical instruments, laboratory equipment, and laboratory supplies
Founded: 1962
Number of Employees: 353
Expertise Needed: Mechanical engineering, electrical engineering, design engineering
Contact: Ms Jennie Pinico
Director of Human Resources

ATLANTIC CITY MEDICAL CENTER
1925 PACIFIC AVENUE
ATLANTIC CITY, NEW JERSEY 08401-6713

Description: Nonprofit private hospital
Founded: 1897
Annual Sales: $249.4 million
Number of Employees: 2,300
Expertise Needed: Registered nursing, occupational therapy, physical therapy
Contact: Ms Karen Cappuccio
Nursing Recruiter
(609) 345-3053

ATWORK CORPORATION
100 EUROPA DRIVE
CHAPEL HILL, NORTH CAROLINA 27514

Description: Designs and develops computer software
Founded: 1981
Annual Sales: $20.0 million
Number of Employees: 115
Expertise Needed: Computer programming
Contact: Ms Debbie Bernard
User Service Manager
(919) 929-1313

AUGUSTA REGIONAL MEDICAL CENTER
3651 WHEELER ROAD
AUGUSTA, GEORGIA 30909-6521

Description: General medical and surgical hospital
Parent Company: Humana, Inc.
Founded: 1968
Annual Sales: $115.6 million
Number of Employees: 1,500
Expertise Needed: Emergency services, pharmacy, physical therapy
Contact: Human Resources

THE AULTMAN HOSPITAL ASSOCIATION
2600 6TH STREET SOUTHWEST
CANTON, OHIO 44710-1702

Description: Public hospital specializing in trauma
Parent Company: Aultman Health Services Association
Annual Sales: $139.6 million
Number of Employees: 3,000
Expertise Needed: Nursing, physical therapy, occupational therapy, respiratory therapy
Contact: Ms Kelli Conley
Human Resources Associate
(216) 452-9911

AUTOMATED HEALTH SYSTEMS, INC.
3545 LAKELAND DRIVE
JACKSON, MISSISSIPPI 39208

Description: Develops and markets computer software for health-care facilities
Founded: 1983

Expertise Needed: Software engineering/development
Contact: Ms Chris Patterson
Office Manager
(601) 932-3704

BAKER CUMMINS PHARMACEUTICALS, INC.
8800 NORTHWEST 36TH STREET
MIAMI, FLORIDA 33178

Description: Pharmaceutical and testing laboratory providing surgical and medical instruments
Number of Employees: 200
Expertise Needed: Electrical engineering, mechanical engineering, chemical engineering, pharmacy, accounting, finance, manufacturing
Contact: Ms Marcia Bucknor
Manager of Human Resources
(305) 590-2200

BAKERSFIELD MEMORIAL HOSPITAL ASSOCIATION
420 34TH STREET
BAKERSFIELD, CALIFORNIA 93301-2237

Description: General medical and surgical hospital
Founded: 1953
Annual Sales: $105.0 million
Number of Employees: 1,258
Contact: Ms Korwin Fuller
Human Resources Administrator
(805) 327-4235

E.G. BALDWIN & ASSOCIATES, INC.
144 EAST 17TH STREET
CLEVELAND, OHIO 44114-2012

Description: Provides x-ray equipment and supplies
Founded: 1925
Annual Sales: $105.6 million
Number of Employees: 210
Expertise Needed: Accounting, marketing, finance, management information systems, sales
Contact: Ms Laura Lewarchick
Benefits Administrator
(216) 621-9599

BALL MEMORIAL HOSPITAL, INC.
2401 WEST UNIVERSITY AVENUE
MUNCIE, INDIANA 47303-3428

Description: Owns and operates hospitals and nursing homes
Parent Company: BMH Health Services, Inc.
Annual Sales: $167.4 million
Number of Employees: 2,108
Expertise Needed: Nursing, licensed practical nursing, physical therapy
Contact: Ms Julie Kevilo
Employment Supervisor
(317) 747-3111

BALLY MANUFACTURING CORPORATION
8700 WEST BRYN MAWR AVENUE
CHICAGO, ILLINOIS 60631-3507

Description: Manufactures gaming equipment, and operates health and fitness centers
Founded: 1931
Annual Sales: $1.3 billion
Number of Employees: 27,000
Expertise Needed: Finance, accounting
Contact: Ms Lois Balodis
Director of Personnel
(312) 399-1300

BAPTIST HOSPITAL OF MIAMI, INC.
8900 SOUTHWEST 88TH STREET
MIAMI, FLORIDA 33176-2118

Description: General medical and surgical hospital
Founded: 1956
Annual Sales: $202.2 million
Number of Employees: 3,300
Expertise Needed: Occupational therapy, physical therapy, nursing, laboratory technology, management, medical records, social work, pharmacy
Contact: Ms Mary Beth Rousses
Director of Human Resources
(305) 596-1960

BAPTIST HOSPITALS, INC.
4007 KRESGE WAY
LOUISVILLE, KENTUCKY 40207-4604

Description: General hospital
Founded: 1918
Annual Sales: $376.9 million
Number of Employees: 6,173
Expertise Needed: Administration, nursing, computer science, computer programming
Contact: Ms Maureen Voss
Employee Relations Specialist
(502) 896-5000

BARBERTON CITIZENS HOSPITAL, INC.
155 5TH STREET NORTHEAST
BARBERTON, OHIO 44203

Description: Provides health-care services
Founded: 1915
Annual Sales: $71.7 million
Number of Employees: 1,400
Number of Managerial and Professional Employees Hired 1993: 50
Expertise Needed: Occupational therapy, physical therapy, nursing, pharmacy, anesthesiology, medical technology
Contact: Ms Judy Bishop
Manager of Employment
(216) 745-1611

BARCO OF CALIFORNIA
350 WEST ROSECRANS AVENUE
GARDENA, CALIFORNIA 90248

Description: Manufactures medical linens and apparel
Founded: 1929
Annual Sales: $25.0 million
Number of Employees: 240
Expertise Needed: Manufacturing engineering, accounting
Contact: Ms Lora DeLaro
Human Resources Manager
(213) 770-1012

C. R. BARD, INC.
730 CENTRAL AVENUE
MURRAY HILL, NEW JERSEY 07974-1139

Description: Develops and manufactures cardiovascular, surgical, and urological products
Founded: 1907
Annual Sales: $990.2 million
Number of Employees: 8,850
Expertise Needed: Sales, chemical engineering, biomedical engineering, quality control, clinical psychology
Contact: Mr Mark Sickles
Vice President of Human Resources
(908) 277-8000

BARD ACCESS SYSTEMS
5425 WEST AMELIA EARHART DRIVE
SALT LAKE CITY, UTAH 84116

Description: Manufactures and markets implantables, tubing, and catheters
Parent Company: C.R. Bard, Inc.
Number of Employees: 350
Number of Managerial and Professional Employees Hired 1993: 10
Expertise Needed: Marketing, quality control, law
Contact: Ms Robin Nielsen
Human Resources Administrator
(801) 595-0700

BARD CARDIOPULMONARY DIVISION
25 COMPUTER DRIVE
HAVERHILL, MASSACHUSETTS 01832

Description: Manufactures blood processing equipment, cardiovascular accessories, and medical supplies
Parent Company: C.R. Bard, Inc.
Number of Employees: 600
Expertise Needed: Biology, chemistry, manufacturing engineering, research and development, blood bank, laboratory technology, quality control, plastics engineering
Contact: Human Resources Department
(508) 373-1000

BARD PATIENT CARE DIVISION

111 SPRING STREET
MURRAY HILL, NEW JERSEY 07974

Description: Manufactures patient care products
Parent Company: C.R. Bard, Inc.
Number of Employees: 300
Expertise Needed: Sales, marketing, advertising

Contact: Mr Dan Bunce
　　　Manager of Human Resources
　　　(908) 277-8000

BARD UROLOGICAL DIVISION

8195 INDUSTRIAL BOULEVARD
COVINGTON, GEORGIA 30209

Description: Manufactures urological equipment and
　　supplies
Parent Company: C.R. Bard, Inc.
Founded: 1908
Number of Employees: 1,350
Expertise Needed: Mechanical engineering,
　　manufacturing engineering, accounting

Contact: Mr Mike Hourihan
　　　Manager of Personnel
　　　(404) 784-6100

BARNES HOSPITAL

BARNES HOSPITAL PLAZA
ST. LOUIS, MISSOURI 63110

Description: Public hospital
Founded: 1890
Annual Sales: $451.0 million
Number of Employees: 5,358
Expertise Needed: Nursing, occupational therapy,
　　physical therapy

Contact: Ms Carol Esrock
　　　Manager of Recruitment
　　　(314) 362-5000

BARONESS ERLANGER HOSPITAL

975 EAST 3RD STREET
CHATTANOOGA, TENNESSEE 37403-2112

Description: Public hospital
Founded: 1899
Annual Sales: $272.8 million
Number of Employees: 3,500
Expertise Needed: Nursing, licensed practical nursing,
　　allied health

Contact: Ms Valerie Sauceman
　　　Director of Nurse Recruitment
　　　(615) 778-6517

BARR LABORATORIES, INC.

2 QUAKER ROAD
POMONA, NEW YORK 10970-2930

Description: Manufactures and sells prescription drugs
Annual Sales: $58.0 million
Number of Employees: 375

Number of Managerial and Professional Employees Hired
　1993: 59
Expertise Needed: Chemistry, mechanical engineering,
　　electrical engineering, industrial engineering

Contact: Mr Steven Sheehy
　　　Human Resources Specialist
　　　(914) 362-1100

MARY IMOGENE BASSETT HOSPITAL

1 ATWELL ROAD
COOPERSTOWN, NEW YORK 13326-1301

Description: Hospital affiliated with outreach clinics
Founded: 1924
Annual Sales: $98.0 million
Number of Employees: 1,900
Expertise Needed: Pharmacy, nursing, certified nursing
　　and nursing assistance, respiratory therapy, mental
　　health

Contact: Mr Bruce Wilhelm
　　　Director of Personnel
　　　(607) 547-3120

BATON ROUGE HEALTH CARE

134 MCGEHEE DRIVE
BATON ROUGE, LOUISIANA 70815-5012

Description: Home health-care agency
Founded: 1979
Annual Sales: $29.7 million
Number of Employees: 1,250
Expertise Needed: Physical therapy, occupational therapy,
　　speech therapy, social work

Contact: Ms Linda Burns
　　　Human Resources Manager
　　　(504) 273-4120

BAUSCH & LOMB, INC.

1 CHASE SQUARE
ROCHESTER, NEW YORK 14604

Description: Diversified manufacturer of optical
　　products
Founded: 1853
Annual Sales: $1.7 billion
Number of Employees: 15,000
Expertise Needed: Sales, marketing, finance, human
　　resources, manufacturing engineering

Contact: Ms Marge Boehme
　　　Vice President of Human Resources
　　　(716) 338-6000

BAUSCH & LOMB PHARMACEUTICAL DIVISION

8500 HIDDEN RIVER PARKWAY
TAMPA, FLORIDA 33637

Description: Pharmaceuticals manufacturer
Founded: 1972
Number of Employees: 1,450
Number of Managerial and Professional Employees Hired
　1993: 38

Expertise Needed: Chemistry, manufacturing engineering, chemical engineering, biology, production control, pharmaceutical, quality control, microbiology

Contact: Ms Pat D'Urso
  Staffing Coordinator
  (813) 975-7700

BAXA CORPORATION
13760 EAST ARAPAHOE ROAD
ENGLEWOOD, COLORADO 80112

Description: Manufactures and distributes pharmaceutical supplies, pumps, syringes, and needles
Number of Employees: 150
Number of Managerial and Professional Employees Hired 1993: 20
Expertise Needed: Mechanical engineering
Contact: Ms Heather Dackow
  Human Resources Manager
  (303) 690-4204

BAXTER BIOTECH, HYLAND DIVISION
550 NORTH BRAND BOULEVARD
GLENDALE, CALIFORNIA 91203

Description: Manufactures biological products, blood, and blood products
Parent Company: Baxter International, Inc.
Founded: 1947
Number of Employees: 325
Expertise Needed: Mechanical engineering, design engineering, hematology
Contact: Human Resources
  (818) 956-3200

BAXTER DIAGNOSTICS
9750 NORTHWEST 25TH STREET
MIAMI, FLORIDA 33152

Description: Researches and develops medical and clinical diagnostic products
Parent Company: Baxter International, Inc.
Founded: 1948
Number of Employees: 2,000
Expertise Needed: Manufacturing engineering, design engineering, mechanical engineering, industrial engineering, sales, marketing, finance, information systems
Contact: Ms Pam Basinger
  Manager of Human Resources
  (305) 592-2311

BAXTER HEALTHCARE CORPORATION
1 BAXTER PARKWAY
DEERFIELD, ILLINOIS 60015-4625

Description: Manufactures and distributes health-care products
Parent Company: Baxter International, Inc.
Founded: 1931

Annual Sales: $6.2 billion
Number of Employees: 36,300
Expertise Needed: Pharmacology, biomedical engineering, computer science, pharmacy, biology, electronics/electronics engineering, plastics engineering, chemistry, credit management, life sciences
Contact: Ms Sylvia Grote
  Manager
  (708) 948-4126

BAXTER INTERNATIONAL, INC.
1 BAXTER PARKWAY
DEERFIELD, ILLINOIS 60015-4625

Description: Manufactures and distributes products to hospitals and clinical laboratories
Founded: 1931
Annual Sales: $8.9 billion
Number of Employees: 60,400
Expertise Needed: Information systems, engineering, finance, chemistry, biology, marketing, sales, credit management
Contact: Ms Sylvia Grote
  Manager of Staffing
  (708) 546-4126

BAY MEDICAL CENTER
1900 COLUMBUS AVENUE
BAY CITY, MICHIGAN 48708-6831

Description: General medical and surgical hospital
Parent Company: Bay Health Systems
Founded: 1972
Annual Sales: $103.9 million
Number of Employees: 1,600
Expertise Needed: Physical therapy
Contact: Department of Human Resources
  (517) 894-3000

BAYSTATE MEDICAL CENTER, INC.
759 CHESTNUT STREET
SPRINGFIELD, MASSACHUSETTS 01199-0001

Description: General medical and surgical hospital
Founded: 1883
Annual Sales: $231.5 million
Number of Employees: 4,800
Expertise Needed: Accounting, data processing, licensed practical nursing, occupational therapy, registered nursing, radiology, physical therapy
Contact: Ms. Cynthia Suopis
  Director of Staffing & Recruiting
  (800) 767-6612

BEAR MEDICAL SYSTEMS, INC.
2085 RUSTIN AVENUE
RIVERSIDE, CALIFORNIA 92507

Description: Manufactures and distributes ventilators and monitors for patient care
Number of Employees: 250

Bear Medical Systems, Inc. (continued)

Number of Managerial and Professional Employees Hired 1993: 12

Expertise Needed: Mechanical engineering, product design and development

Contact: Ms Kay Wagner
Human Resources Specialist

WILLIAM BEAUMONT HOSPITAL

3601 WEST 13 MILE ROAD
ROYAL OAK, MICHIGAN 48073-6712

Description: General hospital
Founded: 1949
Annual Sales: $602.2 million
Number of Employees: 8,850
Expertise Needed: Registered nursing, licensed practical nursing, accounting, data processing, cardiology, physical therapy, occupational therapy, respiratory therapy

Contact: Ms Carolyn Thompson
Nursing Recruiter
(313) 551-5000

BECKMAN INSTRUMENTS, INC.

2500 NORTH HARBOR BOULEVARD
FULLERTON, CALIFORNIA 92635-2607

Description: Manufactures laboratory and research instruments
Founded: 1934
Annual Sales: $908.8 million
Number of Employees: 6,879
Expertise Needed: Biology, finance, physics, marketing, chemistry, law, accounting, sales

Contact: Ms Maureen Groudas
Employment Manager
(719) 993-8584

BECTON DICKINSON & COMPANY

1 BECTON DRIVE
FRANKLIN LAKES, NEW JERSEY 07417-1815

Description: Manufactures medical and surgical products and antibiotics
Founded: 1897
Annual Sales: $2.4 billion
Number of Employees: 19,100
Expertise Needed: Accounting, marketing, sales, mechanical engineering, manufacturing engineering, chemical engineering, chemistry, biomedical technology

Contact: Human Resources Department
(201) 847-6800

BECTON DICKINSON, ACUTECARE DIVISION

1 BECTON DRIVE
FRANKLIN LAKES, NEW JERSEY 07417-1815

Description: Develops and manufactures disposable operating room surgical supplies

Parent Company: Becton Dickinson & Company
Founded: 1987
Number of Employees: 1,300
Expertise Needed: Sales, marketing, design engineering, manufacturing engineering, industrial engineering, mechanical engineering

Contact: Mr Larry Kleinman
Manager of Human Resources
(201) 847-6900

BECTON DICKINSON, CONSUMER PRODUCTS DIVISION

1 BECTON DRIVE
FRANKLIN LAKES, NEW JERSEY 07417-1815

Description: Manufactures dressings, bandages, thermometers, gloves, syringes, and needles
Parent Company: Becton Dickinson & Company
Founded: 1984
Number of Employees: 350
Expertise Needed: Accounting, sales, marketing, chemical engineering, manufacturing engineering, industrial engineering, mechanical engineering

Contact: Ms Ruth Jenkins
Human Resources Representative
(201) 847-7100

BEHRING DIAGNOSTICS

151 UNIVERSITY AVENUE
WESTWOOD, MASSACHUSETTS 02090

Description: Markets and distributes diagnostic instruments
Number of Employees: 200
Expertise Needed: Biology, chemistry, biochemistry

Contact: Human Resources Department
(617) 320-3000

BENNET GROUP

2200 FARADAY AVENUE
CARLSBAD, CALIFORNIA 92008

Description: Manufactures and markets medical equipment and supplies
Founded: 1956
Number of Employees: 800
Expertise Needed: Manufacturing engineering, design engineering, mechanical engineering

Contact: Ms. Barbara Colbert
Manager of Human Resources
(619) 929-4000

BENNETT X-RAY CORPORATION

445 OAK STREET
COPIAGUE, NEW YORK 11726-2719

Description: Manufactures diagnostic X-ray equipment and radiographic imaging systems
Founded: 1958
Annual Sales: $31.9 million
Number of Employees: 200

Expertise Needed: Accounting, marketing, finance, management information systems, sales

Contact: Ms Lori Loughlin
      Personnel Director
      (516) 691-6100

BENSON EYECARE CORPORATION
555 THEODORE FREMD AVENUE
RYE, NEW YORK 10580-2050

Description: Operates ophthalmological dispensaries and sells eyecare products
Founded: 1992
Annual Sales: $29.9 million
Number of Employees: 480
Expertise Needed: Optics, optometry, data processing, health care

Contact: Personnel Department
      (914) 967-9400

BENSON OPTICAL COMPANY, INC.
10900 RED CIRCLE DRIVE
MINNETONKA, MINNESOTA 55343

Description: Operates optical laboratories and dispensaries
Founded: 1913
Annual Sales: $35.0 million
Number of Employees: 600
Expertise Needed: Optics, optometry, ophthalmological engineering, data processing, accounting, finance, sales

Contact: Human Resources Department
      (612) 546-1460

BERGAN MERCY MEDICAL CENTER
7500 MERCY ROAD
OMAHA, NEBRASKA 68124-2319

Description: Health-care clinic
Parent Company: Mercy Midlands
Founded: 1961
Annual Sales: $123.8 million
Number of Employees: 2,319
Expertise Needed: Registered nursing, certified nursing and nursing assistance, licensed practical nursing, physical therapy, medical technology, radiation technology, occupational therapy, respiratory therapy

Contact: Ms Gail Hafer
      Employment Manager
      (402) 398-6060

BERGEN BRUNSWIG CORPORATION
4000 WEST METROPOLITAN DRIVE
ORANGE, CALIFORNIA 92668-3502

Description: Distributes pharmaceuticals, health-care products, and cosmetics
Founded: 1947
Annual Sales: $5.8 billion
Number of Employees: 2,965

Number of Managerial and Professional Employees Hired 1993: 115
Expertise Needed: Accounting, sales, computer programming, finance

Contact: Ms Teresa Baber
      Manager of Human Resources
      (714) 385-4000

BERLEX LABORATORIES, INC.
300 FAIRFIELD ROAD
WAYNE, NEW JERSEY 07927-2007

Description: Manufactures pharmaceuticals
Parent Company: Schering Berlin, Inc.
Founded: 1979
Annual Sales: $190.1 million
Number of Employees: 1,229
Expertise Needed: Marketing, finance, sales, pharmacology, computer programming

Contact: Ms Toni Dolecki
      Human Resource Associate
      (201) 694-4100

BESTCARE, INC.
3000 HEMPSTEAD TURNPIKE
LEVITTOWN, NEW YORK 11756-1396

Description: Home health-care agency
Annual Sales: $15.0 million
Number of Employees: 800
Expertise Needed: Nursing, licensed practical nursing, home health care

Contact: Mr Garfield Vassell
      Employment Manager
      (516) 731-3770

THE BETH ISRAEL HOSPITAL ASSOCIATION
330 BROOKLINE AVENUE
BOSTON, MASSACHUSETTS 02215-5400

Description: Nonprofit private hospital specializing in acute and trauma care
Founded: 1915
Annual Sales: $337.1 million
Number of Employees: 4,600
Expertise Needed: Registered nursing, physical therapy, occupational therapy, respiratory therapy, networking

Contact: Ms Mary Ellen Kiley
      Nurse Recruiter
      (617) 735-2000

BETH ISRAEL MEDICAL CENTER
FIRST AVENUE AT 16TH STREET
NEW YORK, NEW YORK 10003

Description: General medical and surgical hospital
Annual Sales: $559.0 million
Number of Employees: 6,000

Beth Israel Medical Center (continued)

Expertise Needed: Nursing, licensed practical nursing, physical therapy

Contact: Ms Mae Concannon
      Nursing Recruiter
      (212) 387-6900

BETHESDA HEALTHCARE CORPORATION
2815 SOUTH SEACREST BOULEVARD
BOYNTON BEACH, FLORIDA 33435-7934

Description: Provides hospital and health-care consulting and ambulance services
Annual Sales: $102.5 million
Number of Employees: 1,600
Expertise Needed: Nursing, physical therapy, nuclear medicine
Contact: Ms Lisa Bossman
      Human Resource Development
      (407) 737-7733

BETHESDA HOSPITAL, INC.
619 OAK STREET
CINCINNATI, OHIO 45206-1613

Description: Owns and operates general medical and surgical hospitals
Founded: 1896
Annual Sales: $200.8 million
Number of Employees: 4,100
Expertise Needed: Registered nursing
Contact: Department of Human Resources
      (513) 569-6111

BEVERLY CALIFORNIA CORPORATION
1200 SOUTH WALDRON ROAD
FORT SMITH, ARKANSAS 72903-2591

Description: Manufactures medical equipment and supplies
Parent Company: Beverly Enterprises, Inc.
Founded: 1964
Annual Sales: $423.0 million
Expertise Needed: Accounting, finance, nursing, management information systems
Contact: Mr Bill Barrett
      Manager of Recruiting
      (501) 452-6712

BEVERLY ENTERPRISES, INC.
1200 SOUTH WALDRON ROAD
FORT SMITH, ARKANSAS 72913-3324

Description: Owns and operates nursing homes, pharmacies, and retirement living centers and manufactures medical equipment
Founded: 1964
Annual Sales: $3.0 billion
Number of Employees: 90,564

Expertise Needed: Auditing, accounting, finance, marketing, quality control, law, data processing, nursing
Contact: Mr Bill Barrett
      Manager of Recruiting
      (501) 452-6712

BIG B, INC.
2600 MORGAN ROAD
BESSEMER, ALABAMA 35023

Description: Operates a chain of drug stores and rents home health-care equipment
Founded: 1968
Annual Sales: $502.7 million
Number of Employees: 4,500
Expertise Needed: Sales, accounting, finance, marketing, data processing
Contact: Mr Charles Underwood
      Corporate Recruiter
      (205) 424-3421

BIG SUN HEALTHCARE SYSTEMS
131 SOUTHWEST 15TH STREET
OCALA, FLORIDA 34474-4029

Description: Nonprofit private hospital providing general health-care services
Founded: 1927
Annual Sales: $105.2 million
Number of Employees: 1,350
Expertise Needed: Nursing, respiratory therapy, radiology
Contact: Ms Jan Hutchinson
      Employment
      (904) 351-7273

BINDLEY WESTERN INDUSTRIES
4212 WEST 71ST STREET
INDIANAPOLIS, INDIANA 46268

Description: Wholesale distributor of prescription drugs
Founded: 1968
Annual Sales: $2.9 billion
Number of Employees: 628
Expertise Needed: Finance, accounting, purchasing, operations
Contact: Ms Kathy Messick
      Director of Personnel
      (317) 298-9900

BIOCRAFT LABORATORIES, INC.
1801 RIVER ROAD
FAIRLAWN, NEW JERSEY 07410-1202

Description: Manufactures human and veterinary pharmaceuticals
Founded: 1964
Annual Sales: $113.2 million
Number of Employees: 720

Expertise Needed: Chemistry, analysis, biology, chemical engineering

Contact: Mr Robert Rooney
Director of Human Resources
(201) 703-0400

BIOGEN, INC.
14 CAMBRIDGE CENTER
CAMBRIDGE, MASSACHUSETTS 02142-1481

Description: Researches and develops pharmaceutical products
Founded: 1978
Annual Sales: $135.1 million
Number of Employees: 350
Expertise Needed: Chemical engineering, chemistry, biology, biochemistry, microbiology
Contact: Mr Stephen Hobbs
Employment Manager
(617) 252-9200

BIOMEDICAL APPLICATIONS MANAGEMENT
1601 TRAPELO ROAD
WALTHAM, MASSACHUSETTS 02154-7353

Description: Owns and operates kidney dialysis centers
Parent Company: National Medical Care, Inc.
Founded: 1971
Annual Sales: $285.7 million
Number of Employees: 5,000
Expertise Needed: Accounting, finance, computer programming, biomedical technology, business management
Contact: Department of Human Resources
(617) 466-9850

BIOMET, INC.
AIRPORT INDUSTRIAL PARK
WARSAW, INDIANA 46581

Description: Develops and manufactures orthopedic products and reconstructive devices
Founded: 1977
Annual Sales: $274.8 million
Number of Employees: 1,606
Number of Managerial and Professional Employees Hired 1993: 5
Expertise Needed: Marketing, sales, finance, accounting, research and development
Contact: Ms Darlene Whaley
Director of Personnel
(219) 267-6639

BIONAIRE, INC.
222 LAKEVIEW AVENUE
WEST PALM BEACH, FLORIDA 33401

Description: Manufactures air and water filtration products and systems
Founded: 1977
Annual Sales: $59.5 million
Number of Employees: 135

Expertise Needed: Mechanical engineering, manufacturing engineering, industrial engineering

Contact: Mr Tom Keyser
Vice President of Management
(407) 820-0100

BIO-REFERENCE LABORATORIES, INC.
481 EDWARD H. ROSS DRIVE
ELMWOOD PARK, NEW JERSEY 07407

Description: Operates chemical diagnostic testing laboratories
Annual Sales: $16.3 million
Number of Employees: 260
Expertise Needed: Laboratory technology, biology, accounting, hematology
Contact: Ms Carmela Mulligan
Manager of Personnel
(201) 791-3600

BIOSPHERICS, INC.
12051 INDIAN CREEK COURT
BELTSVILLE, MARYLAND 20705

Description: Testing laboratory and commercial physical research company
Founded: 1967
Annual Sales: $16.7 million
Number of Employees: 492
Expertise Needed: Environmental engineering, safety engineering
Contact: Ms Mary Jo Lavorata
Director of Personnel
(301) 419-3900

BIOSYM TECHNOLOGIES, INC.
9685 SCRANTON ROAD
SAN DIEGO, CALIFORNIA 92121-3752

Description: Provides computer programming services
Parent Company: Corning, Inc.
Annual Sales: $42.0 million
Number of Employees: 220
Expertise Needed: Computer programming, program analysis
Contact: Ms Kimberly Ellstrom
Human Resources Director
(619) 458-9990

BIOTEST DIAGNOSTICS CORPORATION
66 FORD ROAD
DENVILLE, NEW JERSEY 07834

Description: Distributes blood products, diagnostic reagents, and testing equipment
Founded: 1946
Number of Employees: 100
Expertise Needed: Sales, distribution
Contact: Mr Robert Perry
President
(201) 625-1300

BIOWHITTAKER, INC.
8830 BIGGS FORD ROAD
WALKERSVILLE, MARYLAND 21793-0127

Description: Manufactures and markets clinical
   diagnostic products
Founded: 1947
Annual Sales: $51.6 million
Number of Employees: 510
Expertise Needed: Manufacturing engineering, design
   engineering, chemistry, packaging engineering,
   distribution, biological engineering, biochemistry
Contact: Ms Joyce Dennis
      Human Resources Administrator
      (301) 898-7025

BIRD MEDICAL TECHNOLOGIES, INC.
1100 BIRD CENTER DRIVE
PALM SPRINGS, CALIFORNIA 92262

Description: Manufactures respiratory care and
   infection control products
Annual Sales: $43.9 million
Number of Employees: 300
Expertise Needed: Electrical engineering, mechanical
   engineering, physics, biology, chemistry
Contact: Ms Stella Adams
      Human Resources Administrator
      (619) 778-7200

BIRTCHER MEDICAL SYSTEMS, INC.
50 TECHNOLOGY DRIVE
IRVINE, CALIFORNIA 92718

Description: Manufactures and markets medical devices
   and surgical products
Founded: 1938
Annual Sales: $52.4 million
Number of Employees: 140
Expertise Needed: Mechanical engineering, industrial
   engineering, design engineering, research and
   development, quality control, sales
Contact: Ms Paula Stevens
      Human Resources Manager
      (714) 753-9400

BISSELL HEALTHCARE CORPORATION
2345 WALKER AVENUE NORTHWEST
GRAND RAPIDS, MICHIGAN 49504-2516

Description: Manufactures and sells physical therapy
   and orthopedic products
Parent Company: Bissell, Inc.
Founded: 1976
Annual Sales: $85.2 million
Number of Employees: 1,117
*Number of Managerial and Professional Employees Hired
   1993:* 8

Expertise Needed: Marketing, social service, product
   engineering, chemistry, credit/credit analysis, sales,
   mechanical engineering
Contact: Mr Thomas McInerney
      Director of Human Resources
      (616) 453-4451

BLOCK DRUG COMPANY, INC.
257 CORNELISON AVENUE
JERSEY CITY, NEW JERSEY 07302-3113

Description: Distributes pharmaceuticals, dental
   supplies, and toiletries
Founded: 1907
Annual Sales: $624.8 million
Number of Employees: 3,505
Expertise Needed: Marketing, sales, finance, pharmacy,
   biology, physics, accounting, chemical engineering,
   environmental engineering, law
Contact: Ms Mary Shevlia
      Senior Personnel Administrator
      (201) 434-3000

BLOCK MEDICAL
5957 LANDAU COURT
CARLSBAD, CALIFORNIA 92008

Description: Manufactures home infusion devices
Annual Sales: $30.0 million
Number of Employees: 260
Expertise Needed: Manufacturing engineering, design
   engineering, mechanical engineering
Contact: Ms Anna Maria Grace
      Human Resources Manager
      (619) 431-1501

BLOOD SYSTEMS, INC.
6210 EAST OAK STREET
SCOTTSDALE, ARIZONA 85257-1101

Description: Nonprofit blood bank and plasma facility
Founded: 1943
Annual Sales: $99.0 million
Number of Employees: 1,700
Expertise Needed: Registered nursing, licensed practical
   nursing
Contact: Mr Larry Reese
      Director of Human Resources
      (602) 946-4201

BLOOMINGTON HOSPITAL, INC.
601 WEST 2ND STREET
BLOOMINGTON, INDIANA 47403-2317

Description: Public general hospital
Founded: 1905
Annual Sales: $89.4 million
Number of Employees: 2,100

Expertise Needed: Physical therapy, nursing, pharmacy
Contact: Mr John Lee
   Director of Human Resources
   (812) 336-9535

BLUE CARE NETWORK, EAST MICHIGAN
4200 FASHION SQUARE
SAGINAW, MICHIGAN 48603-1247

Description: Health maintenance organization
Parent Company: Blue Cross & Blue Shield of Michigan
Annual Sales: $95.8 million
Number of Employees: 462
Expertise Needed: Registered nursing, health care, finance, accounting
Contact: Ms April Williamson
   Human Resources Specialist
   (517) 791-3200

BLUE CARE NETWORK, HEALTH CENTRAL
1403 SOUTH CREYTS ROAD
LANSING, MICHIGAN 48917-8507

Description: Health maintenance organization
Parent Company: Blue Cross & Blue Shield of Michigan
Founded: 1979
Annual Sales: $101.5 million
Number of Employees: 471
Expertise Needed: Business management, finance, accounting, marketing, health care
Contact: Ms Joyce Kindt
   Recruitment & EEO Officer
   (517) 322-8000

BLUE CROSS & BLUE SHIELD MUTUAL OF OHIO
2060 EAST 9TH STREET
CLEVELAND, OHIO 44115-1304

Description: Provides health-care insurance services
Founded: 1945
Annual Sales: $1.5 billion
Number of Employees: 2,900
Expertise Needed: Systems analysis, computer programming, accounting, sales, registered nursing, claims processing/management, and administration, customer service and support
Contact: Ms Cindy Cardwell
   Manager of Employee Relations
   (216) 687-7000

BLUE CROSS & BLUE SHIELD OF ALABAMA
450 RIVERCHASE PARKWAY EAST
BIRMINGHAM, ALABAMA 35298-2858

Description: Provides health-care insurance services
Founded: 1934
Annual Sales: $2.1 billion
Number of Employees: 2,200

Expertise Needed: Accounting, actuarial, finance, marketing, computer programming, sales
Contact: Ms Elizabeth Hanlin
   Manager of Employment
   (205) 988-2100

BLUE CROSS & BLUE SHIELD OF ARKANSAS
601 GAINES
LITTLE ROCK, ARKANSAS 72201-4041

Description: Provides health-care insurance services
Founded: 1949
Annual Sales: $424.3 million
Number of Employees: 1,500
Expertise Needed: Nursing, licensed practical nursing, computer programming, accounting
Contact: Ms Theresa Smith
   Recruiting Coordinator
   (501) 378-2000

BLUE CROSS & BLUE SHIELD OF COLORADO
700 BROADWAY
DENVER, COLORADO 80203-3421

Description: Provides health-care insurance services
Annual Sales: $116.8 million
Number of Employees: 2,135
Expertise Needed: Finance, accounting, actuarial, claims adjustment/examination
Contact: Ms Sharon Anderson
   Manager of Compensation and Executive Recruiting
   (303) 831-2131

BLUE CROSS & BLUE SHIELD OF CONNECTICUT
370 BASSETT ROAD
NORTH HAVEN, CONNECTICUT 06473-4201

Description: Provides health-care insurance services
Founded: 1937
Annual Sales: $1.4 billion
Number of Employees: 2,500
Expertise Needed: Sales, health insurance, actuarial, mathematics, human resources, computer programming, network analysis, law
Contact: Ms Sheila Vallombroso
   Staffing Consultant
   (203) 239-4911

BLUE CROSS & BLUE SHIELD OF FLORIDA
532 RIVERSIDE AVENUE
JACKSONVILLE, FLORIDA 32202-4914

Description: Provides health-care insurance services
Founded: 1944
Annual Sales: $1.7 billion
Number of Employees: 5,427

Blue Cross & Blue Shield of Florida (continued)

Expertise Needed: Accounting, finance, actuarial, underwriting, real estate, law, nursing

Contact: Mr Robert Croteau
Director of Human Resources
(904) 791-6111

BLUE CROSS & BLUE SHIELD OF GEORGIA

3350 PEACHTREE ROAD NORTHEAST
ATLANTA, GEORGIA 30326-1040

Description: Provides health-care insurance services
Founded: 1937
Annual Sales: $915.8 million
Number of Employees: 1,800
Expertise Needed: Claims adjustment/examination

Contact: Mr Jim Burns
Director of Employment
(404) 842-8000

BLUE CROSS & BLUE SHIELD OF KANSAS

1133 SOUTHWEST TOPEKA BOULEVARD
TOPEKA, KANSAS 66629-0001

Description: Provides health-care insurance services
Annual Sales: $602.1 million
Number of Employees: 2,000
Expertise Needed: Accounting, finance, data processing, nursing, licensed practical nursing, law

Contact: Mr Mike Valdivia
Manager of Personnel
(913) 291-7000

BLUE CROSS & BLUE SHIELD OF MARYLAND

10455 MILL RUN CIRCLE
OWINGS MILLS, MARYLAND 21117-4208

Description: Provides health-care insurance services
Founded: 1950
Expertise Needed: Computer programming, accounting, customer service and support, marketing, finance, clinical services

Contact: Ms Kay Keim
Human Resources Assistant
(410) 581-3000

BLUE CROSS & BLUE SHIELD OF MASSACHUSETTS

100 SUMMER STREET
BOSTON, MASSACHUSETTS 02110-2103

Description: Provides health-care insurance services
Founded: 1937
Annual Sales: $3.4 billion
Number of Employees: 5,323
Expertise Needed: Actuarial, real estate, underwriting, law, accounting, finance

Contact: Human Resources Department
(617) 956-2090

BLUE CROSS & BLUE SHIELD OF MICHIGAN

600 EAST LAFAYETTE BOULEVARD
DETROIT, MICHIGAN 48226-2927

Description: Provides health-care insurance services
Founded: 1939
Annual Sales: $6.2 billion
Number of Employees: 8,521
Expertise Needed: Business management, finance, computer programming, accounting, marketing, sales

Contact: Ms Mary Smith
Human Resources Representative
(313) 255-9000

BLUE CROSS & BLUE SHIELD OF MINNESOTA

3535 BLUE CROSS ROAD
SAINT PAUL, MINNESOTA 55164-1154

Description: Provides health-care insurance services
Founded: 1972
Annual Sales: $580.3 million
Number of Employees: 2,923
Expertise Needed: Computer programming, sales, law, marketing, claims adjustment/examination

Contact: Human Resources Department
(612) 456-8048

BLUE CROSS & BLUE SHIELD OF MISSOURI

1831 CHESTNUT STREET
SAINT LOUIS, MISSOURI 63103

Description: Provides health-care insurance services
Founded: 1936
Annual Sales: $788.9 million
Number of Employees: 1,761
Expertise Needed: Underwriting, actuarial, customer service and support, data processing, physicians, nursing, human resources, finance

Contact: Ms Kalyn Brantley-McNeil
Director of Employee Services
(314) 923-4444

BLUE CROSS & BLUE SHIELD OF NATIONAL CAPITOL AREA

550 12TH STREET SOUTHWEST
WASHINGTON, DC 20024-2104

Description: Provides health-care insurance services
Founded: 1939
Annual Sales: $1.5 billion
Number of Employees: 2,500
Expertise Needed: Computer programming, finance, accounting, marketing

Contact: Ms Dana Tayag
Manager of Recruitment
(202) 479-8000

BLUE CROSS & BLUE SHIELD OF NEW JERSEY

33 WASHINGTON STREET
NEWARK, NEW JERSEY 07102-3107

Description: Provides health-care insurance services
Founded: 1932
Annual Sales: $1.6 billion
Number of Employees: 3,200
Number of Managerial and Professional Employees Hired 1993: 150
Expertise Needed: Law, actuarial, operations, finance, communications, accounting, marketing, sales, auditing
Contact: Mr Kenneth Goodman
Recruiter
(201) 466-4000

BLUE CROSS & BLUE SHIELD OF NORTH CAROLINA

5901 DURHAM CHAPEL HILL BOULEVARD
DURHAM, NORTH CAROLINA 27702

Description: Provides health-care insurance services
Founded: 1968
Annual Sales: $907.5 million
Number of Employees: 2,090
Number of Managerial and Professional Employees Hired 1993: 300
Expertise Needed: Computer programming, allied health, accounting, sales, actuarial, underwriting, registered nursing, human resources
Contact: Mr Mike Plueddemann
Manager of Employee Relations
(919) 489-7431

BLUE CROSS & BLUE SHIELD OF OREGON

100 SOUTHWEST MARKET STREET
PORTLAND, OREGON 97201-5747

Description: Provides health-care insurance services
Founded: 1941
Annual Sales: $1.1 billion
Number of Employees: 2,110
Number of Managerial and Professional Employees Hired 1993: 150
Expertise Needed: Nursing, claims adjustment/examination, accounting, data processing, computer programming
Contact: Ms Connie Schweppe
Supervisor of Employee Relations
(503) 225-5221

BLUE CROSS & BLUE SHIELD OF ROCHESTER AREA

150 EAST MAIN STREET
ROCHESTER, NEW YORK 14604-1618

Description: Provides health-care insurance services
Founded: 1934
Annual Sales: $797.5 million
Number of Employees: 1,340

Expertise Needed: Claims adjustment/examination, actuarial, mathematics, computer science
Contact: Ms Ruth Petrich
Recruiter
(716) 454-1700

BLUE CROSS & BLUE SHIELD OF SOUTH CAROLINA

I-20 EAST AT ALPINE ROAD
COLUMBIA, SOUTH CAROLINA 29219

Description: Provides health-care insurance services
Founded: 1946
Annual Sales: $256.9 million
Number of Employees: 3,200
Expertise Needed: Computer programming, registered nursing
Contact: Ms May Rhea
Supervisor of Recruiting
(803) 699-3792

BLUE CROSS & BLUE SHIELD OF TENNESSEE

801 PINE STREET
CHATTANOOGA, TENNESSEE 37402-2520

Description: Provides health-care insurance services
Founded: 1945
Annual Sales: $1.2 billion
Number of Employees: 1,900
Expertise Needed: Business administration, computer science, accounting
Contact: Human Resources Department
(615) 755-5961

BLUE CROSS & BLUE SHIELD OF TEXAS, INC.

901 SOUTH CENTRAL EXPRESSWAY
RICHARDSON, TEXAS 75080-7302

Description: Provides health-care insurance services
Founded: 1939
Annual Sales: $1.3 billion
Number of Employees: 4,100
Number of Managerial and Professional Employees Hired 1993: 200
Expertise Needed: Computer programming, marketing, nursing, accounting, actuarial, mathematics, data processing, underwriting
Contact: Mr Ed Toogood
Director of Employment
(214) 766-6900

BLUE CROSS & BLUE SHIELD OF UTICA/ WATERTOWN, INC.

12 RHOADS ROAD
UTICA, NEW YORK 13502-6306

Description: Provides health-care insurance services
Founded: 1937
Annual Sales: $226.8 million

Blue Cross & Blue Shield of Utica/Watertown, Inc. (continued)

Number of Employees: 345

Expertise Needed: Actuarial, accounting, claims adjustment/examination, mathematics, computer programming, administration

Contact: Mr Alan O'Brien
Director of Human Resources
(315) 798-4200

BLUE CROSS & BLUE SHIELD OF VERMONT
1 EAST ROAD
MONTPELIER, VERMONT 05602

Description: Provides health-care insurance services

Annual Sales: $175.7 million

Number of Employees: 295

Expertise Needed: Accounting, finance, data processing, law

Contact: Ms Louisa Neveau
Human Resources Assistant
(802) 223-6131

BLUE CROSS & BLUE SHIELD OF VIRGINIA
2015 STAPLES MILL ROAD
RICHMOND, VIRGINIA 23279-3108

Description: Provides health-care insurance services

Annual Sales: $2.2 billion

Number of Employees: 3,600

Number of Managerial and Professional Employees Hired 1993: 300

Expertise Needed: Actuarial, underwriting, law, claims adjustment/examination, information services

Contact: Ms Lyn Runnett
Manager of Staffing
(804) 354-3358

BLUE CROSS & BLUE SHIELD OF WESTERN NEW YORK
1901 MAIN STREET
BUFFALO, NEW YORK 14240

Description: Provides health-care insurance services

Founded: 1939

Annual Sales: $1.1 billion

Number of Employees: 2,156

Number of Managerial and Professional Employees Hired 1993: 10

Expertise Needed: Program analysis, statistics, nursing, marketing, accounting, administration

Contact: Mr Paul Marohn
Manager of Human Resources
(716) 887-6900

BLUE CROSS & BLUE SHIELD UNITED OF WISCONSIN
401 WEST MICHIGAN STREET
MILWAUKEE, WISCONSIN 53203-2804

Description: Provides health-care insurance services

Founded: 1939

Annual Sales: $850.0 million

Number of Employees: 1,435

Expertise Needed: Accounting, finance, data processing, nursing, licensed practical nursing

Contact: Ms Leslie Lynch
Manager of Recruitment
(414) 226-5000

BLUE CROSS OF IDAHO HEALTH SERVICE
1501 FEDERAL WAY
BOISE, IDAHO 83705-2550

Description: Provides health-care insurance services

Founded: 1945

Annual Sales: $230.6 million

Number of Employees: 370

Expertise Needed: Accounting, finance, business administration, nursing, licensed practical nursing, data processing

Contact: Ms Cece Schnuerle
Human Resources Administrator
(208) 345-4550

BLUE CROSS OF WESTERN PENNSYLVANIA
5TH AVENUE PLACE
PITTSBURGH, PENNSYLVANIA 15222-0001

Description: Provides health-care insurance services

Founded: 1937

Annual Sales: $1.9 billion

Number of Employees: 2,300

Expertise Needed: Utilization review, quality control, customer service and support, marketing, medical records, case management, customer service and support, claims adjustment/examination, sales

Contact: Mr Wayne Nelson
Corporate Vice President of Human Resources
(412) 255-7000

BMC INDUSTRIES, INC.
2 APPLETREE SQUARE
MINNEAPOLIS, MINNESOTA 55425

Description: Manufactures ophthalmic goods and electronic components

Founded: 1907

Annual Sales: $180.8 million

Number of Employees: 1,983

Expertise Needed: Manufacturing engineering, design engineering, industrial engineering, sales, accounting

Contact: Ms Mary O'Connell
Director of Compensation/Benefits
(612) 851-6000

BOEHRINGER INGELHEIM PHARMACEUTICALS

900 RIDGEBURY ROAD
RIDGEFIELD, CONNECTICUT 06877

Description: Manufactures and sells pharmaceutical products

Parent Company: Boehringer Ingelheim Corporation

Founded: 1971

Annual Sales: $384.6 million

Number of Employees: 1,963

Expertise Needed: Laboratory technology, chemistry, research and development, toxicology

Contact for College Students and Recent Graduates:
Mr Jim Conklin
Associate Director of Human Resources
(203) 798-5364

Contact for All Other Candidates:
Mr. John Petraglia
Senior Human Resources Specialist
(203) 798-9988

BOEHRINGER MANNHEIM CORPORATION

9115 HAGUE ROAD
INDIANAPOLIS, INDIANA 46250

Description: Researches and develops medical instruments and produces hospital supplies

Number of Employees: 700

Expertise Needed: Chemical engineering, mechanical engineering, software engineering/development

Contact: Ms Vanessa Scott
Manager of Human Resources
(317) 845-2000

BON SECOURS HEALTH SYSTEMS

1505 MARRIOTTSVILLE ROAD
MARRIOTTSVILLE, MARYLAND 21104-1301

Description: Provides acute-care services

Annual Sales: $541.6 million

Number of Employees: 10,000

Expertise Needed: Accounting, finance, law, marketing, business administration, hospital administration, training and development

Contact: Ms Virginia Rounsaville
Personnel Administrator
(410) 442-5511

BOOTS PHARMACEUTICALS, INC.

300 TRI STATE INTERNATIONAL CENTER
LINCOLNSHIRE, ILLINOIS 60069-4413

Description: Develops and manufactures pharmaceuticals to treat infections, wounds, and pain

Founded: 1977

Annual Sales: $270.0 million

Number of Employees: 941

Expertise Needed: Chemistry, bi○

Contact: Mr Joseph Vinci
Manager of Staffing and De
(708) 405-7400

BOSTON METAL PRODUCTS CORPOR

400 RIVERSIDE AVENUE
MEDFORD, MASSACHUSETTS 02155

Description: Manufactures storage fixtures and carts for hospitals and clinics

Founded: 1937

Number of Employees: 220

Expertise Needed: Accounting, finance, marketing, sales, design engineering, mechanical engineering, production engineering

Contact: Ms Lisa Donaldson
Human Resources Assistant
(617) 395-7417

BOSTON SCIENTIFIC CORPORATION

480 PLEASANT STREET
WATERTOWN, MASSACHUSETTS 02172-2407

Description: Manufactures medical devices and equipment

Founded: 1979

Annual Sales: $315.2 million

Number of Employees: 2,100

Expertise Needed: Manufacturing engineering, clinical technology, biomedical engineering, management, medical technology, design engineering, research and development, marketing, finance, accounting

Contact: Mr Don Potter
Manager of Human Resources
(617) 923-1720

BOTSFORD GENERAL HOSPITAL

28050 GRAND RIVER AVENUE
FARMINGTON HILLS, MICHIGAN 48336-5919

Description: Community-based osteopathic teaching hospital

Annual Sales: $66.2 million

Number of Employees: 1,955

Expertise Needed: Physical therapy, medical technology, nursing

Contact: Ms Barbara Giorgio
Human Resources Coordinator
(313) 471-8834

THE BRIAN CENTER CORPORATION

1331 4TH STREET DRIVE NORTHWEST
HICKORY, NORTH CAROLINA 28601-2523

Description: Provides nursing home and retirement home care services

Annual Sales: $167.8 million

Number of Employees: 6,000

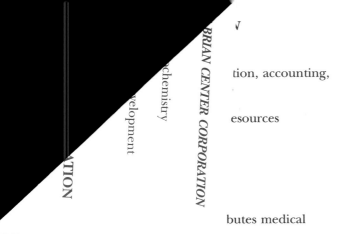

BRIAN CENTER CORPORATION

tion, accounting,

esources

butes medical

Founded: 1950
Annual Sales: $15.0 million
Number of Employees: 305
Number of Managerial and Professional Employees Hired 1993: 60
Expertise Needed: Accounting, computer programming, marketing, sales
Contact: Ms Linda Hill
Human Resources Coordinator
(515) 274-9227

BRIGHAM AND WOMEN'S HOSPITAL, INC.
75 FRANCIS STREET
BOSTON, MASSACHUSETTS 02115-6195

Description: Nonprofit surgical hospital
Founded: 1962
Annual Sales: $467.6 million
Number of Employees: 7,800
Expertise Needed: Nursing, licensed practical nursing, physical therapy, occupational therapy
Contact: Ms Susan Gomley
Manager of Employment
(617) 732-5500

BRIM, INC.
305 NE 102ND AVENUE
PORTLAND, OREGON 97220-4170

Description: Provides administrative personnel services for the health-care industry
Annual Sales: $75.1 million
Number of Employees: 1,000
Expertise Needed: Administration, business, nursing management and administration
Contact: Ms Toni Grabler
Vice President of Human Resources
(503) 256-2070

BRINKMAN INSTRUMENTS, INC.
1 CANTIAGUE ROAD
WESTBURY, NEW YORK 11590-0207

Description: Markets and distributes laboratory instruments and devices
Founded: 1941
Annual Sales: $70.0 million
Number of Employees: 296

Expertise Needed: Sales, distribution
Contact: Ms Maureen Smith
Human Resource Administrator
(516) 334-7500

BRISTOL-MYERS SQUIBB COMPANY
345 PARK AVENUE
NEW YORK, NEW YORK 10154-0001

Description: Manufactures pharmaceutical, medical, and health-care products, toiletries, and beauty aids
Founded: 1887
Annual Sales: $11.2 billion
Number of Employees: 52,600
Expertise Needed: Business management, biology, finance, mechanical engineering, chemical engineering, chemistry
Contact: Human Resources Department
(212) 546-4000

BRISTOL REGIONAL MEDICAL CENTER
209 MEMORIAL DRIVE
BRISTOL, TENNESSEE 37620-1703

Description: Nonprofit hospital with a regional cancer center and trauma center
Founded: 1923
Annual Sales: $98.5 million
Number of Employees: 2,000
Expertise Needed: Physical therapy, occupational therapy, nursing, nuclear medicine, medical records
Contact: Ms Kim Poore
Employment Coordinator
(615) 968-6070

BRITTHAVEN, INC.
1128 HIGHWAY 258 NORTH
KINGSTON, NORTH CAROLINA 28501

Description: Owns and operates extended-care nursing facilities
Parent Company: Neil Realty Company
Annual Sales: $91.1 million
Number of Employees: 3,500
Expertise Needed: Registered nursing, licensed practical nursing, accounting, finance
Contact: Ms Sue Ball
Human Resources Administrator
(919) 523-9094

BROMENN HEALTHCARE
VIRGINIA & FRANKLIN AVENUE
NORMAL, ILLINOIS 61761

Description: Nonprofit hospital
Founded: 1919
Annual Sales: $97.5 million
Number of Employees: 1,800

Expertise Needed: Dietetics, nursing

Contact: Ms Deborah Dulberson
　　　　Personnel Director
　　　　(309) 454-1000

BRONSON METHODIST HOSPITAL
252 EAST LOVELL STREET
KALAMAZOO, MICHIGAN 49007

Description: Rehabilitation center and general medical
　　and surgical hospital
Annual Sales: $215.5 million
Number of Employees: 2,370
Expertise Needed: Nursing, physical therapy,
　　occupational therapy
Contact: Ms Marilyn Potgiesser
　　　　Professional Staff Recruiter
　　　　(616) 341-6310

BRONX LEBANON HOSPITAL CENTER
1276 FULTON AVENUE
BRONX, NEW YORK 10456-3402

Description: General-care hospital
Founded: 1890
Annual Sales: $302.9 million
Number of Employees: 4,000
Expertise Needed: Physical therapy, occupational therapy,
　　radiation technology, nursing
Contact: Ms Denise Corvina
　　　　Director of Human Resources
　　　　(718) 590-1800

BROOKDALE HOSPITAL
LINDEN BOULEVARD & BROOKDALE PLACE
BROOKLYN, NEW YORK 11212

Description: General medical and surgical hospital
Parent Company: Linroc Community Services
　　Corporation
Annual Sales: $259.0 million
Number of Employees: 3,800
Expertise Needed: Respiratory therapy, occupational
　　therapy, physical therapy, registered nursing
Contact: Ms Melisa Fiech
　　　　Employment Manager
　　　　(718) 240-5000

BROOKLYN HOSPITAL CENTER, INC.
121 DEKALB AVENUE
BROOKLYN, NEW YORK 11201-5425

Description: General medical and surgical hospital
Founded: 1845
Annual Sales: $239.3 million
Number of Employees: 3,200
Expertise Needed: Operating room, registered nursing,
　　tax accounting, certified nursing and nursing
　　assistance
Contact: Human Resources
　　　　(718) 250-8000

BRYAN MEMORIAL HOSPITAL, INC.
1600 SOUTH 48TH STREET
LINCOLN, NEBRASKA 68506-1227

Description: General hospital
Founded: 1926
Annual Sales: $123.5 million
Number of Employees: 2,015
Expertise Needed: Physical therapy, occupational therapy,
　　nuclear technology, medical technology, radiation
　　technology, management information systems
Contact: Ms Deb Komenda
　　　　Employment Specialist
　　　　(402) 489-0200

BRYN MAWR HOSPITAL, INC.
130 SOUTH BRYN MAWR AVENUE
BRYN MAWR, PENNSYLVANIA 19010-3121

Description: Community hospital
Founded: 1892
Annual Sales: $154.2 million
Number of Employees: 2,825
Expertise Needed: Physical therapy, occupational therapy,
　　nursing
Contact: Ms Sharon Johnson
　　　　Professional Recruiter
　　　　(215) 526-8666

BUCKEYE DISCOUNT, INC.
1020 FORD STREET
MAUMEE, OHIO 43537-1820

Description: Drug store chain
Parent Company: Seaway Food Town, Inc.
Annual Sales: $103.1 million
Number of Employees: 791
Expertise Needed: Sales, marketing, management
Contact: Mr Charles North
　　　　Director of Human Resources
　　　　(419) 893-9401

BUFFALO GENERAL HOSPITAL
100 HIGH STREET
BUFFALO, NEW YORK 14203-1154

Description: General medical and surgical hospital and
　　nursing home
Parent Company: General Care Corporation
Annual Sales: $227.6 million
Number of Employees: 4,249
Expertise Needed: Physical therapy, nursing,
　　administration
Contact: Ms Bonnie Hackford
　　　　Human Resources Director
　　　　(716) 845-5600

BURROUGHS WELLCOME COMPANY
3030 CORNWALLIS ROAD
RESEARCH TRIANGLE PARK, NORTH
CAROLINA 27709-2700

Description: Manufactures pharmaceutical products
Founded: 1924
Annual Sales: $1.4 billion
Number of Employees: 5,000
Expertise Needed: Pharmacy, chemistry, computer
    programming, research, data processing, biology,
    biochemistry
Contact: Ms Ann Jones
        Manager of Human Resources
        (919) 315-8347

THE BURROWS COMPANY
230 WEST PALATINE ROAD
WHEELING, ILLINOIS 60090-5825

Description: Distributes medical products
Founded: 1962
Annual Sales: $225.0 million
Number of Employees: 400
Expertise Needed: Accounting, finance, data processing
Contact: Mr Scott Schoeder
        Accounting Manager
        (708) 537-7300

BUTTERWORTH HEALTH CORPORATION
100 BOSTWICK AVENUE
GRAND RAPIDS, MICHIGAN 49503-2560

Description: Nonprofit hospital
Annual Sales: $346.4 million
Number of Employees: 4,400
Expertise Needed: Nursing, occupational therapy,
    physical therapy, respiratory therapy, radiology
Contact: Ms Lucy Duggan
        Manager of Employment
        (616) 774-1774

CABARRUS MEMORIAL HOSPITAL
920 CHURCH STREET NORTH
CONCORD, NORTH CAROLINA 28025-2927

Description: Private hospital
Founded: 1937
Annual Sales: $89.1 million
Number of Employees: 1,500

Expertise Needed: Nursing, physical therapy, radiology
Contact: Ms Dottie Settlemyer
        Employment Coordinator
        (704) 786-2111

CABOT MEDICAL CORPORATION
2021 CABOT BOULEVARD WEST
LANGHORNE, PENNSYLVANIA 19047-1841

Description: Designs and manufactures surgical devices
Annual Sales: $55.0 million
Number of Employees: 404
*Number of Managerial and Professional Employees Hired
    1993:* 10
Expertise Needed: Accounting, finance, data processing,
    mechanical engineering, electrical engineering
Contact: Ms Judy Smoyer
        Director of Human Resources
        (215) 752-8300

CALIFORNIA PACIFIC MEDICAL CENTER
3700 CALIFORNIA STREET
SAN FRANCISCO, CALIFORNIA 94118-1618

Description: Provides hospital services
Parent Company: California Healthcare System
Founded: 1885
Annual Sales: $387.6 million
Number of Employees: 4,000
Expertise Needed: Nursing, licensed practical nursing,
    pharmacy, nutrition, accounting, finance, electrical
    engineering, computer science
Contact: Ms Robin Berkman
        Manager of Nursing Recruitment
        (415) 750-6117

CALIFORNIA PHYSICIANS SERVICE
2 NORTH POINT STREET
SAN FRANCISCO, CALIFORNIA 94133-1598

Description: Provides medical insurance services
Founded: 1939
Annual Sales: $3.7 billion
Number of Employees: 3,997
Expertise Needed: Systems analysis, accounting, finance,
    marketing, sales, health care, administration
Contact: Ms Deborah LeFevre
        Manager of Human Resources
        (415) 445-5000

CAMBREX CORPORATION

1 MEADOWLANDS PLAZA
EAST RUTHERFORD, NEW JERSEY 07073-2137

Description: Manufactures specialty chemical products
for pharmaceutical, herbicide, and pesticide
companies
Annual Sales: $179.5 million
Number of Employees: 750
Expertise Needed: Chemical engineering, chemistry
Contact: Ms Jeanne Patterson
Manager of Human Resources
(201) 804-3000

CAMBRIDGE BIOTECH CORPORATION

365 PLANTATION STREET
WORCESTER, MASSACHUSETTS 01605-2388

Description: Develops and manufactures diagnostic,
vaccine, and therapeutic products for infectious
diseases
Founded: 1981
Annual Sales: $38.1 million
Number of Employees: 348
Expertise Needed: Biology, chemistry, physics, business
administration, data processing, accounting
Contact: Ms Mattie Schadt
Senior Technical Recruiter
(508) 797-5777

CAMP INTERNATIONAL, INC.

744 WEST MICHIGAN AVENUE
JACKSON, MICHIGAN 49201

Description: Manufactures orthotic products
Founded: 1908
Number of Employees: 500
Expertise Needed: Marketing, sales, advertising
Contact: Mr Dennis Donnellan
Manager of Human Resources
(517) 787-1600

CANDELA LASER CORPORATION

530 BOSTON POST ROAD
WAYLAND, MASSACHUSETTS 01778-1833

Description: Designs and manufactures laser systems
and related accessories
Founded: 1970
Annual Sales: $33.2 million
Number of Employees: 224
Expertise Needed: Electronics/electronics engineering,
mechanical engineering, computer science
Contact: Ms Rachel Dupuis
Manager of Human Resources
(508) 358-7637

CANDLER HOSPITAL, INC.

5353 REYNOLDS STREET
SAVANNAH, GEORGIA 31405-6005

Description: General medical and surgical hospital
Parent Company: Candler Health System, Inc.
Annual Sales: $95.1 million
Number of Employees: 1,600
Expertise Needed: Physical therapy, occupational therapy,
radiation technology, nuclear medicine
Contact: Ms Arlene King
Recruiter
(912) 692-6219

CAPE COD HOSPITAL

27 PARK STREET
HYANNIS, MASSACHUSETTS 02601-5203

Description: Regional referral hospital
Founded: 1919
Annual Sales: $95.5 million
Number of Employees: 1,350
Expertise Needed: Occupational therapy, physical
therapy, registered nursing
Contact: Mr Francis Matthews
Director of Personnel
(508) 771-1800

CAPE CORAL MEDICAL CENTER, INC.

636 DEL PRADO BOULEVARD
CAPE CORAL, FLORIDA 33990

Description: Public hospital
Founded: 1977
Annual Sales: $83.5 million
Number of Employees: 1,400
Expertise Needed: Nursing, physical therapy
Contact: Mr John Mantica
Manager of Employment
(813) 574-0123

CAPITAL AREA COMMUNITY HEALTH PLAN

1201 TROY SCHENECTADY ROAD
LATHAM, NEW YORK 12110-1014

Description: Health maintenance organization
Founded: 1975
Annual Sales: $305.0 million
Number of Employees: 2,000
Expertise Needed: Advertising, marketing, finance, sales,
accounting
Contact: Ms Rose Marie Reichenbach
Manager of Employment
(518) 783-3110

CAPITAL BLUE CROSS, INC.

2500 ELMERTON AVENUE
HARRISBURG, PENNSYLVANIA 17110-9763

Description: Provides health-care insurance services
Founded: 1938
Annual Sales: $1.0 billion

Capital Blue Cross, Inc. (continued)

Number of Employees: 1,772

Expertise Needed: Claims adjustment/examination, accounting, market research, program analysis, systems analysis

Contact: Ms Deb Cohen
Manager of Employee Relations
(717) 541-7000

CARBOMEDICS, INC.

1300 EAST ANDERSON LANE
AUSTIN, TEXAS 78752-1799

Description: Manufactures heart valves

Annual Sales: $50.0 million

Number of Employees: 564

Number of Managerial and Professional Employees Hired 1993: 25

Expertise Needed: Mechanical engineering, quality engineering, materials science, ceramic engineering

Contact: Ms Theresa Folmar
Employment Specialist
(512) 873-3200

CARDINAL GLENNON CHILDREN'S HOSPITAL

1465 SOUTH GRAND BOULEVARD
SAINT LOUIS, MISSOURI 63104-1003

Description: Pediatric hospital

Founded: 1949

Annual Sales: $100.4 million

Number of Employees: 1,600

Expertise Needed: Occupational therapy, physical therapy

Contact: Ms Mary Jane Brecklin
Manager of Employment
(314) 577-5300

CARDINAL HEALTH, INC.

655 METRO PLACE SOUTH
DUBLIN, OHIO 43017-3377

Description: Wholesales and distributes pharmaceuticals and health and beauty aids

Founded: 1979

Annual Sales: $2.0 billion

Number of Employees: 1,600

Expertise Needed: Accounting, finance, data processing, law, pharmacology

Contact: Mr Ted Diabisi
Director of Human Resources
(614) 761-8700

CARE GROUP, INC.

1 HOLLOW LANE
NEW HYDE PARK, NEW YORK 11042-1215

Description: Provides home health-care services

Annual Sales: $28.3 million

Number of Employees: 1,852

Expertise Needed: Registered nursing, licensed practical nursing, physical therapy, occupational therapy, social work, certified nursing and nursing assistance

Contact: Ms Gilda Schechter
Manager of Employment
(516) 869-8383

CAREMARK INTERNATIONAL, INC.

2215 SANDERS ROAD
NORTHBROOK, ILLINOIS 60062-6114

Description: Provides outpatient care and managed care services

Number of Employees: 6,100

Expertise Needed: Registered nursing, occupational therapy, physical therapy, information systems, marketing, finance, accounting

Contact: Mr Kent Delucenay
Vice President of Human Resources
(708) 559-4700

CAREMET, INC.

1690 SOUTH COUNTY FARM
WARSAW, INDIANA 46580-8248

Description: Owns and operates nursing homes

Annual Sales: $92.5 million

Number of Employees: 2,807

Expertise Needed: Accounting, marketing, health insurance, finance

Contact: Mr Gene Bone
Senior Employee Relations Manager
(219) 267-7211

CARILION HEALTH SYSTEM

1212 3RD STREET SOUTHWEST
ROANOKE, VIRGINIA 24016-4612

Description: Health-care facility

Annual Sales: $513.9 million

Number of Employees: 8,338

Expertise Needed: Cardiac care, oncology, emergency services

Contact: Ms Becky Allen
Employment Specialist
(703) 981-7900

CARLE CLINIC ASSOCIATION

602 WEST UNIVERSITY AVENUE
URBANA, ILLINOIS 61801-2530

Description: Hospital-affiliated clinic

Founded: 1931

Annual Sales: $169.8 million

Number of Employees: 1,950

Expertise Needed: Physical therapy, occupational therapy, nursing, pharmacy

Contact: Ms Cathy McCasky
Manager of Employment
(217) 383-3066

THE CARLE FOUNDATION
611 WEST PARK STREET
URBANA, ILLINOIS 61801-2529

Description: Public general hospital
Founded: 1946
Annual Sales: $94.6 million
Number of Employees: 1,800
Expertise Needed: Nursing, physical therapy, occupational therapy, pharmacy, respiratory therapy, accounting, management information systems
Contact: Ms Jodi Swearingen
      Nursing Recruiter
      (217) 383-3311

CARRIER FOUNDATION, INC.
601 COUNTY ROAD
BELLE MEAD, NEW JERSEY 08502

Description: Provides mental health counseling and psychiatric treatment services
Founded: 1977
Annual Sales: $40.2 million
Number of Employees: 854
Expertise Needed: Accounting, finance, marketing, clinical psychology, counseling, psychiatry, psychotherapy, psychiatric social work
Contact: Ms Nancy DaLonzo
      Manager of Recruitment
      (908) 281-1000

CARRINGTON LABORATORIES, INC.
2001 WALNUT HILL LANE
IRVING, TEXAS 75038

Description: Manufactures wound-care products
Founded: 1974
Annual Sales: $20.1 million
Number of Employees: 240
Number of Managerial and Professional Employees Hired 1993: 30
Expertise Needed: Law, marketing, sales, laboratory technology
Contact: Ms Pamela Mitchell
      Human Resources Director
      (214) 518-1300

CARTER-WALLACE, INC.
1345 AVENUE OF THE AMERICAS
NEW YORK, NEW YORK 10105-0302

Description: Manufactures health-care and pharmaceutical products
Founded: 1880
Annual Sales: $653.5 million
Number of Employees: 4,020

Expertise Needed: Manufacturing engineering, sales, accounting, finance, data processing, pharmaceutical chemistry, pharmacology, chemical engineering
Contact: Ms Tina Scudere
      Representative for Recruitment
      (212) 339-5000

CATHOLIC HEALTHCARE WEST
1700 MONTGOMERY STREET
SAN FRANCISCO, CALIFORNIA 94111-1021

Description: Owns and operates hospitals and medical centers
Annual Sales: $1.2 billion
Number of Employees: 14,000
Expertise Needed: Accounting, business administration
Contact: Ms Irene Tonogan
      Corporate Recruiter
      (415) 397-9000

CATHOLIC MEDICAL CENTER
100 MCGREGOR STREET
MANCHESTER, NEW HAMPSHIRE 03102-3730

Description: General hospital
Parent Company: Fidelity Health Alliance
Annual Sales: $107.9 million
Number of Employees: 1,350
Expertise Needed: Registered nursing, licensed practical nursing, physical therapy, respiratory therapy
Contact: Mr Pete Doolittle
      Recruitment
      (603) 668-3545

CEDARS MEDICAL CENTER, INC.
1400 NORTHWEST 12TH AVENUE
MIAMI, FLORIDA 33136-1003

Description: Not-for-profit medical and surgical hospital
Founded: 1959
Annual Sales: $124.5 million
Number of Employees: 2,466
Expertise Needed: Occupational therapy, physical therapy
Contact: Ms Santra Lush
      Manager of Recruitment
      (305) 325-5511

CEDARS-SINAI MEDICAL CENTER
22 ALDEN DRIVE
LOS ANGELES, CALIFORNIA 90048

Description: General medical and surgical hospital
Founded: 1902
Annual Sales: $593.1 million
Number of Employees: 6,000

Cedars-Sinai Medical Center (continued)

Expertise Needed: Nursing, allied health, laboratory technology, research and development, finance, information services

Contact: Ms Jeanne Flores
Director of Employee Recruitment
(310) 967-8230

CENTER FOR HEALTH CARE SERVICE

3031 INTERSTATE HIGHWAY 10 WEST
SAN ANTONIO, TEXAS 78204

Description: Community mental health organization
Founded: 1965
Annual Sales: $25.8 million
Number of Employees: 420
Expertise Needed: Registered nursing, licensed practical nursing, social work, accounting, physical therapy

Contact: Mr C E Jackson
Director of Human Resources
(210) 731-1300

CENTOCOR, INC.

200 GREAT VALLEY PARKWAY
MALVERN, PENNSYLVANIA 19355-1307

Description: Develops diagnostic and therapeutic products
Founded: 1979
Annual Sales: $44.3 million
Number of Employees: 1,400
Expertise Needed: Chemical engineering, chemistry, biochemistry, biomedical engineering, allied therapy

Contact: Ms. Kathy Costello
Human Resources Secretary
(215) 651-6000

CENTRAL MASSACHUSETTS HEALTH CARE

100 FRONT STREET
WORCESTER, MASSACHUSETTS 01608-1402

Description: Health maintenance organization
Founded: 1973
Annual Sales: $137.4 million
Number of Employees: 200
Expertise Needed: Registered nursing, administration, health care, licensed practical nursing, sales, claims adjustment/examination, claims processing/ management, and administration, health science

Contact: Human Resources Department
(508) 798-8667

CENTRAL PHARMACEUTICALS, INC.

120 EAST 3RD STREET
SEYMOUR, INDIANA 47274

Description: Manufactures and markets pharmaceuticals
Founded: 1904
Number of Employees: 300

Expertise Needed: Manufacturing engineering, chemistry, laboratory technology, accounting, marketing, sales

Contact: Mr Daniel Desmond
President
(812) 522-3915

CENTRASTATE MEDICAL CENTER

901 WEST MAIN STREET
FREEHOLD, NEW JERSEY 07728-2537

Description: Nonprofit hospital specializing in acute care
Parent Company: Centrastate Healthcare System
Annual Sales: $84.2 million
Number of Employees: 1,500
Expertise Needed: Registered nursing

Contact: Ms Pat Ahearn
Director of Employee Relations
(908) 294-2904

CERNER CORPORATION

2800 ROCK CREEK PARKWAY
KANSAS CITY, MISSOURI 64117-2530

Description: Develops software and provides clinical information systems
Founded: 1979
Annual Sales: $101.1 million
Number of Employees: 525
Number of Managerial and Professional Employees Hired 1993: 20
Expertise Needed: Software engineering/development, computer programming

Contact: Mr Michael Bunch
Recruitment Team Leader
(816) 221-1024

CHARLESTON AREA MEDICAL CENTER

3200 MACCORKLE
CHARLESTON, WEST VIRGINIA 25305

Description: General hospital
Parent Company: Camcare, Inc.
Annual Sales: $329.2 million
Number of Employees: 4,740
Expertise Needed: Medical technology, respiratory therapy, occupational therapy, physical therapy, oncology, orthopedics, obstetrics, neurology, gynecology, cardiology

Contact: Ms Jean Campbell
Employment Specialist
(304) 348-5432

CHARLOTTE MECKLENBURG HOSPITAL AUTHORITY

1012 SOUTH KINGS ROAD
CHARLOTTE, NORTH CAROLINA 28203-5812

Description: Provides hospital administration services
Founded: 1943
Annual Sales: $459.8 million

Number of Employees: 6,300
Expertise Needed: Cardiology, nursing, oncology, physical therapy, occupational therapy
Contact: Mr Judd Tillett
　　　Director of Human Resources
　　　(704) 355-2000

CHARLTON MEMORIAL HOSPITAL
363 HIGHLAND AVENUE
FALL RIVER, MASSACHUSETTS 02720-3703

Description: General medical and surgical hospital
Founded: 1900
Annual Sales: $106.8 million
Number of Employees: 1,344
Expertise Needed: Nursing, occupational therapy, medical records, food science
Contact: Human Resources Department
　　　(508) 679-3131

CHARTER FAIRMOUNT INSTITUTE
561 FAIRTHORNE AVENUE
PHILADELPHIA, PENNSYLVANIA 19128-2412

Description: Psychiatric hospital
Parent Company: Charter Medical Corporation
Annual Sales: $21.7 million
Number of Employees: 275
Expertise Needed: Psychiatry, psychology, nursing, therapy
Contact: Ms Maureen Keeney
　　　Director of Human Resources
　　　(215) 487-4000

CHARTER HOSPITAL OF CORPUS CHRISTI
3126 RODD FIELD ROAD
CORPUS CHRISTI, TEXAS 78414-3901

Description: Psychiatric hospital
Parent Company: Charter Medical Corporation
Annual Sales: $24.5 million
Number of Employees: 170
Expertise Needed: Accounting, finance, data processing, social work, registered nursing, licensed practical nursing, psychiatric social work, counseling, chemical dependency, marketing
Contact: Human Resources Department
　　　(512) 993-8893

CHARTER LAKESIDE HOSPITAL, INC.
1550 FIRST COLONY BOULEVARD
SUGAR LAND, TEXAS 77479-4000

Description: Psychiatric hospital
Parent Company: Charter Medical Corporation
Annual Sales: $20.4 million
Number of Employees: 125

Expertise Needed: Accounting, data processing, finance, nursing management and administration, registered nursing, licensed practical nursing, occupational therapy, physical therapy, radiology
Contact: Ms Mary Winne
　　　Manager of Human Resources
　　　(713) 980-4000

CHARTER LAKESIDE HOSPITAL, INC.
2911 BRUNSWICK ROAD
MEMPHIS, TENNESSEE 38133-4105

Description: Psychiatric hospital
Parent Company: Charter Medical Corporation
Founded: 1973
Annual Sales: $37.8 million
Number of Employees: 489
Expertise Needed: Nursing management and administration, health care, registered nursing, licensed practical nursing, occupational therapy, physical therapy, radiology, respiratory care
Contact: Human Resources Department
　　　(901) 377-4700

CHARTER MEDICAL CORPORATION
577 MULBERRY STREET
MACON, GEORGIA 31201-2742

Description: Owns and operates psychiatric and acute-care hospitals
Founded: 1969
Annual Sales: $1.3 billion
Number of Employees: 12,800
Expertise Needed: Accounting, finance, marketing, computer programming, data processing
Contact: Mr Al Joyner
　　　Employment Manager
　　　(912) 742-1161

CHARTER REAL, INC.
8550 HUEBNER ROAD
SAN ANTONIO, TEXAS 78240-1803

Description: Psychiatric hospital
Parent Company: Charter Medical Corporation
Annual Sales: $21.9 million
Number of Employees: 180
Expertise Needed: Psychiatry, psychology, social work
Contact: Mr Lee Wise
　　　Director of Human Resources
　　　(210) 699-8585

CHARTER WESTBROOK HOSPITAL
1500 WESTBROOK AVENUE
RICHMOND, VIRGINIA 23227-3312

Description: Psychiatric hospital
Parent Company: Charter Medical Corporation
Founded: 1970
Annual Sales: $40.1 million
Number of Employees: 290

Expertise Needed: Information systems, psychiatry, psychology

Contact: Mr. Lee Byrd
Director of Human Resources
(804) 201-7178

CHASE PHARMACEUTICAL COMPANY

280 CHESTNUT STREET
NEWARK, NEW JERSEY 07105

Description: Manufactures pharmaceuticals
Founded: 1929
Number of Employees: 350
Number of Managerial and Professional Employees Hired 1993: 50
Expertise Needed: Chemistry, research and development, chemical engineering, manufacturing engineering, accounting, marketing, sales

Contact: Mr Greg Danzer
Human Resources Manager
(201) 589-8181

CHASE SCIENTIFIC GLASS

6760 JIMMY CARTER BOULEVARD
NORCROSS, GEORGIA 30071

Description: Manufactures laboratory glassware
Founded: 1929
Number of Employees: 280
Number of Managerial and Professional Employees Hired 1993: 5
Expertise Needed: Mechanical engineering, accounting, management information systems

Contact: Ms Becky Sherriff
Corporate Controller
(404) 729-7400

CHATTANOOGA GROUP, INC.

4717 ADAMS ROAD
HIXSON, TENNESSEE 37343-4001

Description: Manufactures physical therapy and rehabilitation equipment, and specialty tables and chairs
Founded: 1968
Annual Sales: $32.3 million
Number of Employees: 425
Expertise Needed: Mechanical engineering, electrical engineering, data processing, accounting, finance

Contact: Mr Dan Lawlor
Director of Personnel
(615) 870-2281

CHELSEA LAB, INC.

2021 EAST ROOSEVELT BOULEVARD
MONROE, NORTH CAROLINA 28111

Description: Manufactures pharmaceuticals
Parent Company: Rugby-Darby Group Companies
Annual Sales: $34.0 million

Number of Employees: 275
Expertise Needed: Chemistry
Contact: Mr Carl Chapman
Manager of Human Resources
(704) 289-5531

CHEMD, INC.

14281 WELCH ROAD
DALLAS, TEXAS 75244-3932

Description: Operates chain of pharmacy stores
Annual Sales: $50.0 million
Number of Employees: 350
Expertise Needed: Pharmacy
Contact: Ms Karen Koether
Manager of Employment
(214) 960-9000

CHICAGO HMO, LTD.

540 NORTH LASALLE STREET
CHICAGO, ILLINOIS 60610-4217

Description: Health maintenance organization
Parent Company: HMO America, Inc. (NV)
Annual Sales: $216.7 million
Number of Employees: 333
Expertise Needed: Finance, marketing, accounting
Contact: Ms. Josie Bautista
Human Resources Representative
(312) 751-4460

CHILDREN'S HEALTH SYSTEM, INC.

601 CHILDREN'S LANE
NORFOLK, VIRGINIA 23507-1905

Description: Pediatric hospital
Annual Sales: $80.4 million
Number of Employees: 1,211
Expertise Needed: Physical therapy, respiratory therapy, laboratory technology, medical technology
Contact for College Students and Recent Graduates:
Mr Lynn Baucom
Personnel Generalist/Nurse Recruiter
(804) 668-7000
Contact for All Other Candidates:
Ms Martha Wright
Personnel Generalist
(804) 668-7000

CHILDREN'S HOSPITAL AND MEDICAL CENTER

4800 SAND POINT WAY NORTHEAST
SEATTLE, WASHINGTON 98105-3916

Description: Nonprofit pediatric hospital
Parent Company: Coh-Care, Inc.
Founded: 1907
Annual Sales: $128.6 million
Number of Employees: 2,375

Expertise Needed: Nursing, physical therapy, pediatrics

Contact: Ms Kathy Schumer
Manager of Employment
(206) 526-2000

CHILDREN'S HOSPITAL ASSOCIATION

1056 EAST 19TH AVENUE
DENVER, COLORADO 80218-1007

Description: Pediatric hospital
Parent Company: Children's Health Corporation
Annual Sales: $141.4 million
Number of Employees: 2,300
Expertise Needed: Nursing, occupational therapy, physical therapy, respiratory therapy

Contact: Ms Kay Swepston
Recruitment Manager
(303) 861-6480

CHILDREN'S HOSPITAL, INC.

700 CHILDREN'S DRIVE
COLUMBUS, OHIO 43205-2666

Description: Pediatric general hospital
Founded: 1974
Annual Sales: $177.8 million
Number of Employees: 2,390
Expertise Needed: Hospital administration, social work, medical records, registered nursing, licensed practical nursing, physical therapy, occupational therapy

Contact: Human Resources Department
(614) 722-2000

CHILDREN'S HOSPITAL OF SAN DIEGO

3020 CHILDREN'S WAY
SAN DIEGO, CALIFORNIA 92123-4224

Description: Private pediatric hospital
Founded: 1925
Annual Sales: $136.2 million
Number of Employees: 2,200
Expertise Needed: Registered nursing, physical therapy, occupational therapy

Contact: Mr Larry Schou
Director of Nursing
(619) 576-1700

CHILDREN'S MEMORIAL HOSPITAL

8301 DODGE STREET
OMAHA, NEBRASKA 68114-4114

Description: Pediatric general hospital
Founded: 1943
Annual Sales: $54.0 million
Number of Employees: 716
Expertise Needed: Registered nursing, licensed practical nursing, emergency services, triage, operating room, computer programming, pediatric nursing

Contact: Department of Human Resources

CHILDREN'S MEMORIAL HOSPITAL

2300 NORTH CHILDREN'S PLAZA
CHICAGO, ILLINOIS 60614-3318

Description: Private pediatric hospital
Parent Company: Children's Memorial Medical Center
Annual Sales: $173.8 million
Number of Employees: 2,750
Expertise Needed: Nursing, physical therapy

Contact: Ms Sue Quillin
Director of Employment
(312) 880-4000

CHILDREN'S HEALTH CORPORATION

1056 EAST 19TH AVENUE
DENVER, COLORADO 80218-1007

Description: Nonprofit pediatric hospital
Annual Sales: $140.9 million
Number of Employees: 2,500
Expertise Needed: Nursing, physical therapy, occupational therapy

Contact: Ms Kay Swepston
Manager of Recruitment
(303) 861-6449

CHILDREN'S HEALTH SERVICES OF TEXAS

1935 MOTOR STREET
DALLAS, TEXAS 75235-7794

Description: Nonprofit private pediatric hospital
Annual Sales: $130.0 million
Number of Employees: 1,713
Expertise Needed: Nursing, allied health

Contact: Ms Angie Rhodes
Human Resources Team Leader/Generalist
(214) 640-6099

CHILDREN'S HOSPITAL & MEDICAL CENTER

3333 BURNET AVENUE
CINCINNATI, OHIO 45229-3026

Description: Public pediatric hospital
Founded: 1973
Annual Sales: $216.3 million
Number of Employees: 3,700
Expertise Needed: Registered nursing, social work, physical therapy, pharmacology, business

Contact: Ms Beth Dobrovsi
Manager of Human Resources
(513) 559-4200

CHILDREN'S HOSPITAL & MEDICAL CENTER

1 PERKINS SQUARE
AKRON, OHIO 44308-1063

Description: Pediatric general hospital
Founded: 1891
Annual Sales: $113.8 million
Number of Employees: 1,919

Children's Hospital & Medical Center (continued)

Expertise Needed: Nursing, pharmacy, physical therapy, occupational therapy

Contact: Human Resources Department
(216) 379-8098

CHILDREN'S HOSPITAL & MEDICAL CENTER OF NORTHERN CALIFORNIA

747 52ND STREET
OAKLAND, CALIFORNIA 94609-1809

Description: Pediatric hospital
Founded: 1912
Annual Sales: $136.6 million
Number of Employees: 2,000
Expertise Needed: Registered nursing, speech pathology, pharmacology

Contact: Ms Yvette Williams
Manager of Human Resources
(510) 428-3420

CHILDREN'S HOSPITAL OF ALABAMA

1600 7TH AVENUE SOUTH
BIRMINGHAM, ALABAMA 35233-1711

Description: Pediatric general hospital
Founded: 1960
Annual Sales: $143.0 million
Number of Employees: 1,715
Expertise Needed: Nursing, pediatrics, radiology, medical records, medical technology, physical therapy, occupational therapy, pharmacy

Contact: Employment Office
(205) 939-9100

CHILDREN'S HOSPITAL OF BUFFALO, INC.

219 BRYANT STREET
BUFFALO, NEW YORK 14222-2006

Description: Pediatric hospital
Parent Company: Children's & Women's Health
Annual Sales: $102.8 million
Number of Employees: 2,200
Expertise Needed: Pediatric care, licensed practical nursing, registered nursing, maternity nursing

Contact: Ms. Anne Stonebreaker
Personnel Department
(716) 878-7000

CHILDREN'S HOSPITAL OF MICHIGAN

3901 BEAUBIEN STREET
DETROIT, MICHIGAN 48201-2119

Description: Pediatric general hospital
Parent Company: The Detroit Medical Center
Annual Sales: $166.3 million
Number of Employees: 2,310

Expertise Needed: Physical therapy, occupational therapy, laboratory technology, medical technology

Contact: Mr Vince Garrasi
Human Resources Specialist
(313) 745-5364

CHILDREN'S HOSPITAL OF PHILADELPHIA

34TH STREET & CIVIC CENTER BOULEVARD
PHILADELPHIA, PENNSYLVANIA 19104-4399

Description: Pediatric general hospital
Founded: 1855
Annual Sales: $213.4 million
Number of Employees: 3,000
Expertise Needed: Laboratory technology, medical technology, biology, chemistry, genetics, research

Contact: Department of Medical Affairs
(215) 590-1000

CHILDREN'S HOSPITAL OF PITTSBURGH

3705 5TH AVENUE
PITTSBURGH, PENNSYLVANIA 15213-2524

Description: Private hospital specializing in pediatrics
Founded: 1887
Annual Sales: $153.6 million
Number of Employees: 1,772
Expertise Needed: Registered nursing, physical therapy, research

Contact: Ms Gloria Ferguson
Recruiter
(800) 692-5009

CHILDREN'S HOSPITAL OF WISCONSIN

9000 WEST WISCONSIN AVENUE
MILWAUKEE, WISCONSIN 53226-3518

Description: Pediatric hospital
Founded: 1894
Annual Sales: $130.1 million
Number of Employees: 2,000
Expertise Needed: Emergency services, radiology, respiratory therapy, cardiology, accounting, medical technology

Contact: Human Resources Department
(414) 266-2732

CHILDREN'S MEDICAL CENTER OF DAYTON, OHIO

1 CHILDREN'S PLAZA
DAYTON, OHIO 45404-1898

Description: Pediatric general hospital
Founded: 1919
Annual Sales: $76.4 million
Number of Employees: 1,200
Expertise Needed: Nursing
Contact: Ms Rose Crouch
Human Resources Specialist
(513) 226-8300

CHILDREN'S SPECIALIZED HOSPITAL
150 NEW PROVIDENCE ROAD
MOUNTAINSIDE, NEW JERSEY 07092-2590

Description: Nonprofit private pediatric hospital
Founded: 1891
Annual Sales: $28.9 million
Number of Employees: 550
Expertise Needed: Physical therapy, registered nursing, certified nursing and nursing assistance, speech therapy
Contact: Mr William J. Dwyer
Vice President of Human Resources
(908) 233-3720

CHIRON CORPORATION
4560 HORTON STREET
EMERYVILLE, CALIFORNIA 94608-2916

Description: Develops and sells therapeutic, diagnostic, ophthalmic, and vaccine products
Founded: 1981
Annual Sales: $118.5 million
Number of Employees: 1,510
Expertise Needed: Ophthalmological engineering, chemical engineering, chemistry, manufacturing engineering, design engineering
Contact: Human Resources Department
(510) 655-8730

CHIRON VISION, INC.
9342 JERONIMO ROAD
IRVINE, CALIFORNIA 92718-1903

Description: Manufactures interoptical lenses
Parent Company: Chiron Corporation
Annual Sales: $90.0 million
Number of Employees: 600
Expertise Needed: Mechanical engineering, electrical engineering, industrial engineering, optics
Contact: Ms Susan Astroth
Human Resources Manager
(714) 768-4690

CHOICE DRUG SYSTEMS, INC.
2930 WASHINGTON BOULEVARD
BALTIMORE, MARYLAND 21230

Description: Distributes prescription drugs, medication carts, and computerized tracking systems
Founded: 1973
Annual Sales: $42.6 million
Number of Employees: 400
Expertise Needed: Data processing, accounting, finance, computer programming, sales
Contact: Ms Kim Belford
Director of Personnel
(410) 646-7373

CHRIST HOSPITAL
176 PALISADE AVENUE
JERSEY CITY, NEW JERSEY 07306-1121

Description: General hospital
Parent Company: Christ Hospital Health Services Corporation
Annual Sales: $120.0 million
Number of Employees: 1,200
Expertise Needed: Nursing, physical therapy, cardiac care, oncology, intensive care, home health care, information systems
Contact: Ms Eileen Maloney
Manager of Employment
(201) 795-8200

CHRISTIAN HEALTH CARE CENTER
301 SICOMAC AVENUE
WYCKOFF, NEW JERSEY 07481

Description: Provides nursing and psychiatric care services
Founded: 1911
Annual Sales: $21.1 million
Number of Employees: 550
Expertise Needed: Nursing, licensed practical nursing, psychiatry, psychology, social service, occupational therapy
Contact: Ms Nancy Soto
Recruiter
(201) 848-5200

CHRISTIAN HEALTH SERVICES DEVELOPMENT CORPORATION
11133 DUNN ROAD
ST. LOUIS, MISSOURI 63136

Description: Owns and manages hospitals
Annual Sales: $407.8 million
Number of Employees: 7,362
Expertise Needed: Physical therapy, occupational therapy, nursing
Contact: Mr Craig Venneman
Manager of Human Resources
(314) 355-2300

CHRISTIAN HOMES, INC.
200 NORTH POSTVILLE DRIVE
LINCOLN, ILLINOIS 62656-1978

Description: Owns and operates nursing homes
Founded: 1962
Annual Sales: $37.5 million
Number of Employees: 1,600
Expertise Needed: Accounting, physical therapy, occupational therapy
Contact: Mr Dave Miller
Director of Human Resources
(217) 732-9651

CHRISTIAN HOSPITAL NORTHEAST-NORTHWEST
11133 DUNN ROAD
ST. LOUIS, MISSOURI 63136-6119

Description: General medical and surgical hospital
Parent Company: Christian Health Services
   Development Corporation
Annual Sales: $184.8 million
Number of Employees: 2,777
Expertise Needed: Physical therapy, licensed practical
   nursing, occupational therapy, nursing
Contact: Human Resources Department
   (314) 355-2300

CIBA-GEIGY CORPORATION
444 SAW MILL RIVER ROAD
ARDSLEY, NEW YORK 10502-2600

Description: Manufactures pharmaceuticals, chemicals,
   plastics, and vision-care products
Founded: 1903
Annual Sales: $4.5 billion
Number of Employees: 16,200
Expertise Needed: Computer science, finance, law,
   human resources, communications
Contact: Ms Janine Petroro
   Human Resources Department
   (914) 479-5000

CIBA VISION CORPORATION
11460 JOHNS CREEK PARKWAY
DULUTH, GEORGIA 30136-1518

Description: Manufactures vision-care products and
   pharmaceuticals
Parent Company: Ciba-Geigy Corporation
Annual Sales: $126.9 million
Number of Employees: 2,000
Expertise Needed: Mechanical engineering, electrical
   engineering, design engineering, project
   engineering
Contact: Ms Joyce Bishop
   Staffing Specialist
   (404) 448-1200

CIGNA CORPORATION
1601 CHESTNUT STREET
PHILADELPHIA, PENNSYLVANIA 19192

Description: Provides life, health, and accident
   insurance
Assets: $18.8 billion
Number of Employees: 53,250
Expertise Needed: Accounting, finance, marketing,
   actuarial
Contact: Ms Mary Ellen Morris
   Director of Corporate Staffing
   (215) 761-1000

CIGNA HEALTH PLANS OF CALIFORNIA
505 NORTH BRAND BOULEVARD
GLENDALE, CALIFORNIA 91203

Description: Provides health-care insurance services
Parent Company: Connecticut General Corporation
Annual Sales: $3.0 billion
Number of Employees: 7,557
Expertise Needed: Physicians, registered nursing, licensed
   practical nursing, human resources, accounting,
   information systems, data processing, accounting
Contact: Ms Adele Lazar
   Director of Human Resources
   (818) 500-6262

CIGNA HEALTHPLAN OF TEXAS, INC., NORTH TEXAS DIVISION
600 LAS COLINAS BOULEVARD
IRVING, TEXAS 75039-5616

Description: Provides health-care insurance services
Parent Company: Cigna Healthcare, Inc.
Annual Sales: $191.5 million
Number of Employees: 300
Expertise Needed: Claims adjustment/examination,
   accounting, finance
Contact: Human Resources Department
   (214) 401-5330

CIRCON CORPORATION
460 WARD DRIVE
SANTA BARBARA, CALIFORNIA 93111-2310

Description: Manufactures medical diagnostic and
   surgical equipment
Founded: 1977
Annual Sales: $83.5 million
Number of Employees: 800
Expertise Needed: Mechanical engineering, optics
Contact: Ms Alyce Dana
   Corporate Recruiter
   (203) 357-8300

CIS TECHNOLOGIES, INC.
ONE WARREN PLACE, 6100 SOUTH YALE
TULSA, OKLAHOMA 74136-1930

Description: Provides billing and claims management
   software to hospitals
Founded: 1982
Number of Employees: 360
Expertise Needed: Marketing, accounting, finance,
   computer programming, sales
Contact: Mr Larry Jefferson
   Human Resources Department
   (918) 496-2451

CLARKSON HOSPITAL

44TH & DEWEY AVENUE
OMAHA, NEBRASKA 68105

Description: Hospital
Annual Sales: $171.0 million
Number of Employees: 1,621
Expertise Needed: Nursing, therapy

Contact: Ms Ann Siewert
　　　　Employment Coordinator

CLAY-PARK LABORATORIES, INC.

1700 BATHGATE AVENUE
BRONX, NEW YORK 10457-7512

Description: Clinical laboratory
Founded: 1975
Annual Sales: $38.0 million
Number of Employees: 450
Expertise Needed: Laboratory technology, life sciences, chemistry

Contact: Mr Steve Edinger
　　　　Manager of Employment
　　　　(718) 901-2800

CLEVELAND CLINIC FOUNDATION

9500 EUCLID AVENUE
CLEVELAND, OHIO 44195-0001

Description: Owns and operates hospitals and medical centers
Founded: 1921
Annual Sales: $887.6 million
Number of Employees: 8,800
Expertise Needed: Accounting, business administration, registered nursing

Contact: Ms Amy Clark
　　　　Director of Human Resources Services
　　　　(216) 444-2200

CLINTEC INTERNATIONAL, INC.

3 PARKWAY NORTH
DEERFIELD, ILLINOIS 60015-2567

Description: Manufactures pharmacuticals and diagnostic substances
Parent Company: Baxter Healthcare Corporation
Annual Sales: $150.0 million
Number of Employees: 400
Expertise Needed: Marketing, sales, advertising

Contact: Ms Sandy Gallegos
　　　　Manager of Staffing
　　　　(708) 317-2800

COASTAL EMERGENCY SERVICES OF THE WEST

1504 FRANKLIN STREET
OAKLAND, CALIFORNIA 94612-2819

Description: Provides contract physician staffing and management services
Annual Sales: $66.0 million

Number of Employees: 60
Expertise Needed: Human resources, hospital administration, nursing, allied health, physicians, emergency services

Contact: Human Resources Department
　　　　(510) 893-7667

COASTAL HEALTHCARE GROUP, INC.

2828 CROASDAILE DRIVE
DURHAM, NORTH CAROLINA 27704

Description: Provides physician contract services to hospitals and other health-care institutions
Founded: 1977
Annual Sales: $475.0 million
Number of Employees: 4,000
Expertise Needed: Sales, marketing, accounting, management information systems, computer programming

Contact: Vice President of Recruiting and Employment
　　　　(919) 383-0355

COBB HOSPITAL, INC.

3950 AUSTELL ROAD
AUSTELL, GEORGIA 30001-1121

Description: Public hospital
Parent Company: Northwest Georgia Health Systems
Annual Sales: $101.7 million
Number of Employees: 1,311
Expertise Needed: Nursing, licensed practical nursing, physical therapy, occupational therapy

Contact: Ms Denise Benifield
　　　　Manager of Employment
　　　　(404) 732-4000

COBE LABORATORIES, INC.

1185 OAK STREET
LAKEWOOD, COLORADO 80215-4407

Description: Manufactures dialysis and surgical support equipment
Annual Sales: $364.5 million
Number of Employees: 2,700
Expertise Needed: Mechanical engineering, electrical engineering, civil engineering, industrial engineering, metallurgical engineering, biology, microbiology, management, laboratory chemistry, research

Contact: Human Resources Department
　　　　(303) 231-4440

COLE VISION CORPORATION

18903 SOUTH MILES ROAD
CLEVELAND, OHIO 44128-4245

Description: Manufactures eyeglasses and eyewear
Parent Company: Cole National Corporation
Annual Sales: $203.4 million
Number of Employees: 2,450

Cole Vision Corporation (continued)

Expertise Needed: Accounting, computer programming, sales, marketing

Contact: Mr Jeff Thompson
Human Resources Representative
(216) 475-8925

COLLAGEN CORPORATION
2500 FABER PLACE
PALO ALTO, CALIFORNIA 94303-3329

Description: Develops and manufactures collagen-based products for implant into human tissue
Founded: 1975
Annual Sales: $49.7 million
Number of Employees: 325
Expertise Needed: Biology, molecular biology, manufacturing engineering, quality control, chemistry, chemical engineering

Contact: Ms Leslie Holderby
Human Resources Representative
(415) 856-0200

COLONIAL LIFE & ACCIDENT INSURANCE
1215 AVERYT ROAD
COLUMBIA, SOUTH CAROLINA 29210

Description: Provides employee benefit and supplemental insurance services
Parent Company: Colonial Companies, Inc.
Founded: 1937
Annual Sales: $343.6 million
Number of Employees: 1,191
Expertise Needed: Sales, product design and development, marketing, customer service and support, human resources

Contact: Mr Robert Douglas
Assistant Vice President of Staffing Services
(803) 798-7000

COLUMBIA HCA HEALTH CARE CORPORATION
777 MAIN STREET
LOUISVILLE, KENTUCKY 40201-7433

Description: Owns and operates general, acute care, and specialty hospital and related facilities
Founded: 1987
Annual Sales: $499.4 million
Number of Employees: 5,000
Expertise Needed: Accounting, business management, systems engineering, hospital administration

Contact: Mr Sam Colter
Director of Field Recruiting
(502) 572-2000

COLUMBIA HOSPITAL, INC.
2025 EAST NEWPORT AVENUE
MILWAUKEE, WISCONSIN 53211-2906

Description: Private hospital
Parent Company: Columbia Health System, Inc.
Founded: 1909
Annual Sales: $111.3 million
Number of Employees: 1,750
Expertise Needed: Physical therapy, occupational therapy

Contact: Ms Sally Brenner
Nursing Recruiter
(414) 961-3719

COMMON BROTHERS, INC.
55 HUNTER LANE
ELMSFORD, NEW YORK 10523-1307

Description: Manufactures pharmaceuticals and druggists' sundries
Annual Sales: $500.0 million
Number of Employees: 370
Expertise Needed: Accounting, marketing, finance, management information systems

Contact: Mr Harry Cocozzo
Payroll Supervisor
(914) 347-5505

COMMUNITY HEALTH CARE PLAN
221 WHITNEY AVENUE
NEW HAVEN, CONNECTICUT 06511-3760

Description: Health maintenance organization
Founded: 1967
Annual Sales: $100.0 million
Number of Employees: 600
Expertise Needed: Accounting, finance, administration, customer service and support, marketing

Contact: Mr Jim Carl
Manager of Human Resources
(203) 781-4100

COMMUNITY HOSPICE CARE, INC.
505 SOUTH VILLA REAL
ANAHEIM, CALIFORNIA 92807-3442

Description: Provides hospice care and home health-care services
Annual Sales: $25.0 million
Number of Employees: 590
Expertise Needed: Nursing, physicians, social work

Contact: Ms Donna Dutton
Assistant to Human Resources Recruiter
(714) 283-2273

COMMUNITY HOSPICE, INC.
340 EAST PALM LANE
PHOENIX, ARIZONA 85004

Description: Provides hospice care services
Annual Sales: $24.0 million

Number of Employees: 490
Expertise Needed: Registered nursing, accounting, social work
Contact: Personnel Department
(602) 252-2273

COMMUNITY HOSPITAL ASSOCIATION, INC.
1100 BALSAM AVENUE
BOULDER, COLORADO 80304-3404

Description: Nonprofit hospital
Founded: 1922
Annual Sales: $80.0 million
Number of Employees: 1,100
Expertise Needed: Registered nursing, licensed practical nursing, certified nursing and nursing assistance, physical therapy, occupational therapy
Contact: Ms Lisa Randall
Nursing Recruiter
(303) 440-2273

COMMUNITY HOSPITAL OF INDIANA, EAST
1500 NORTH RITTER AVENUE
INDIANAPOLIS, INDIANA 46219-3027

Description: General medical and surgical hospital
Founded: 1952
Annual Sales: $286.7 million
Number of Employees: 5,088
Expertise Needed: Physical therapy, occupational therapy, pharmacy, laboratory technology, registered nursing
Contact: Mr. Tim O'Connell
Human Resources Representative
(317) 355-5581

COMMUNITY HOSPITALS OF CENTRAL CALIFORNIA
FRESNO AND A STREETS
FRESNO, CALIFORNIA 93721

Description: Hospital with acute-care facilities
Founded: 1945
Annual Sales: $233.4 million
Number of Employees: 4,000
Expertise Needed: Networking, physical therapy, pharmacology
Contact: Ms Cathy Gegenhuber
Employment Manager
(209) 442-6000

COMMUNITY PSYCHIATRIC CENTERS
24502 PACIFIC PARK DRIVE
ALISO VIEJO, CALIFORNIA 92656-3035

Description: Owns and operates psychiatric hospitals
Founded: 1961
Annual Sales: $392.9 million
Number of Employees: 6,586

Expertise Needed: Administration
Contact: Mr Ronald Ooley
Senior Vice President of Human Resources
(714) 831-1166

COMPLETE HEALTH SERVICES, INC.
2160 HIGHLAND AVENUE SOUTH
BIRMINGHAM, ALABAMA 35205-4015

Description: Health maintenance organization
Annual Sales: $185.6 million
Number of Employees: 508
Expertise Needed: Actuarial, accounting, underwriting
Contact: Human Resources Department

COMPRECARE HEALTH CARE SERVICES
12100 EAST ILIFF AVENUE
AURORA, COLORADO 80014-1249

Description: Health maintenance organization
Parent Company: Comprecare Management Services
Annual Sales: $206.4 million
Number of Employees: 310
Expertise Needed: Claims adjustment/examination, accounting
Contact: Ms Audrey Seavault
Employment Manager
(303) 695-6685

COMPREHENSIVE ADDICTION PROGRAMS
8000 TOWER CRESCENT DRIVE
VIENNA, VIRGINIA 22182

Description: Owns and operates substance abuse treatment facilities
Founded: 1989
Annual Sales: $33.0 million
Number of Employees: 395
Expertise Needed: Accounting, marketing, counseling
Contact: Ms Janet Mark
Director of Human Resources
(703) 847-2600

COMPUCHEM LABORATORIES, INC.
3308 CHAPEL HILL NELSON HIGHWAY
RESEARCH TRIANGLE PARK, NORTH CAROLINA 27709

Description: Drug-testing laboratory
Parent Company: Roche Compuchem, Inc.
Annual Sales: $25.5 million
Number of Employees: 490
Expertise Needed: Chemistry, medical technology, sales, marketing, management information systems
Contact: Ms Ann Bradshaw
Staffing Director
(919) 549-8263

COMPUNET CLINICAL LABORATORIES
2308 SANDRIDGE DRIVE
DAYTON, OHIO 45439-1856

Description: Clinical laboratory
Annual Sales: $15.7 million
Number of Employees: 275
Expertise Needed: Phlebotomy, technical, laboratory technology
Contact: Human Resources Department
    (513) 296-0844

MOSES H. CONE MEMORIAL HOSPITAL, WOMEN'S HOSPITAL OF GREENSBORO
1200 NORTH ELM STREET
GREENSBORO, NORTH CAROLINA 27401-1004

Description: Public hospital
Founded: 1911
Annual Sales: $204.3 million
Number of Employees: 3,500
Expertise Needed: Registered nursing, occupational therapy, physical therapy, respiratory therapy
Contact: Ms Ann North
    Employment
    (910) 574-7000

CONEMAUGH VALLEY MEMORIAL HOSPITAL
1086 FRANKLIN STREET
JOHNSTOWN, PENNSYLVANIA 15905-4305

Description: Public hospital specializing in trauma and cardiac care
Founded: 1889
Annual Sales: $110.2 million
Number of Employees: 2,200
Expertise Needed: Nursing, physical therapy
Contact: Ms Susan Benya
    Manager of Employment
    (814) 533-9130

CONMED CORPORATION
310 BROAD STREET
UTICA, NEW YORK 13501-1203

Description: Distributes medical supplies
Founded: 1970
Annual Sales: $42.6 million
Number of Employees: 660
Expertise Needed: Chemical engineering, mechanical engineering, electrical engineering, pharmaceutical, marketing, accounting, finance
Contact: Ms Elizabeth Bowers
    Director of Human Resources
    (315) 797-8375

CONNAUGHT LABORATORIES, INC.
ROUTE 611
SWIFTWATER, PENNSYLVANIA 18370-9726

Description: Develops and manufactures vaccines
Founded: 1977
Annual Sales: $123.6 million
Number of Employees: 560
Expertise Needed: Quality control, microbiology, chemistry, biochemistry, marketing, sales, process engineering, chemical engineering, mechanical engineering, electrical engineering
Contact: Mr Mark Schilling
    Manager of Recruiting
    (717) 839-7187

CONSERVCO, INC.
3903 NORTHDALE BOULEVARD
TAMPA, FLORIDA 33624-1864

Description: Provides medical care management services
Parent Company: The Travelers Insurance Company
Annual Sales: $29.8 million
Number of Employees: 1,600
Expertise Needed: Computer programming, accounting
Contact: Ms Susan Right
    Manager of Human Resources
    (813) 969-0701

CONTINENTAL HEALTH AFFILIATES, INC.
900 SYLVAN AVENUE
ENGLEWOOD CLIFFS, NEW JERSEY 07632

Description: Provides health-care services and operates nursing homes
Annual Sales: $61.3 million
Number of Employees: 1,198
Expertise Needed: Health care, clinical nursing, nursing, hospice care
Contact: Human Resources Department
    (201) 567-4600

CONTINENTAL MEDICAL SYSTEMS
600 WILSON LANE
MECHANICSBURG, PENNSYLVANIA 17055-4440

Description: Operates rehabilitation hospitals and outpatient clinics and provides contract therapy services
Annual Sales: $901.4 million
Number of Employees: 10,000
Expertise Needed: Accounting, health care, licensed practical nursing, computer programming, nursing, finance, design engineering, civil engineering, data processing
Contact: Ms Vicki Yahn
    Recruiter
    (717) 790-8300

CONTINENTAL X-RAY CORPORATION
2000 SOUTH 25TH AVENUE
BROADVIEW, ILLINOIS 60153

Description: Manufactures medical X-ray equipment
Founded: 1934
Number of Employees: 200
Expertise Needed: X-ray technology, radiological
   technology
Contact: Mr Leif Farney
   Vice President of Customer Relations
   (708) 345-3050

COOK-FORT WORTH CHILDREN'S MEDICAL CENTER
801 7TH AVENUE
FORT WORTH, TEXAS 76104-2733

Description: Private pediatric hospital
Founded: 1918
Annual Sales: $91.8 million
Number of Employees: 1,200
Expertise Needed: Physical therapy, occupational therapy,
   radiation technology, pharmacy, nursing
Contact: Ms Kate Kirby
   Employment Specialist
   (817) 885-4000

COOK GROUP, INC.
300 FOUNTAIN SQUARE, SUITE 300
BLOOMINGTON, INDIANA 47401

Description: Manufactures radiology and cardiology
   products
Founded: 1963
Annual Sales: $151.5 million
Number of Employees: 1,800
Expertise Needed: Physicians, medical technology
Contact: Ms Jackie Wickle
   Vice President of Personnel
   (812) 339-2235

COOPER DEVELOPMENT COMPANY
2420 SANDHILL ROAD
MENLO PARK, CALIFORNIA 94025

Description: Manufactures pharmaceuticals
Annual Sales: $32.0 million
Number of Employees: 202
Expertise Needed: Marketing, sales, law, finance
Contact: Ms Carol Kauffman
   Vice President and Chief Administrative
      Officer
   (415) 969-9030

COOPER HOSPITAL UNIVERSITY MEDICAL CENTER
1 COOPER PLAZA
CAMDEN, NEW JERSEY 08103-1438

Description: Public general hospital
Founded: 1875

Annual Sales: $265.2 million
Number of Employees: 3,000
Expertise Needed: Registered nursing, physical therapy,
   occupational therapy, dietetics
Contact: Human Resources Department
   (609) 342-2000

COPLEY PHARMACEUTICALS, INC.
25 JOHN ROAD
CANTON, MASSACHUSETTS 02021-2827

Description: Manufactures ethical and over-the-counter
   pharmaceutical products
Founded: 1972
Annual Sales: $52.0 million
Number of Employees: 400
Expertise Needed: Pharmacy, accounting, finance, data
   processing
Contact: Director of Human Resources
   (617) 821-6111

CORDIS CORPORATION
14201 NORTHWEST 60TH AVENUE
MIAMI LAKES, FLORIDA 33014-2802

Description: Manufactures diagnostic coronary
   angiographic equipment
Founded: 1959
Annual Sales: $255.5 million
Number of Employees: 2,650
Expertise Needed: Production engineering, product
   engineering, industrial engineering, quality
   engineering, manufacturing engineering,
   mechanical engineering
Contact: Mr John DePrima
   Manager of Human Resources Development
   (305) 824-2318

CORNING COSTAR CORPORATION
ONE ALEWIFE CENTER
CAMBRIDGE, MASSACHUSETTS 02140

Description: Designs and develops laboratory products
Founded: 1946
Annual Sales: $140.0 million
Number of Employees: 1,100
Expertise Needed: Biology, biotechnology, biochemistry,
   laboratory technology
Contact: Department of Human Resources
   (617) 868-6200

CORNING LAB SERVICES, INC.
450 PARK AVENUE
NEW YORK, NEW YORK 10022-2605

Description: Provides clinical laboratory and
   environmental testing services
Parent Company: Corning, Inc.
Annual Sales: $1.2 billion
Number of Employees: 15,000

Corning Costar Corporation (continued)

Expertise Needed: Computer programming, laboratory chemistry, customer service and support

Contact: Ms Lisa Sichon
Human Resources Administrator
(201) 393-5341

COROMETRICS MEDICAL SYSTEMS

61 BARNES PARK ROAD
WALLINGFORD, CONNECTICUT 06492-1883

Description: Manufactures electronic instrumentation, diagnostic ultrasound systems, and related accessories

Parent Company: American Home Products Corporation

Founded: 1974

Annual Sales: $75.1 million

Number of Employees: 750

Expertise Needed: Software engineering/development, electrical engineering, biomedical engineering, manufacturing engineering, finance, accounting, marketing

Contact: Mr John Kubilus
Manager of Human Resources
(203) 265-5631

CORPAK, INC.

100 CHADDICK DRIVE
WHEELING, ILLINOIS 60090

Description: Manufactures and markets nutritional products

Founded: 1968

Number of Employees: 200

Expertise Needed: Sales, manufacturing, design engineering

Contact: Ms Darlene Coram
Human Resources Director
(708) 537-4601

CORVEL CORPORATION

1920 MAIN STREET
IRVINE, CALIFORNIA 92714-7212

Description: Provides managed care and cost management services

Annual Sales: $46.9 million

Number of Employees: 1,200

Expertise Needed: Sales, marketing, finance, accounting

Contact: Human Resources Department
(714) 851-1473

CORVEL HEALTHCARE CORPORATION

2121 SOUTHWEST BROADWAY
PORTLAND, OREGON 97201-3182

Description: Provides medical cost containment and managed care services

Annual Sales: $74.0 million

Number of Employees: 1,400

Expertise Needed: Case management, business management, finance

Contact: Human Resources Department
(503) 222-3144

LESTER E. COX MEDICAL CENTER

3801 SOUTH NATIONAL
SPRINGFIELD, MISSOURI 65807

Description: Hospital and medical center

Founded: 1906

Annual Sales: $155.6 million

Number of Employees: 3,785

Expertise Needed: Medical technology, physical therapy, occupational therapy, rehabilitation, speech pathology, nursing, medical records

Contact: Ms Carol Eagleberger
Recruitor/Nursing Specialist
(417) 885-6125

CRESTWOOD HOSPITALS, INC.

4635 GEORGETOWN PLACE
STOCKTON, CALIFORNIA 95207-6203

Description: Nursing care facility

Founded: 1970

Annual Sales: $89.1 million

Number of Employees: 3,400

Expertise Needed: Nursing, physical therapy, administration

Contact: Ms Mary Lou Glantz
Vice President of Human Resources
(209) 478-5291

CRITIKON, INC.

4110 GEORGE ROAD
TAMPA, FLORIDA 33631-3800

Description: Manufactures critical care medical devices

Number of Employees: 700

Expertise Needed: Mechanical engineering, electrical engineering, software engineering/development, accounting, finance, management information systems

Contact: Human Resources Department
(813) 887-2000

CRITTENTON HOSPITAL

1101 WEST UNIVERSITY DRIVE
ROCHESTER, MICHIGAN 48307-1863

Description: General medical and surgical hospital

Parent Company: Crittenton Corporation

Founded: 1967

Annual Sales: $92.3 million

Number of Employees: 1,130

Expertise Needed: Nursing, respiratory therapy, occupational therapy, physical therapy, medical technology

Contact: Ms Donna Pelkey
Vice President of Human Resources
(810) 652-5000

IRVING CROUSE MEMORIAL HOSPITAL
736 IRVING AVENUE
SYRACUSE, NEW YORK 13210-1690

Description: Public hospital
Parent Company: Irving Crouse Companies, Inc.
Founded: 1893
Annual Sales: $164.1 million
Number of Employees: 2,900
Expertise Needed: Registered nursing

Contact: Ms Vicki Loretto
Manager of Wages and Benefits
(315) 470-7111

CSC HEALTHCARE SYSTEMS, INC.
34505 WEST 12 MILE ROAD
FARMINGTON HILLS, MICHIGAN 48331-3258

Description: Provides computer programming services
Parent Company: Computer Sciences Corporation
Annual Sales: $51.9 million
Number of Employees: 250
Expertise Needed: Program analysis, software engineering/development, systems engineering

Contact: Ms Elaine Mills
Recruiter
(810) 553-0900

CUMBERLAND COUNTY HOSPITAL SYSTEMS
1638 OWEN DRIVE
FAYETTE, NORTH CAROLINA 28302-3424

Description: Public hospital
Founded: 1964
Annual Sales: $140.4 million
Number of Employees: 2,300
Expertise Needed: Physical therapy, occupational therapy, networking

Contact: Ms Diane Deboer
Personnel Department
(919) 609-6700

CUMBERLAND HEALTH SYSTEMS, INC.
2100 WEST END AVENUE
NASHVILLE, TENNESSEE 37203-5223

Description: Provides hospital management services
Founded: 1982
Annual Sales: $53.0 million
Number of Employees: 1,100
Expertise Needed: Physicians, therapy, registered nursing

Contact: Ms Ruth Meinke
Director of Physician Recruiting
(615) 327-2200

CURATIVE TECHNOLOGIES, INC.
14 RESEARCH WAY
SETAUKET, NEW YORK 11733-3453

Description: Manufactures biopharmaceuticals
Founded: 1984
Annual Sales: $26.8 million
Number of Employees: 340
Expertise Needed: Biology, chemistry, laboratory technology, biochemistry

Contact: Ms Denise Smith
Employment Manager
(516) 689-7000

CVS, INC.
1 CVS DRIVE
WOONSOCKET, RHODE ISLAND 02895-6146

Description: Distributes health and beauty aids
Parent Company: People's Drug Stores, Inc.
Annual Sales: $221.5 million
Number of Employees: 2,500
Expertise Needed: Sales, accounting, management information systems, finance, marketing

Contact: Ms Janis Stanovich
Human Resources Manager
(401) 765-1500

CYBEX DIVISION
2100 SMITHTOWN AVENUE
RONKONKOMA, NEW YORK 11779

Description: Manufactures business equipment
Parent Company: Lumex Corporation
Founded: 1947
Number of Employees: 700
Expertise Needed: Manufacturing engineering, electrical engineering, mechanical engineering, marketing, accounting, finance, management information systems

Contact: Human Resources Department
(516) 585-9000

CYCARE SYSTEMS, INC.
7001 NORTH SCOTTSDALE ROAD
SCOTTSDALE, ARIZONA 85253

Description: Provides data processing and systems services for physicians
Founded: 1967
Annual Sales: $71.0 million
Number of Employees: 468
Number of Managerial and Professional Employees Hired 1993: 150
Expertise Needed: Data processing, computer science

Contact: Human Resources Department
(319) 556-3131

DAHLBERG, INC.
4101 DAHLBERG DRIVE
GOLDEN VALLEY, MINNESOTA 55422

Description: Manufactures surgical appliances and
supplies
Founded: 1949
Number of Employees: 840
Expertise Needed: Mechanical engineering, design
engineering, sales, marketing, accounting
Contact: Ms Deborah Pender
Director of Human Resources
(612) 520-9500

DALLAS COUNTY HOSPITAL DISTRICT
5201 HARRY HINES BOULEVARD
DALLAS, TEXAS 75235

Description: General public hospital
Founded: 1954
Annual Sales: $305.6 million
Number of Employees: 5,708
Expertise Needed: Nursing, occupational therapy,
physical therapy
Contact: Director of Nursing Recruiting
(800) 927-0333

DARTMOUTH HITCHCOCK MEDICAL CENTER
1 MEDICAL CENTER DRIVE
LEBANON, NEW HAMPSHIRE 03766-2804

Description: Public hospital
Founded: 1946
Annual Sales: $138.0 million
Number of Employees: 1,200
Expertise Needed: Nursing, licensed practical nursing,
registered nursing
Contact: Ms Kit Hood
Manager of Employment
(603) 650-5000

DARWIN MOLECULAR CORPORATION
22025 20TH AVENUE SOUTHEAST
BOTHELL, WASHINGTON 98201

Description: Biomedical and biotechnology research
firm
Number of Employees: 30
*Number of Managerial and Professional Employees Hired
1993:* 15
Expertise Needed: Biological engineering, biochemistry,
molecular biology, chemistry, genetics
Contact: Ms Jennifer Okimoto
Human Resources Representative
(206) 489-8000

DATACHEM LABORATORIES
960 LEVOY DRIVE
SALT LAKE CITY, UTAH 84123-2500

Description: Chemical laboratory providing research
and design analysis services
Annual Sales: $16.0 million
Number of Employees: 250
Expertise Needed: Analysis
Contact: Ms Jill Olson
Director of Human Resources
(801) 266-7700

THE DCH MEDICAL CENTER
809 UNIVERSITY BOULEVARD EAST
TUSCALOOSA, ALABAMA 35401-2029

Description: General hospital
Founded: 1947
Annual Sales: $207.5 million
Number of Employees: 3,114
Expertise Needed: Registered nursing, licensed practical
nursing, physical therapy, occupational therapy,
medical technology
Contact: Ms Pam Mills
Human Resources Assistant
(205) 759-7911

DCI
1600 HAYES STREET
NASHVILLE, TENNESSEE 37203-3028

Description: Manufactures dental equipment
Founded: 1971
Annual Sales: $149.6 million
Number of Employees: 1,800
Expertise Needed: Dialysis, nursing, physicians
Contact: Human Resources Department
(615) 327-3061

DEACONESS HOSPITAL
600 MARY STREET
EVANSVILLE, INDIANA 47710-1658

Description: Nonprofit hospital specializing in acute
care
Founded: 1892
Annual Sales: $135.1 million
Number of Employees: 2,418
Expertise Needed: Registered nursing, licensed practical
nursing, physician assistant
Contact: Ms Roxie Ivy
Nursing Recruiter
(812) 426-3000

DEACONESS MEDICAL CENTER OF BILLINGS
2813 9TH AVENUE NORTH
BILLINGS, MONTANA 59101-0717

Description: Public hospital
Annual Sales: $93.7 million

Number of Employees: 1,100
Expertise Needed: Critical care nursing, intensive care, registered nursing
Contact: Nurse Recruitment Department
(406) 657-4012

DEAN HEALTH PLAN, INC.
2711 ALLEN BOULEVARD
MIDDLETON, WISCONSIN 53562-2215

Description: Health maintenance organization
Parent Company: Dean Medical Center of South Carolina
Annual Sales: $168.3 million
Number of Employees: 190
Expertise Needed: Underwriting, claims adjustment/ examination
Contact: Ms Mary Jo Spiekerman
Manager of Human Resources
(608) 836-1400

DEAN MEDICAL CENTER OF SOUTH CAROLINA
1808 WEST BELTWAY HIGHWAY
MADISON, WISCONSIN 53715-0328

Description: Multi-specialty clinic
Founded: 1969
Annual Sales: $218.4 million
Number of Employees: 1,465
Expertise Needed: Nursing, licensed practical nursing, laboratory technology, physical therapy, occupational therapy, pharmacy, cardiology
Contact: Human Resources Department
(608) 252-5354

DELMAR GARDEN ENTERPRISES, INC.
101 SOUTH HANLEY
SAINT LOUIS, MISSOURI 63105-3406

Description: Provides nursing home care services
Founded: 1975
Annual Sales: $70.0 million
Number of Employees: 2,000
Expertise Needed: Finance, accounting, economics
Contact: Mr Howard Oppenheimer
Executive Vice President of Administration
(314) 862-0045

DELTA DENTAL PLAN OF CALIFORNIA
100 1ST STREET
SAN FRANCISCO, CALIFORNIA 94105-2634

Description: Provides dental insurance services
Founded: 1955
Annual Sales: $1.4 billion
Number of Employees: 1,200

Expertise Needed: Accounting, finance, data processing, dentistry/dental hygiene, law
Contact: Ms Teri Foresgieri
Manager of Employee Relations
(415) 972-8300

DENMAT CORPORATION
2727 SKYWAY DRIVE
SANTA MARIA, CALIFORNIA 93455-4524

Description: Manufactures dental products
Founded: 1972
Annual Sales: $55.0 million
Number of Employees: 500
Expertise Needed: Dentistry/dental hygiene, accounting, finance, data processing, chemistry, pharmacy
Contact: Mr Al Petit
Manager of Personnel
(805) 922-8491

DENTICARE
28202 CABOT ROAD
LAGUNA NIGUEL, CALIFORNIA 92677-1251

Description: Provides dental insurance services
Parent Company: Foundation Health Corporation
Annual Sales: $20.5 million
Number of Employees: 110
Expertise Needed: Marketing, accounting, information systems
Contact: Ms MaryLou Riley
Director of Personnel
(714) 265-8010

DENTSPLY INTERNATIONAL, INC.
570 WEST COLLEGE AVENUE
YORK, PENNSYLVANIA 17404-3886

Description: Manufactures dental equipment, supplies, prosthetics, and disinfectant products
Founded: 1899
Annual Sales: $507.8 million
Number of Employees: 4,200
Expertise Needed: Accounting, sales, data processing, manufacturing engineering
Contact: Ms Gloria McFadden
Vice President of Human Resources
(708) 640-4800

DEPUY, INC.
700 ORTHOPEDIC DRIVE
WARSAW, INDIANA 46581

Description: Manufactures orthopedic products
Parent Company: Boehringer Mannheim Corporation
Annual Sales: $76.5 million
Number of Employees: 1,002

Depuy, Inc. (continued)

Expertise Needed: Materials science, manufacturing engineering, mechanical engineering, accounting, marketing

Contact: Mr Mike Forrest
Manager of Human Resources
(219) 267-8145

DESPATCH INDUSTRIES
63 ST. ANTHONY PARKWAY
MINNEAPOLIS, MINNESOTA 55418

Description: Manufactures heat processing and environmental testing equipment
Founded: 1902
Annual Sales: $38.0 million
Number of Employees: 350
Expertise Needed: Electrical engineering, mechanical engineering

Contact: Ms Gail Kalata
Personnel Manager
(612) 781-5363

DETROIT-MACOMB HOSPITAL CORPORATION
12000 EAST 12 MILE ROAD
WARREN, MICHIGAN 48093-3570

Description: Owns general medical and surgical hospitals
Founded: 1949
Annual Sales: $170.1 million
Number of Employees: 2,666
Expertise Needed: Networking, emergency services, intensive care, geriatrics, operating room, radio frequency engineering, microwave engineering

Contact: Human Resources Department
(313) 499-3000

THE DETROIT MEDICAL CENTER
4201 SAINT ANTOINE STREET
DETROIT, MICHIGAN 48201-2194

Description: Corporate headquarters for public hospitals
Annual Sales: $1.1 billion
Number of Employees: 13,453
Expertise Needed: Computer programming, marketing, finance, accounting, laboratory technology, business administration

Contact: Ms JoAnn Butash
Director of Human Resources
(313) 745-5192

DEVILBISS HEALTH CARE, INC.
1200 EAST MAIN STREET
SOMERSET, PENNSYLVANIA 15501-2100

Description: Manufactures respiratory care equipment
Annual Sales: $95.0 million
Number of Employees: 600

Expertise Needed: Electrical engineering, manufacturing engineering, accounting, finance, data processing

Contact: Ms Debbie Dinning
Human Resources Assistant
(814) 443-4881

DEVON INDUSTRIES, INC.
9530 DESOTO AVENUE
CHATSWORTH, CALIFORNIA 91311

Description: Manufactures medical and surgical instruments
Founded: 1975
Number of Employees: 450
Number of Managerial and Professional Employees Hired 1993: 55
Expertise Needed: Marketing, finance, accounting, sales

Contact: Ms Patrice Poleto
Human Resources Manager
(818) 709-6880

DIABETES TREATMENT CENTERS OF AMERICA
1 BURTON HILLS BOULEVARD
NASHVILLE, TENNESSEE 37215-6104

Description: Provides diabetes treatment services to acute-care hospitals
Parent Company: American Healthcorp, Inc.
Annual Sales: $38.0 million
Number of Employees: 400
Expertise Needed: Management, project engineering, operations, clinical nursing, dietetics, exercise physiology

Contact: Ms Rita Sailor
Vice President of Human Resources and Organizational Development
(615) 665-1133

DIAGNOSTIC PRODUCTS CORPORATION
5700 WEST 96TH STREET
LOS ANGELES, CALIFORNIA 90045-5544

Description: Manufactures diagnostic test kits
Founded: 1971
Annual Sales: $90.1 million
Number of Employees: 434
Expertise Needed: Chemistry, research, biochemistry, biology, biomedical engineering

Contact: Human Resources Department
(213) 776-0180

DIVERSICARE CORPORATION AMERICA
105 REYNOLDS ROAD
FRANKLIN, TENNESSEE 37064-2926

Description: Owns and operates nursing homes
Annual Sales: $93.3 million
Number of Employees: 4,000

Expertise Needed: Accounting, finance, marketing
Contact: Ms Sandy Irvin
　　　Director of Human Relations
　　　(615) 794-3313

DLP/INRAD, INC.
620 WATSON STREET SOUTHWEST
GRAND RAPIDS, MICHIGAN 49504-6340

Description: Manufactures surgical instruments for
　cardiovascular applications
Founded: 1979
Annual Sales: $34.0 million
Number of Employees: 310
Expertise Needed: Manufacturing engineering,
　electronics/electronics engineering, electrical
　engineering, mechanical engineering, design
　engineering, medical technology, sales, marketing,
　product design and development
Contact: Ms Anne Kelbol
　　　Human Resources Specialist
　　　(616) 242-5200

THE DOCTORS' COMPANY
185 GREENWOOD ROAD
NAPA, CALIFORNIA 94558

Description: Provides professional liability insurance for
　physicians
Annual Sales: $125.0 million
Number of Employees: 285
Expertise Needed: Actuarial, insurance, sales
Contact: Ms Joan Bowyer
　　　Senior Human Resources Generalist
　　　(800) 421-2368

DOMINICAN SANTA CRUZ HOSPITAL
1555 SOQUEL DRIVE
SANTA CRUZ, CALIFORNIA 95065-1705

Description: Facility specializing in coronary care
Parent Company: Catholic Healthcare West
Founded: 1950
Annual Sales: $106.9 million
Number of Employees: 1,224
Expertise Needed: Nursing, nuclear medicine
Contact: Mr Charles Mackh,
　　　Director of Human Resources
　　　(408) 462-7700

DRISCOLL CHILDREN'S HOSPITAL
3533 SOUTH ALAMEDA STREET
CORPUS CHRISTI, TEXAS 78411-1721

Description: Nonprofit pediatric hospital
Founded: 1945
Annual Sales: $67.6 million
Number of Employees: 840

Expertise Needed: Registered nursing, licensed practical
　nursing, certified nursing and nursing assistance
Contact: Ms Linda Elliot
　　　Recruiter
　　　(512) 850-5000

DRUG EMPORIUM, INC.
155 HIDDEN RAVINES DRIVE
POWELL, OHIO 43065-8739

Description: Discount drug store chain
Founded: 1977
Annual Sales: $761.6 million
Number of Employees: 5,300
Expertise Needed: Sales, accounting, merchandising, data
　processing
Contact: Ms Laurie Stroman
　　　Manager of Human Resources
　　　(614) 548-7080

DURHAM REGIONAL HOSPITAL
3643 NORTH ROXBORO ROAD
DURHAM, NORTH CAROLINA 27704-2702

Description: Regional nonprofit hospital
Founded: 1971
Annual Sales: $144.6 million
Number of Employees: 2,250
Expertise Needed: Registered nursing, allied health,
　physical therapy, cardiography, clinical technology,
　respiratory therapy, ultrasound technology,
　occupational therapy, speech pathology
Contact: Ms Lynne Downes
　　　Employment Manager
　　　(919) 549-5001

DURR DRUG COMPANY
301 BROWN SPRINGS ROAD
MONTGOMERY, ALABAMA 36117

Description: Distributes pharmaceuticals, medical and
　surgical products, and veterinary products
Parent Company: Bergen Brunswig Corporation
Founded: 1992
Annual Sales: $950.5 million
Number of Employees: 1,311
Expertise Needed: Sales, marketing
Contact: Ms Diane Blackwell
　　　Human Resources Representative
　　　(205) 213-8800

EAGLESTON HOSPITAL FOR CHILDREN
1405 CLIFTON ROAD NORTHEAST
ATLANTA, GEORGIA 30322-1101

Description: Children's hospital
Founded: 1928
Annual Sales: $95.5 million
Number of Employees: 1,930

Eagleston Hospital for Children (continued)

Expertise Needed: Pediatric care, radiation technology, medical technology, registered nursing, licensed practical nursing

Contact: Ms Joy Roark
Employment Recruiter
(404) 325-6000

EASTMAN KODAK HEALTH GROUP

343 STATE STREET
ROCHESTER, NEW YORK 14650

Description: Manufactures and markets pharmaceuticals, laboratory products, reagents and test kits, and X-ray film

Expertise Needed: Health science, health care, health insurance, research and development

Contact: Ms Sandy Rother
Staffing and College Relations
(716) 724-4000

EASTON HOSPITAL

250 SOUTH 21ST STREET
EASTON, PENNSYLVANIA 18042-3851

Description: General hospital
Founded: 1890
Annual Sales: $125.9 million
Number of Employees: 1,425
Expertise Needed: Medical technology, physical therapy, occupational therapy, nursing

Contact: Ms Sharon Carney
Professional Recruiting
(215) 250-4000

ECKERD DRUGS OF TEXAS, INC.

8333 BRYAN DAIRY ROAD
LARGO, FLORIDA 34647

Description: Drug store chain
Annual Sales: $598.4 million
Number of Employees: 6,745
Expertise Needed: Marketing, accounting, sales, retail, pharmacy

Contact: Ms Luisa Hollingworth
Manager of Human Resources
(813) 399-6000

EDWARD HOSPITAL

801 SOUTH WASHINGTON STREET
NAPERVILLE, ILLINOIS 60540-7430

Description: Private hospital
Parent Company: Edward Health Services Corporation
Annual Sales: $98.0 million
Number of Employees: 1,400
Expertise Needed: Physical therapy, allied health, nursing

Contact: Ms Linda Hagen
Nursing Recruiter
(708) 355-0450

EG&G, INC.

45 WILLIAM STREET
WELLESLEY, MASSACHUSETTS 02181-4004

Description: Manufactures electronic, scientific, engineering, nuclear, and geophysical products and performs biomedical research
Founded: 1947
Annual Sales: $2.8 billion
Number of Employees: 34,487
Expertise Needed: Manufacturing engineering, chemical engineering, electrical engineering

Contact: Mr Peter Murphy
Director of Corporate Training and Development
(617) 237-5100

EL CAMINO HEALTH CARE SYSTEMS

2500 GRANT ROAD
MOUNTAIN VIEW, CALIFORNIA 94040-4378

Description: General medical and surgical hospital
Founded: 1961
Annual Sales: $166.9 million
Number of Employees: 2,000
Expertise Needed: Registered nursing, licensed practical nursing, occupational therapy, physical therapy, radiology, cardiovascular, critical care nursing, nursing management and administration, emergency nursing, intensive care nursing

Contact: Human Resources Department
(415) 940-7246

ELAN PHARMACEUTICAL RESEARCH CORPORATION

1300 GOULD DRIVE
GAINESVILLE, GEORGIA 30504-3947

Description: Manufactures oral drug delivery systems
Annual Sales: $26.3 million
Number of Employees: 215
Expertise Needed: Business, pharmacology, research and development

Contact: Mr. David Kelley
Director of Human Resources
(404) 534-8239

ELECTRO-BIOLOGY, INC.

6 UPPER POND ROAD
PARSIPPANY, NEW JERSEY 07054-1051

Description: Manufactures orthopedic equipment and disposable devices
Parent Company: Biomet, Inc.
Annual Sales: $72.5 million
Number of Employees: 380
Expertise Needed: Electrical engineering, accounting, marketing, finance, information systems

Contact: Ms Nancy Meehan
Director of Human Resources
(201) 299-9022

ELECTROMEDICS, INC.
18501 EAST PLAZA DRIVE
PARKER, COLORADO 80134

Description: Manufactures autotransfusion equipment
and disposable devices
Founded: 1974
Annual Sales: $39.1 million
Number of Employees: 350
Expertise Needed: Clinical services, cardiology, registered
nursing, licensed practical nursing
Contact: Ms Susie Perlman
        Director of Human Resources
        (303) 840-4000

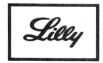

ELI LILLY AND COMPANY
LILLY CORPORATE CENTER, DC 1811
INDIANAPOLIS, INDIANA 46285

Description: Develops, manufactures, and markets
pharmaceutical products and animal health
products
Founded: 1876
Annual Sales: $6.4 billion
Number of Employees: 29,800
*Number of Managerial and Professional Employees Hired
1993:* 300
Expertise Needed: Research and development,
management information systems, marketing, sales,
chemical engineering
Contact: Mr Ron L Anglea
        Manager of Corporate Recruitment
        (800) 428-4592

CORPORATE STATEMENT

Eli Lilly and Company, a world leader in the
pharmaceutical industry, develops, manufactures, and
markets pharmaceuticals, medical instruments, diagnostic
products, and animal health products. Headquartered
in Indianapolis, Indiana, Lilly is a multinational research-
based corporation with a focus on the life sciences.

ELIZABETH GENERAL MEDICAL CENTER
925 EAST JERSEY STREET
ELIZABETH, NEW JERSEY 07201-2728

Description: Public hospital
Parent Company: Jersey Healthcare Services
Founded: 1982
Annual Sales: $192.8 million
Number of Employees: 2,000
Expertise Needed: Registered nursing, physical therapy,
occupational therapy
Contact: Ms Jodi Mesack
        Employment Manager
        (908) 289-8600

ELKHART GENERAL H
600 EAST BOULEVARD
ELKHART, INDIANA 46514-2483

Description: General medical and surg
Founded: 1909
Annual Sales: $71.9 million
Number of Employees: 1,300
Expertise Needed: Physical therapy, networking, sp
therapy, occupational therapy, radiation technolo
respiratory therapy
Contact: Ms Laura Perkins
        Medical Staff Recruiter
        (219) 294-2621

ELKINS-SINN, INC.
2 ESTERBROOK LANE
CHERRY HILL, NEW JERSEY 08003-4002

Description: Develops pharmaceuticals for veterinary
applications
Parent Company: American Home Products
Corporation
Annual Sales: $92.0 million
Number of Employees: 725
Expertise Needed: Pharmaceutical, pharmacology,
biomedical engineering, medical technology,
research and development, sales, biochemistry,
marketing
Contact: Ms Patricia Kraol
        Manager of Personnel
        (609) 424-3700

ELLIOT HOSPITAL
955 AUBURN STREET
MANCHESTER, NEW HAMPSHIRE 03103-3503

Description: General hospital
Parent Company: Elliot Health System, Inc.
Annual Sales: $124.0 million
Number of Employees: 1,306
Expertise Needed: Nursing, licensed practical nursing,
respiratory therapy, laboratory technology, physical
therapy, occupational therapy, program analysis,
medical records, phlebotomy
Contact: Mr Robert Miller
        Director of Employment
        (603) 669-5300

EMCARE, INC.
1717 MAIN STREET
DALLAS, TEXAS 75201-7365

Description: Provides contract emergency room
management services
Annual Sales: $91.0 million
Number of Employees: 85
Expertise Needed: Human resources
Contact: Human Resources
        (214) 761-9200

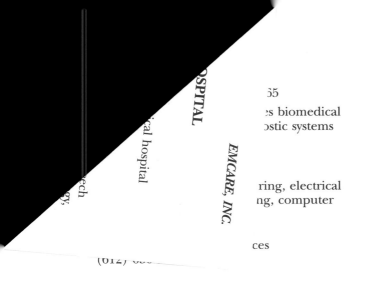

... 55

... es biomedical
... ostic systems

... ring, electrical
... ng, computer

... ces

(612) ...

EMPIRE BLUE CROSS & BLUE SHIELD
622 3RD AVENUE
NEW YORK, NEW YORK 10017-6707

Description: Provides health-care insurance services
Founded: 1935
Annual Sales: $6.6 billion
Number of Employees: 9,678
Expertise Needed: Accounting, finance, data processing,
  computer programming, management information
  systems
Contact: Ms Lisa Engelson
  Human Resources Recruiter
  (212) 476-1117

EMPIRE VISION CENTER
2921 ERIE BOULEVARD EAST
SYRACUSE, NEW YORK 13224-1430

Description: Manufactures eyewear
Founded: 1976
Annual Sales: $30.0 million
Number of Employees: 450
Expertise Needed: Ophthalmology, business, finance,
  retail
Contact: Mr Tom Ferris
  Vice President of Administration
  (315) 446-3145

EMPLOYEE BENEFIT PLANS, INC.
435 FORD ROAD
MINNEAPOLIS, MINNESOTA 55426-4912

Description: Provides third-party benefits administration
  services
Annual Sales: $218.6 million
Number of Employees: 1,488
Expertise Needed: Claims adjustment/examination,
  actuarial
Contact: Mr Joe Gasik
  Employee Relations Representative
  (612) 546-4353

EMPLOYERS HEALTH INSURANCE COMPANY
1100 EMPLOYERS BOULEVARD
GREEN BAY, WISCONSIN 54344

Description: Provides health-care insurance services
Parent Company: Lincoln National Corporation
Annual Sales: $1.2 billion
Number of Employees: 2,402
Expertise Needed: Accounting, finance, law, management
  information systems, sales
Contact: Ms Lynn Adamczak
  Recruiter
  (414) 337-7969

EMSI
111 WEST MOCKINGBIRD LANE
DALLAS, TEXAS 75247

Description: Provides medical insurance claims
  management services
Parent Company: Examination Management Services,
  Inc., America
Founded: 1976
Annual Sales: $65.1 million
Number of Employees: 2,000
Expertise Needed: Computer science, management
  information systems, accounting, customer service
  and support, medical technology
Contact: Personnel Department
  (214) 638-3629

ENCORE ASSOCIATES, INC.
4354 SHERWOOD FOREST
BATON ROUGE, LOUISIANA 70816

Description: Designs and develops medical management
  software systems
Founded: 1970
Expertise Needed: Computer programming, program
  analysis
Contact: Ms Barbara Borkland
  Order Manager
  (504) 291-7080

ENGLEWOOD HOSPITAL
350 ENGLE STREET
ENGLEWOOD, NEW JERSEY 07631-1808

Description: Public hospital
Parent Company: Englewood Healthcare Foundation
Founded: 1888
Annual Sales: $144.1 million
Number of Employees: 2,200
Expertise Needed: Registered nursing, occupational
  therapy, physical therapy
Contact: Ms Carol Krisson
  Assistant Recuitment Manager
  (201) 894-3000

N.T. ENLOE MEMORIAL HOSPITAL
WEST 5TH AVENUE AND ESPLANADE
CHICO, CALIFORNIA 95926

Description: General medical and surgical hospital
Parent Company: Superior California Medical Center
Annual Sales: $184.6 million
Number of Employees: 1,787
Expertise Needed: Licensed practical nursing, registered
    nursing, management
Contact: Ms Jane Mulkey
        Director of Personnel
        (916) 891-7300

ENSCO, INC.
5400 PORT ROYAL ROAD
SPRINGFIELD, VIRGINIA 22151-2301

Description: Develops industrial laboratory testing
    equipment and computer hardware and software
Annual Sales: $30.4 million
Number of Employees: 407
Expertise Needed: Software engineering/development,
    hardware engineering, computer science, computer
    engineering
Contact: Mr William Moore
        Professional Recruiter
        (703) 321-9000

ENZO BIOCHEM, INC.
60 EXECUTIVE BOULEVARD
FARMINGDALE, NEW YORK 11735-4710

Description: Provides biomolecular research and
    development and diagnostic imaging services
Founded: 1976
Annual Sales: $20.5 million
Number of Employees: 300
Expertise Needed: Biology, chemistry
Contact: Ms June Tedesco
        Manager of Human Resources
        (516) 755-5500

EPI CORPORATION
9707 SHELBYVILLE ROAD
LOUISVILLE, KENTUCKY 40223-2976

Description: Owns and operates nursing homes
Founded: 1973
Annual Sales: $33.5 million
Number of Employees: 1,800
Expertise Needed: Home health care, accounting,
    marketing, finance, law
Contact: Mr John Snyder
        President
        (502) 426-2242

EPISCOPAL HOSPITAL
100 EAST LEHIGH AVENUE
PHILADELPHIA, PENNSYLVANIA 19125

Description: General hospital
Founded: 1851
Annual Sales: $133.5 million
Number of Employees: 1,200
Expertise Needed: Registered nursing, licensed practical
    nursing, respiratory technology, physical therapy,
    radiation technology, anesthesiology
Contact: Ms Ruth Alden
        Professional Recruiting
        (215) 427-7000

ETHIX HEALTHCARE CORPORATION
888 SOUTHWEST 5TH AVENUE
PORTLAND, OREGON 97204-2020

Description: Provides medical insurance claims
    management services
Annual Sales: $250.3 million
Number of Employees: 650
Expertise Needed: Claims adjustment/examination,
    actuarial, accounting, sales, marketing
Contact: Personnel Department
        (503) 225-9548

EVANGELICAL HEALTH SYSTEMS
2025 WINDSOR DRIVE
OAK BROOK, ILLINOIS 60521

Description: Owns and operates hospitals and nursing
    homes
Number of Employees: 10,200
Expertise Needed: Registered nursing, licensed practical
    nursing, physicians, clinical engineering, law
Contact: Mr Ben Grigaliounas
        Senior Vice President of Human Resources
        (708) 572-9393

EVANGELICAL LUTHERAN GOOD SAMARITAN
1000 WEST AVENUE NORTH
SIOUX FALLS, SOUTH DAKOTA 57104-1332

Description: Provides long-term health-care and
    retirement living services
Founded: 1922
Annual Sales: $403.6 million
Number of Employees: 16,588
Expertise Needed: Analog engineering, accounting,
    physical therapy
Contact: Ms Sonja Norine
        Manager of Employment
        (605) 336-2998

EVANS, GRIFFITHS & HART, INC.
55 WALTHAM STREET
LEXINGTON, MASSACHUSETTS 02173

Description: Designs and develops computer software
for medical and industrial applications
Founded: 1970
Expertise Needed: Computer science, software
engineering/development, computer programming
Contact: Ms Martha Scott
Human Resources Department
(617) 861-0670

EVERGREEN HEALTHCARE, LTD.
11350 NORTH MERIDIAN STREET
CARMEL, INDIANA 46032-4563

Description: Manages nursing homes
Annual Sales: $60.5 million
Number of Employees: 4,300
Expertise Needed: Home health care, nursing, licensed
practical nursing, certified nursing and nursing
assistance
Contact: Mr Greg Smith
Human Resources Manager
(317) 580-8585

EXTREL CORPORATION
575 EPILON DRIVE
PITTSBURGH, PENNSYLVANIA 15238

Description: Manufactures analytical instruments
Founded: 1967
Number of Employees: 100
Expertise Needed: Manufacturing engineering,
mechanical engineering, electrical engineering
Contact: Ms Gloria DeBiasio
Human Resources Representative
(412) 963-7530

EYE CARE CENTERS OF AMERICA
11103 WEST AVENUE
SAN ANTONIO, TEXAS 78213-1373

Description: Owns and operates retail stores selling
eyewear, and optical products
Parent Company: Desai Capital Management, Inc.
Annual Sales: $125.0 million
Number of Employees: 1,700
Expertise Needed: Management, sales
Contact: Ms Evelyn Gonzales
Vice President of Human Resources
(210) 340-3531

E-Z-EM, INC.
717 MAIN STREET
WESTBURY, NEW YORK 11590

Description: Manufactures and markets diagnostic
imaging products
Founded: 1961
Number of Employees: 500

*Number of Managerial and Professional Employees Hired
1993:* 10
Contact: Ms Sandra Baron
Director of Human Resources
(516) 333-8230

FAIRVIEW HOSPITAL HEALTHCARE SERVICES
2450 RIVERSIDE AVENUE
MINNEAPOLIS, MINNESOTA 55454-1450

Description: Public hospital specializing in trauma and
acute care
Founded: 1905
Annual Sales: $432.4 million
Number of Employees: 8,654
Expertise Needed: Occupational therapy, physical therapy
Contact: Ms Chery Isham
Human Resources Representative
(612) 672-6300

FALLON HEALTH CARE SYSTEM
630 PLANTATION STREET
WORCESTER, MASSACHUSETTS 01605-2038

Description: Multi-specialty health maintenance
organization
Founded: 1966
Annual Sales: $82.6 million
Number of Employees: 1,200
*Number of Managerial and Professional Employees Hired
1993:* 25
Expertise Needed: Physicians, nursing, physical therapy,
administration, computer programming,
management information systems
Contact: Mr Augustin Auffant
Professional Medical Recruiter
(508) 852-0600

FAMILY AIDES, INC.
120 WEST JOHN STREET
HICKSVILLE, NEW YORK 11801-1016

Description: Provides home health-care services
Founded: 1972
Annual Sales: $40.0 million
Number of Employees: 3,000
Expertise Needed: Home health care, registered nursing,
health care, physical therapy, occupational therapy,
speech therapy, home health care, social work
Contact: Mr William C Schnell
President
(516) 681-2300

FAMILY HOME CARE
6910 5TH AVENUE
BROOKLYN, NEW YORK 11209-1507

Description: Provides home health-care services
Annual Sales: $44.8 million
Number of Employees: 1,800

Expertise Needed: Accounting
Contact: Mr John Purcell
Assistant Director of Personnel
(718) 238-4700

FAMILY VISION CENTERS, INC.
3061 MARKET AVENUE
FAYETTEVILLE, ARKANSAS 72703-3561

Description: Manufactures and distributes eyewear
Founded: 1966
Annual Sales: $40.0 million
Number of Employees: 500
Expertise Needed: Optometry, optics, sales, marketing
Contact: Ms Stachia Trice
Manager of Human Resources
(501) 444-2400

FERNO-WASHINGTON, INC.
70 WEIL WAY
WILMINGTON, OHIO 45177-9371

Description: Manufactures orthopedic devices, patient systems, and rehabilitation equipment
Founded: 1956
Annual Sales: $56.2 million
Number of Employees: 650
Expertise Needed: Mechanical engineering, electrical engineering, accounting, data processing, finance, design engineering, marketing, production
Contact: Mr Robert Ginter
Vice President of Human Resources
(513) 382-1451

FHP TAKECARE
5725 MARK DABLING BOULEVARD
COLORADO SPRINGS, COLORADO 80919

Description: Health maintenance organization and managed care provider
Annual Sales: $129.7 million
Number of Employees: 475
Expertise Needed: Nursing, accounting, finance, marketing
Contact: Ms Marilyn Reed
Administrative Assistant
(719) 522-6000

FIDELITY
3832 KETTERING BOULEVARD
DAYTON, OHIO 45439-2032

Description: Provides home health-care services
Annual Sales: $21.1 million
Number of Employees: 1,000
Expertise Needed: Occupational therapy, physical therapy, speech therapy, registered nursing, licensed practical nursing, home health care
Contact: Mr Wayne Waite
Vice President of Human Resources
(513) 496-6400

MILLARD FILLMORE HOSPITAL
3 GATES CIRCLE
BUFFALO, NEW YORK 14209-1120

Description: General hospital
Founded: 1872
Annual Sales: $187.7 million
Number of Employees: 2,860
Expertise Needed: Social work, bilingual social work, X-ray technology, radiation technology
Contact: Ms Michelle Frick
Employment Coordinator
(716) 887-4600

FIRST HOSPITAL CORPORATION
240 CORPORATE BOULEVARD
NORFOLK, VIRGINIA 23502-4948

Description: Provides mental health services and substance abuse treatment
Annual Sales: $155.0 million
Number of Employees: 3,000
Expertise Needed: Accounting, finance, marketing, economics, data processing
Contact: Ms Catherine Callahan
Corporate Director of Human Resources
(804) 459-5100

FIRST HOSPITAL CORPORATION OF PORTSMOUTH
301 FORT LANE
PORTSMOUTH, VIRGINIA 23704-2221

Description: Manages residential treatment and mental health programs
Parent Company: First Hospital Corporation
Annual Sales: $25.0 million
Number of Employees: 800
Expertise Needed: Registered nursing, licensed practical nursing, occupational therapy, physical therapy, radiology, nursing management and administration, cardiology, certified nursing and nursing assistance
Contact: Human Resources Department
(804) 393-0061

FIRST HOSPITAL WYOMING VALLEY
149 DANA STREET
WILKES BARRE, PENNSYLVANIA 18702-4825

Description: Provides administrative management services and operates a psychiatric clinic
Annual Sales: $26.9 million
Number of Employees: 200
Expertise Needed: Registered nursing, licensed practical nursing, occupational therapy, physical therapy, radiology, accounting, finance
Contact: Ms Debbie Piontkowski
Director of Human Resources
(717) 829-7900

FISCHER IMAGING CORPORATION

12300 GRANT STREET
DENVER, COLORADO 80241-3120

Description: Manufactures medical X-ray equipment
Founded: 1910
Annual Sales: $67.1 million
Number of Employees: 568
Number of Managerial and Professional Employees Hired 1993: 15
Expertise Needed: Accounting, sales, design engineering, mechanical engineering, software engineering/development
Contact: Ms Dru Yokum
Human Resources Representative
(303) 452-6800

FISHER HAMILTON SCIENTIFIC, INC.

1316 18TH STREET
TWO RIVERS, WISCONSIN 54241

Description: Manufactures laboratory equipment, furniture, and fixtures
Founded: 1880
Number of Employees: 800
Number of Managerial and Professional Employees Hired 1993: 75
Expertise Needed: Laboratory technology, mechanical engineering, sales, marketing
Contact: Mr Chris Klages
Manager of Human Resources
(414) 793-1121

FISONS CORPORATION

755 JEFFERSON ROAD
ROCHESTER, NEW YORK 14623-3233

Description: Manufactures ethical pharmaceuticals
Founded: 1973
Annual Sales: $153.1 million
Number of Employees: 1,200
Expertise Needed: Chemistry, biology, pharmacology, clinical research, marketing, process engineering
Contact: Mr James Weltzer
Director of Employee Relations
(716) 475-9000

FISONS INSTRUMENTS, INC.

55 CHERRY HILL DRIVE
BEVERLY, MASSACHUSETTS 01915

Description: Manufactures analytical instruments
Founded: 1979
Number of Employees: 250
Expertise Needed: Computer science, biology, life sciences, chemistry, systems analysis, sales, customer service and support
Contact: Human Resources Department
(508) 524-1000

F&M DISTRIBUTORS, INC.

25800 SHERWOOD
WARREN, MICHIGAN 48091-4160

Description: Manufactures and distributes health and beauty aids, stationery products, and pet food
Founded: 1956
Annual Sales: $760.0 million
Number of Employees: 4,600
Number of Managerial and Professional Employees Hired 1993: 240
Expertise Needed: Pharmacy, management, retail
Contact: Mr Mark Brabaw
Manager of Recruiting and Training
(313) 758-1400

FOCUS HEALTHCARE MANAGEMENT

7101 EXECUTIVE CENTER
BRENTWOOD, TENNESSEE 37027-5236

Description: Provides medical cost management services
Parent Company: United Healthcare
Founded: 1986
Annual Sales: $86.0 million
Number of Employees: 350
Expertise Needed: Physicians, human resources, claims processing/management, and administration
Contact: Ms Judy Lofurno
Human Resources Representative
(615) 377-9936

HENRY FORD HEALTH SYSTEM

3011 WEST GRAND BOULEVARD
DETROIT, MICHIGAN 48202-3008

Description: General hospital
Annual Sales: $597.4 million
Number of Employees: 16,300
Expertise Needed: Medical technology, registered nursing, licensed practical nursing, occupational therapy, physical therapy, accounting, finance, marketing, data processing, computer programming
Contact: Ms Dolores Hunt
Director of Employment
(313) 876-8450

FOREST PHARMACEUTICALS, INC.

13622 LAKEFRONT DRIVE
HAZELWOOD, MISSOURI 63045-1403

Description: Distributes pharmaceutical products
Parent Company: Forest Laboratories, Inc.
Annual Sales: $150.0 million
Number of Employees: 300
Expertise Needed: Pharmacy, sales, marketing, accounting, finance
Contact: Ms Joan Alalof
Director of Human Resources
(314) 344-8870

FORREST COUNTY GENERAL HOSPITAL
6051 US HIGHWAY 49
HATTIESBURG, MISSISSIPPI 39401-7332

Description: Public hospital
Founded: 1952
Annual Sales: $127.4 million
Number of Employees: 2,000
Expertise Needed: Physical therapy, occupational therapy, medical technology, licensed practical nursing, registered nursing
Contact: Ms Susan Kelly
Health Care Recruiter
(601) 288-7000

FORUM GROUP, INC.
8900 KEYSTONE CROSSING
INDIANAPOLIS, INDIANA 46240-2112

Description: Provides long-term health-care services
Founded: 1967
Annual Sales: $84.7 million
Number of Employees: 3,500
Expertise Needed: Accounting, nursing management and administration, management, purchasing
Contact: Ms Nancy Connally
Manager of Human Resources
(317) 575-1333

FOSTER MEDICAL SUPPLY, INC.
275 WYMAN STREET
WALTHAM, MASSACHUSETTS 02154-1209

Description: Distributes medical supplies and equipment to hospitals and physicians
Annual Sales: $165.0 million
Number of Employees: 700
Expertise Needed: Accounting, marketing, finance
Contact: Ms Carla Savchuk
Personnel Manager
(617) 890-4848

FOUNDATION HEALTH
3400 DATA DRIVE
RANCHO CORDOVA, CALIFORNIA 95670-7956

Description: Health maintenance organization
Founded: 1975
Annual Sales: $439.3 million
Number of Employees: 854
Expertise Needed: Nursing, claims adjustment/ examination, actuarial, management information systems, finance, computer programming, program analysis
Contact: Ms Deborah Taylor
Director of Human Resources
(916) 631-5000

FOXMEYER CORPORATION
1220 SENLAC DRIVE
CARROLLTON, TEXAS 75006

Description: Wholesale distributor of pharmaceuticals and health and beauty aids
Annual Sales: $3.1 billion
Number of Employees: 3,000
Expertise Needed: Pharmacy
Contact: Ms Sandra Stevens
Vice President of Human Resources
(214) 446-4800

FRANCISCAN CHILDREN'S HOSPITAL AND REHABILITATION CENTER
30 WARREN STREET
BOSTON, MASSACHUSETTS 02135-3680

Description: Church-operated rehabilitation hospital
Founded: 1949
Annual Sales: $36.7 million
Number of Employees: 555
Expertise Needed: Occupational therapy, medical technology, physical therapy
Contact: Department of Human Resources
(617) 254-3800

FRANCISCAN HEALTH SYSTEM, INC.
1 MACINTYRE DRIVE
ASTON, PENNSYLVANIA 19014-1122

Description: Owns and operates hospitals
Annual Sales: $1.0 billion
Number of Employees: 12,307
Expertise Needed: Accounting, marketing, finance, management information systems, business management
Contact: Director of Human Resources
(215) 358-3950

FRANTZ MEDICAL DEVELOPMENT, LTD.
595 MADISON AVENUE
NEW YORK, NEW YORK 10022-1907

Description: Develops and manufactures endoscopy and disposable health-care products
Founded: 1980
Annual Sales: $30.2 million
Number of Employees: 360
Expertise Needed: Accounting, finance, data processing, mechanical engineering, chemical engineering
Contact: Mr Mark Frantz
President
(212) 308-4860

FRAZIER REHABILITATION CENTER
220 ABRAHAM FLEXNER WAY
LOUISVILLE, KENTUCKY 40202-1818

Description: Not-for-profit rehabilitation hospital
Founded: 1953
Annual Sales: $21.7 million

Frazier Rehabilitation Center (continued)

Number of Employees: 335
Expertise Needed: Occupational therapy, physical therapy, nursing, rehabilitation
Contact: Department of Human Resources
(502) 582-7400

DANIEL FREEMAN HOSPITALS, INC.
333 NORTH PRAIRIE AVENUE
INGLEWOOD, CALIFORNIA 90301-4501

Description: General and surgical Hospital
Parent Company: Carondelet Health Care Corporation
Annual Sales: $192.7 million
Number of Employees: 1,400
Expertise Needed: Physical therapy, occupational therapy, respiratory therapy, nursing, medical records
Contact: Ms Gaynell Carter
Allied Health Recruiter
(310) 419-8373

FRESENIUS USA, INC.
2637 SHADELANDS DRIVE
WALNUT CREEK, CALIFORNIA 94598-2512

Description: Manufactures hemodialysis equipment
Founded: 1974
Annual Sales: $128.6 million
Number of Employees: 845
Number of Managerial and Professional Employees Hired 1993: 150
Expertise Needed: Mechanical engineering, chemical engineering, electrical engineering, industrial engineering, sales, marketing, registered nursing, licensed practical nursing, computer science
Contact: Mr Dick Groben
Director of Human Resources
(510) 295-0200

FROEDTERT MEMORIAL LUTHERAN HOSPITAL
9200 WEST WISCONSIN AVENUE
MILWAUKEE, WISCONSIN 53226-3522

Description: Private general hospital
Founded: 1965
Annual Sales: $129.2 million
Number of Employees: 1,346
Expertise Needed: Networking, licensed practical nursing, respiratory therapy, social service
Contact: Ms Nancy Heisler
Assistant Vice President of Human Resources
(414) 259-3000

FUJI MEDICAL SYSTEMS USA
333 LUDLOW STREET
STAMFORD, CONNECTICUT 06902-6982

Description: Distributes medical imaging materials and related products
Parent Company: Fujifilm America, Inc.

Annual Sales: $120.0 million
Number of Employees: 250
Expertise Needed: Government affairs/relations, law, marketing, importing/exporting
Contact: Personnel Department
(203) 353-0300

FUJISAWA USA, INC.
3 PARKWAY NORTH
DEERFIELD, ILLINOIS 60015-2537

Description: Manufactures critical care pharmaceuticals
Annual Sales: $250.0 million
Number of Employees: 1,226
Expertise Needed: Packaging engineering, chemical engineering, mechanical engineering, computer programming, accounting, marketing
Contact: Ms Mary Ann Schroeder
Recruiter
(708) 317-8800

FULTON DEKALB HOSPITAL AUTHORITY
80 BUTLER STREET SOUTHEAST
ATLANTA, GEORGIA 30303-3050

Description: Owns and operates hospitals
Founded: 1945
Annual Sales: $235.9 million
Number of Employees: 6,000
Expertise Needed: Nursing, physical therapy, occupational therapy, medical technology, physician assistant
Contact: Human Resources - Employment Department
(404) 616-1900

GARDEN STATE REHABILITATION HOSPITAL
14 HOSPITAL DRIVE
TOMS RIVER, NEW JERSEY 08755-6402

Description: Private hospital
Parent Company: National Medical Enterprises
Annual Sales: $31.2 million
Number of Employees: 400
Expertise Needed: Licensed practical nursing, registered nursing, physical therapy, occupational therapy
Contact: Ms Mary Mickens
Human Resources Manager
(908) 244-9366

GASTON MEMORIAL HOSPITAL, INC.
2525 COURT DRIVE
GASTONIA, NORTH CAROLINA 28054-2141

Description: General medical and surgical hospital
Parent Company: Gaston Health Care, Inc.
Founded: 1945
Annual Sales: $98.2 million
Number of Employees: 1,654

Expertise Needed: Coronary care, orthopedics, emergency services, psychology

Contact: Ms Deborah Jolley
    Professional Recruiter
    (704) 834-2000

GAYMAR INDUSTRIES, INC.
10 CENTRE DRIVE
ORCHARD PARK, NEW YORK 14127-2280

Description: Manufactures medical supplies
Founded: 1956
Annual Sales: $40.0 million
Number of Employees: 300
Expertise Needed: Manufacturing engineering, design engineering, electrical engineering, mechanical engineering, marketing, computer programming

Contact: Mr Paul Kunkemoeller
    Employment Administrator
    (716) 662-2551

GC AMERICA COMPANY
3737 WEST 127TH STREET
CHICAGO, ILLINOIS 60658

Description: Manufactures Dental Equipment
Founded: 1928
Number of Employees: 140
Expertise Needed: Data processing, quality control, marketing

Contact: Human Resources Department
    (708) 597-0900

GEISINGER MEDICAL CENTER
100 NORTH ACADAMY AVENUE
DANVILLE, PENNSYLVANIA 17822

Description: General medical and surgical hospital
Founded: 1915
Annual Sales: $227.9 million
Number of Employees: 3,872
Expertise Needed: Registered nursing, licensed practical nursing, radiology, physical therapy, occupational therapy, physicians, physician assistant, general surgery

Contact: Mr James Cleary
    Senior Vice President of Human Resources
    (717) 271-6202

GEN-PROBE, INC.
9880 CAMPUS POINT DRIVE
SAN DIEGO, CALIFORNIA 92121-1514

Description: Manufactures medical diagnostic kits
Annual Sales: $42.8 million
Number of Employees: 288

Expertise Needed: Accounting, finance, mechanical engineering, data processing, chemistry, biology, chemical engineering

Contact: Ms Leslie Tobias
    Employment Relations Manager
    (619) 546-8000

GENENTECH, INC.
460 POINT SAN BRUNO BOULEVARD
SOUTH SAN FRANCISCO, CALIFORNIA 94080-4918

Description: Develops and manufactures pharmaceutical products
Parent Company: Roche Holdings, Inc.
Founded: 1976
Annual Sales: $391.0 million
Number of Employees: 2,331
Number of Managerial and Professional Employees Hired 1993: 300
Expertise Needed: Biology, chemistry, physics, chemical engineering

Contact: Human Resources Department
    (415) 225-1000

GENERAL HOSPITAL CENTER AT PASSAIC
350 BOULEVARD
PASSAIC, NEW JERSEY 07055-2840

Description: Public community hospital
Parent Company: Health Care Continuum, Inc.
Annual Sales: $110.5 million
Number of Employees: 1,450
Expertise Needed: Respiratory therapy, X-ray technology, registered nursing

Contact: Ms Yolanda Green
    Manager of Employment
    (201) 365-4513

GENERAL INJECTIBLES & VACCINES
HIGHWAY 21-52 TERRACE HILL
BASTIAN, VIRGINIA 24314

Description: Manufactures pharmaceuticals
Annual Sales: $72.1 million
Number of Employees: 250
Expertise Needed: Marketing, distribution, telecommunications

Contact: Mr Larry Miller
    Supervisor of Personnel
    (703) 688-4121

GENERAL MEDICAL CORPORATION
8741 LANDMARK ROAD
RICHMOND, VIRGINIA 23228-2801

Description: Distributes medical, surgical, and laboratory supplies
Parent Company: Rabco Health Services, Inc.
Annual Sales: $853.6 million
Number of Employees: 2,000

General Medical Corporation (continued)

Expertise Needed: Mechanical engineering, accounting, electrical engineering, manufacturing engineering

Contact: Ms Deborah Vild
Professional Recruiter
(804) 264-7500

GENESIS HEALTH VENTURES

515 FAIRMONT AVENUE
TOWSON, MARYLAND 21286-5466

Description: Owns and operates long-term care facilities and retirement centers
Annual Sales: $63.3 million
Number of Employees: 5,000
Expertise Needed: Administration, nursing

Contact: Director of Human Resources
(410) 296-1000

GENESIS HEALTH VENTURES, INC.

148 WEST STATE STREET
KENNETT SQUARE, PENNSYLVANIA 19348-3021

Description: Owns and operates nursing homes and retirement centers
Annual Sales: $196.3 million
Number of Employees: 6,000
Expertise Needed: Registered nursing, marketing, accounting

Contact: Mr James Tabak
Director of Human Resources
(215) 444-6350

GENESYS REGIONAL MEDICAL CENTER

302 KENSINGTON AVENUE
FLINT, MICHIGAN 48503-2044

Description: Public hospital
Founded: 1920
Annual Sales: $105.2 million
Number of Employees: 4,600
Expertise Needed: Physical therapy, registered nursing

Contact: Mr Phillip Espinosa
Employment Manager
(313) 762-8000

GENETICS INSTITUTE, INC.

87 CAMBRIDGE PARK DRIVE
CAMBRIDGE, MASSACHUSETTS 02140-2311

Description: Research and development laboratory for biopharmaceutical products
Parent Company: American Home Products Corporation
Annual Sales: $82.0 million
Number of Employees: 700
Expertise Needed: Biology, life sciences, pharmacy, chemistry, manufacturing engineering

Contact: Ms Barbara Covel
Senior Director of Human Resources
(617) 876-1170

GENEVA PHARMACEUTICALS, INC.

2555 WEST MIDWAY BOULEVARD
BROOMFIELD, COLORADO 80020-1632

Description: Manufactures generic drugs
Parent Company: Ciba-Geigy Corporation
Annual Sales: $175.0 million
Number of Employees: 814
Expertise Needed: Chemical engineering, computer programming, accounting, sales, chemistry, pharmaceutical

Contact: Mr Thomas Callaway
Vice President of Human Resources
(303) 466-2400

GENICA PHARMACEUTICALS

377 PLANTATION STREET
WORCESTER, MASSACHUSETTS 01605

Description: Biopharmaceutical research company
Number of Employees: 65
Expertise Needed: Biology, chemistry, customer service and support

Contact: Ms Michelle Shoreys
Human Resources Administrator
(508) 756-2886

GENSIA PHARMACEUTICALS, INC.

11025 ROSELLE STREET
SAN DIEGO, CALIFORNIA 92121-1204

Description: Manufactures and distributes pharmaceuticals
Annual Sales: $30.8 million
Number of Employees: 440
Expertise Needed: Chemistry, production, sales, marketing, research

Contact: Human Resources Department
(619) 546-8300

GENVEC

12111 PARKLAWN DRIVE
ROCKVILLE, MARYLAND 20852

Description: Biotechnology research company
Number of Employees: 30
Expertise Needed: Molecular biology, laboratory technology

Contact: Dr Imi Kovesdi
Director of Vector Biology
(301) 816-0396

GENZYME CORPORATION

1 KENDALL SQUARE
CAMBRIDGE, MASSACHUSETTS 02139-1561

Description: Supplies diagnostic products and services
Annual Sales: $180.0 million
Number of Employees: 1,658

Expertise Needed: Biology, chemistry, physics, chemical engineering, electrical engineering, mechanical engineering

Contact: Ms Sue Lynch
Human Resources Administrator
(617) 252-7500

GERIATRIC AND MEDICAL COMPANIES
5601 CHESTNUT STREET
PHILADELPHIA, PENNSYLVANIA 19139-3255

Description: Owns and operates nursing homes and provideshomecare services
Founded: 1957
Annual Sales: $164.4 million
Number of Employees: 4,018
Expertise Needed: Registered nursing, occupational therapy, physical therapy
Contact: Ms Letitia Gill
Nurse Recruiter
(215) 476-2250

GETTYSBURG HEALTH CARE CORPORATION
147 GETTYS STREET
GETTYSBURG, PENNSYLVANIA 17325-2534

Description: Administrative management firm
Annual Sales: $24.2 million
Number of Employees: 700
Contact: Mr William Shipman
Director of Human Resources
(717) 337-4137

GIRLING HEALTH CARE, INC.
4902 GROVER AVENUE
AUSTIN, TEXAS 78756-2629

Description: Home health-care agency
Annual Sales: $46.8 million
Number of Employees: 700
Expertise Needed: Licensed practical nursing, registered nursing, physical therapy
Contact: Mr David McMillan
Director of Human Resources
(512) 452-5781

GLAXO AMERICAS, INC.
499 PARK AVENUE
NEW YORK, NEW YORK 10022-1240

Description: Manufactures pharmaceuticals
Founded: 1972
Annual Sales: $495.0 million
Number of Employees: 3,854

Expertise Needed: Accounting, finance, chemistry, biochemistry, biology
Contact: Mr Don Cashion
Vice President of Human Resources
(212) 308-1210

GLAXO, INC.
5 MOORE DRIVE
RESEARCH TRIANGLE PARK, NORTH CAROLINA 27701-4613

Description: Manufactures pharmaceutical products
Founded: 1977
Annual Sales: $5.4 billion
Number of Employees: 3,854
Expertise Needed: Chemistry, biology, chemical engineering, accounting
Contact: Mr Steve Sons
Director of Human Resources
(919) 248-2100

GLENMARK ASSOCIATES, INC.
1369 STEWARTSTOWN ROAD
MORGANTOWN, WEST VIRGINIA 26505-2951

Description: Owns nursing homes
Annual Sales: $24.6 million
Number of Employees: 1,474
Expertise Needed: Hospital administration, therapy, accounting
Contact: Ms Kathy Gessler
Employment Manager
(304) 599-0395

GLENS FALLS HOSPITAL
100 PARK STREET
GLENS FALLS, NEW YORK 12801-4413

Description: Public hospital
Parent Company: Adirondack Health Services
Annual Sales: $91.1 million
Number of Employees: 2,044
Expertise Needed: Registered nursing, occupational therapy, physical therapy, pharmacy, psychology
Contact: Ms Penny Lorretto
Employment Interviewer
(518) 792-3151

GLYNN BRUNSWICK HOSPITAL AUTHORITY OF SOUTHEAST GEORGIA

3100 KEMBLE AVENUE
BRUNSWICK, GEORGIA 31520-4211

Description: Owns and operates hospitals
Founded: 1954
Annual Sales: $109.7 million
Number of Employees: 1,310
Expertise Needed: Registered nursing, physical therapy, occupational therapy, respiratory therapy
Contact: Ms Rhonda Butts
　　　　Vice President of Human Resources
　　　　(912) 264-7080

GOLDEN STATE HEALTH CENTERS

13347 VENTURA BOULEVARD
SHERMAN OAKS, CALIFORNIA 91423-3912

Description: Owns, operates, and leases convalescent hospital and health-care facilities
Founded: 1968
Annual Sales: $68.4 million
Number of Employees: 2,000
Expertise Needed: Licensed practical nursing, registered nursing, certified nursing and nursing assistance
Contact: Mr Michael Fuksman
　　　　Director of Human Resources
　　　　(818) 986-1550

GOLDLINE LABORATORIES, INC.

1900 WEST COMMERCIAL BOULEVARD
FORT LAUDERDALE, FLORIDA 33309

Description: Distributes pharmaceutical products
Founded: 1972
Number of Employees: 480
Number of Managerial and Professional Employees Hired 1993: 8
Expertise Needed: Sales, marketing, administration
Contact: Ms Susan Haddad
　　　　Human Resources Specialist
　　　　(305) 491-4002

GOOD SAMARITAN HOSPITAL

1000 MONTAUK HIGHWAY
WEST ISLIP, NEW YORK 11795-4927

Description: Community hospital
Founded: 1906
Annual Sales: $114.2 million
Number of Employees: 2,200
Expertise Needed: Nursing, physical therapy
Contact: Ms Marge Restivo
　　　　Nursing Recruiter
　　　　(516) 376-3000

GOOD SAMARITAN HOSPITAL OF SUFFERN

255 LAFAYETTE AVENUE
SUFFERN, NEW YORK 10901-4817

Description: Private hospital specializing in prenatal intensive care
Founded: 1902
Annual Sales: $100.2 million
Number of Employees: 1,500
Expertise Needed: Registered nursing
Contact: Ms Ellen Johnson
　　　　Manager of Employment
　　　　(914) 368-5000

GOOD SHEPHERD MEDICAL CENTER

700 EAST MARSHALL AVENUE
LONGVIEW, TEXAS 75601-6621

Description: Hospital specializing in acute care and cardiology
Founded: 1934
Annual Sales: $86.1 million
Number of Employees: 1,800
Expertise Needed: Nursing, physical therapy, occupational therapy, respiratory therapy, medical technology
Contact: Mr James Klepper
　　　　Human Resources Director
　　　　(903) 236-2000

GRADUATE HOSPITAL

1 GRADUATE PLAZA
PHILADELPHIA, PENNSYLVANIA 19146-1407

Description: Not-for-profit medical and surgical hospital
Founded: 1977
Annual Sales: $176.1 million
Number of Employees: 1,700
Expertise Needed: Hospital administration, marketing
Contact: Human Resources Department
　　　　(215) 892-2200

GRAHAM FIELD, INC.

400 RABRO DRIVE
HAUPPAUGE, NEW YORK 11788-4258

Description: Distributes medical products
Annual Sales: $56.5 million
Number of Employees: 500
Expertise Needed: Accounting, finance, marketing, sales
Contact: Ms Cathy Natalie
　　　　Director of Personnel
　　　　(516) 582-5900

GRANCARE, INC.

300 CORPORATE POINTE
CULVER CITY, CALIFORNIA 90230-7635

Description: Operates a chain of nursing homes, rehabilitation centers, and pharmacies
Founded: 1988
Annual Sales: $174.8 million

Number of Employees: 6,500
Number of Managerial and Professional Employees Hired 1993: 300
Expertise Needed: Licensed practical nursing, pharmacy, therapy, hospital administration, registered nursing, occupational therapy, physical therapy, rehabilitation, respiratory therapy, nursing
Contact: Mr Mark Rubenstein
Vice President of Human Resources
(414) 278-1212

GRANT MEDICAL CENTER
111 SOUTH GRANT AVENUE
COLUMBUS, OHIO 43215-4701

Description: General medical and surgical hospital
Parent Company: U.S. Health Corporation
Annual Sales: $211.8 million
Number of Employees: 2,250
Expertise Needed: Registered nursing, licensed practical nursing, physical therapy, occupational therapy, radiology
Contact: Mr Michael Heys
Director of Human Resources Services
(614) 461-3232

GREAT LAKES REHABILITATION HOSPITAL
143 EAST 2ND STREET
ERIE, PENNSYLVANIA 16507-1501

Description: Private hospital
Parent Company: Rehabilitation Hospital Services Corporation
Annual Sales: $39.7 million
Number of Employees: 350
Expertise Needed: Nursing management and administration, hospital administration, occupational therapy, physical therapy, speech therapy, respiratory therapy, allied therapy, clinical services, cardiovascular therapy, rehabilitation
Contact: Human Resources Department
(814) 878-1200

GREATER ATLANTIC HEALTH SERVICE
3550 MARKET STREET
PHILADELPHIA, PENNSYLVANIA 19104-3329

Description: Health maintenance organization
Annual Sales: $133.4 million
Number of Employees: 350
Expertise Needed: Registered nursing, occupational therapy, physical therapy, physicians, sales
Contact: Ms. Valerie Mettern
Vice President of Human Resources
(215) 823-8600

GREATER BALTIMORE MEDICAL CENTER
6701 NORTH CHARLES STREET
BALTIMORE, MARYLAND 21204-6808

Description: Public hospital
Parent Company: Maryland Healthcorp, Inc.

Annual Sales: $169.2 million
Number of Employees: 2,500
Expertise Needed: Certified nursing a[...] assistance
Contact: Ms Billie Dunn
Personnel Recruiter
(410) 828-2000

GREENERY REHABILITATION GROUP
400 CENTRE STREET
NEWTON, MASSACHUSETTS 02158-2000

Description: Owns and operates rehabilitation and skilled nursing facilities
Annual Sales: $47.4 million
Number of Employees: 6,100
Expertise Needed: Marketing, physical therapy, occupational therapy
Contact: Mr David Levitton
Human Resources Specialist
(617) 244-4744

GREENLEAF HEALTH SYSTEMS, INC.
1 NORTHGATE PARK SOUTH
CHATTANOOGA, TENNESSEE 37415-6912

Description: Hospital management firm
Founded: 1979
Annual Sales: $25.0 million
Number of Employees: 300
Expertise Needed: Psychiatry, counseling, social work
Contact: Mr Gary Silcox
Vice President of Development
(615) 870-5110

GRIFFITH LABORATORIES
ONE GRIFFITH CENTER
ALSIP, ILLINOIS 60658

Description: Manufactures and sells sterilizers and provides contract sterilization services
Founded: 1919
Expertise Needed: Laboratory science, laboratory technology, laboratory chemistry, analysis
Contact: Human Resources Department
(708) 371-0900

GROSSMONT HOSPITAL CORPORATION
5555 GROSSMONT CENTER DRIVE
LA MESA, CALIFORNIA 91942-3019

Description: General hospital
Founded: 1953
Annual Sales: $155.2 million
Number of Employees: 2,800
Expertise Needed: Laboratory assistance, phlebotomy, pharmaceutical technology, occupational therapy, physical therapy, cardiovascular technology, oncology
Contact: Human Resources Department
(619) 450-6240

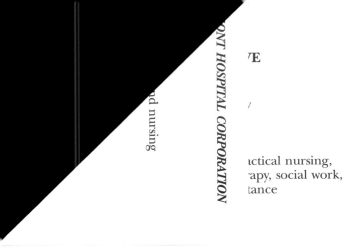

...ont HOSPITAL CORPORATION

...E

...ctical nursing,
...apy, social work,
...tance

GROUP HEALTH COOPERATIVE OF PUGET SOUND

521 WALL STREET
SEATTLE, WASHINGTON 98121-1524

Description: Health maintenance organization
Founded: 1945
Annual Sales: $854.2 million
Number of Employees: 6,670
Expertise Needed: Nursing, pharmacy, data processing,
physics, chemistry, physical therapy
Contact: Mr Peter Humlecker
Manager of Recruitment
(206) 448-5811

GROUP HEALTH NORTHWEST

WEST 5615 SUNSET HIGHWAY
SPOKANE, WASHINGTON 99204-1639

Description: Health maintenance organization
Founded: 1977
Annual Sales: $120.4 million
Number of Employees: 600
*Number of Managerial and Professional Employees Hired
1993:* 25
Expertise Needed: Physicians, computer programming,
maternity nursing, licensed practical nursing,
optometry, marketing, customer service and
support, registered nursing, psychology, therapy
Contact: Mr Don Schoesler
Director of Human Resources
(509) 838-9100

GROVE HILL MEDICAL CENTER

300 KENSINGTON AVENUE
NEW BRITAIN, CONNECTICUT 06051-3916

Description: Private hospital
Founded: 1975
Annual Sales: $30.4 million
Number of Employees: 415
Expertise Needed: Nursing
Contact: Personnel Department
(203) 221-6200

GUARDIAN LIFE INSURANCE COMPANY OF AMERICA

201 PARK AVENUE SOUTH
NEW YORK, NEW YORK 10003-1605

Description: Provides life, health, and disability
insurance services
Founded: 1860
Assets: $6.1 billion
Number of Employees: 4,500
Expertise Needed: Marketing, sales, finance, actuarial,
accounting, underwriting, computer programming,
law
Contact: Mr Brian Silva
Director of Employment
(212) 598-8000

GUARDIAN PRODUCTS, INC.

12800 WENTWORTH STREET
PACOIMA, CALIFORNIA 91331-4331

Description: Manufactures medical walking aids
Parent Company: Sunrise Medical, Inc.
Annual Sales: $49.5 million
Number of Employees: 650
Expertise Needed: Accounting, design engineering,
industrial engineering, manufacturing engineering
Contact: Ms Kim Welch
Director of Human Resources
(818) 504-2820

GULL LABORATORIES, INC.

1011 EAST 4800 SOUTH
SALT LAKE CITY, UTAH 84117-4921

Description: Manufactures and markets medical
diagnostic test kits
Founded: 1974
Expertise Needed: Biology, microbiology
Contact: Human Resources Department
(801) 263-3524

GUNDERSEN CLINIC, LTD.

1836 SOUTH AVENUE
LA CROSSE, WISCONSIN 54601-5429

Description: Nonprofit hospital
Founded: 1930
Annual Sales: $150.0 million
Number of Employees: 1,900
Expertise Needed: Registered nursing, licensed practical
nursing, cardiac care, pediatrics, oncology,
maternity care, human resources, benefits
administration
Contact: Mr Len Vingers
Manager of Personnel
(608) 791-6670

GWINETT HOSPITAL SYSTEM, INC.

1000 MEDICAL CENTER BOULEVARD
LAWRENCEVILLE, GEORGIA 30245-7694

Description: General medical and surgical hospital
Founded: 1956
Annual Sales: $121.2 million
Number of Employees: 1,800
Expertise Needed: Registered nursing, licensed practical nursing, physical therapy, occupational therapy, medical technology, respiratory therapy, radiology
Contact: Ms Diane Bayless
Employment Manager
(404) 995-4562

HACKENSACK MEDICAL CENTER

30 PROSPECT AVENUE
HACKENSACK, NEW JERSEY 07601-1915

Description: Public general hospital
Parent Company: Hillcrest Health Service Systems
Founded: 1888
Annual Sales: $226.6 million
Number of Employees: 4,000
Expertise Needed: Registered nursing
Contact: Ms Lenore Mooney
Senior Recruiter
(201) 996-3601

HAEMONETICS CORPORATION

400 WOOD ROAD
BRAINTREE, MASSACHUSETTS 02184-2486

Description: Designs and manufactures automated systems to collect and process blood and plasma
Annual Sales: $216.3 million
Number of Employees: 1,002
Expertise Needed: Electrical engineering, software engineering/development, mechanical engineering, polymers, biomedical engineering, finance, accounting, life sciences, general nursing, administration
Contact: Ms Susan Tomaski
Director of Staffing
(617) 848-7100

HALSEY DRUG COMPANY, INC.

1827 PACIFIC STREET
BROOKLYN, NEW YORK 11233-3599

Description: Manufactures and sells generic drug products and bulk chemical products
Founded: 1935
Number of Employees: 375
Expertise Needed: Chemistry, accounting
Contact: Ms Beverly Burke
Employment Manager
(718) 467-7500

HAMILTON COMPANY

4970 ENERGY WAY
RENO, NEVADA 89502

Description: Manufactures and markets precision fluid instruments
Founded: 1953
Expertise Needed: Mechanical engineering, industrial engineering, laboratory technology, research and development, phlebotomy
Contact: Ms Edie Harvey
Director of Personnel
(702) 858-3000

HAMOT MEDICAL CENTER

201 STATE STREET
ERIE, PENNSYLVANIA 16507-1426

Description: General medical and surgical hospital
Annual Sales: $142.8 million
Number of Employees: 1,839
Expertise Needed: Registered nursing, licensed practical nursing, physical therapy, occupational therapy
Contact: Mr Al Richards
Employment Manager
(814) 870-6000

G. C. HANFORD MANUFACTURING COMPANY

304 ONEIDA STREET
SYRACUSE, NEW YORK 13201

Description: Pharmaceuticals company
Founded: 1846
Number of Employees: 240
Number of Managerial and Professional Employees Hired 1993: 135
Expertise Needed: Laboratory technology, pharmacy, research and development
Contact: Ms Linda Moore
Manager of Human Resources
(315) 476-7418

HANGER ORTHOPEDIC GROUP, INC.

7700 OLD GEORGETOWN ROAD
BETHESDA, MARYLAND 20814

Description: Manufactures orthopedic and prosthetic devices
Number of Employees: 600
Number of Managerial and Professional Employees Hired 1993: 150
Expertise Needed: Orthopedics, prosthetics, accounting, management information systems
Contact: Ms Ada Brady
Director of Human Resources
(301) 986-0701

HANNAFORD BROTHERS
145 PLEASANT HILL ROAD
SCARBOROUGH, MAINE 04074-8768

Description: Operates a chain of drug stores
Parent Company: Hannaford Brothers Company
Founded: 1967
Annual Sales: $177.0 million
Number of Employees: 681
Expertise Needed: Marketing, accounting
Contact: Mr Norman Brackett
      Vice President of Human Resources
      (207) 883-2911

HARBOR HOSPITAL CENTER, INC.
3001 SOUTH HANOVER STREET
BALTIMORE, MARYLAND 21225-1233

Description: General medical and surgical hospital
Founded: 1903
Annual Sales: $96.5 million
Number of Employees: 1,450
Expertise Needed: Registered nursing, licensed practical nursing, physical therapy, occupational therapy, radiology
Contact: Ms Susan Stein
      Employment Coordinator
      (301) 347-3200

HARDWOOD PRODUCTS COMPANY
SCHOOL STREET
GUILFORD, MAINE 04443

Description: Manufactures metal products for the medical industry
Founded: 1919
Number of Employees: 330
Number of Managerial and Professional Employees Hired 1993: 10
Expertise Needed: Mechanical engineering, electrical engineering, nursing, accounting, finance, sales
Contact: Mr Jerry Noble
      Management Supervisor
      (207) 876-3311

HARLAN SPRAGUE DAWLEY, INC.
298 SOUTH COUNTY LINE ROAD EAST
INDIANAPOLIS, INDIANA 46229

Description: Breeds commercial and laboratory animals
Founded: 1931
Number of Employees: 300
Expertise Needed: Accounting, laboratory technology, operations
Contact: Ms Cheryl Breslin
      Director of Human Resources
      (317) 891-8382

HARMAC MEDICAL PRODUCTS, INC.
2201 BAILEY AVENUE
BUFFALO, NEW YORK 14211

Description: Manufactures plastic disposable medical products
Number of Employees: 500
Number of Managerial and Professional Employees Hired 1993: 150
Expertise Needed: Project engineering, electrical engineering, accounting, sales, marketing
Contact: Ms Donna Ciulis
      Human Resources Manager
      (716) 897-4500

HARRIS COUNTY HOSPITAL DISTRICT
2525 HOLLY HALL
HOUSTON, TEXAS 77054-4124

Description: Public hospital operating community clinics and trauma center
Founded: 1965
Annual Sales: $532.8 million
Number of Employees: 5,232
Expertise Needed: Registered nursing, medical technology, physical therapy, respiratory therapy, occupational therapy, nursing
Contact: Ms Jennie Carmouche
      Director of Employment
      (713) 746-6435

HARRIS LABS
624 PEACH STREET
LINCOLN, NEBRASKA 68502

Description: Performs scientific testing for the pharmaceutical industry
Founded: 1933
Number of Employees: 500
Expertise Needed: Technical engineering, laboratory technology, chemistry, accounting, marketing, sales
Contact: Ms Mary Crook
      Manager of Human Resources
      (402) 476-2811

HARRIS METHODIST FORT WORTH
1301 PENNSYLVANIA AVENUE
FORT WORTH, TEXAS 76104-2122

Description: Public hospital
Founded: 1930
Annual Sales: $364.8 million
Number of Employees: 3,049
Expertise Needed: Registered nursing
Contact: Ms Jan Hoffman
      Manager of Employment
      (817) 882-2000

HARRIS METHODIST HEB

1600 HOSPITAL PARKWAY
BEDFORD, TEXAS 76022-6913

Description: General hospital
Founded: 1967
Annual Sales: $97.9 million
Number of Employees: 1,200
Expertise Needed: Medical technology, laboratory technology, physical therapy, radiology, occupational therapy, anesthesiology
Contact: Ms Kelley Jacobson
       Employment Specialist
       (817) 685-4000

HARTFORD HOSPITAL

80 SEYMOUR STREET
HARTFORD, CONNECTICUT 06102-5037

Description: Public hospital specializing in acute and trauma care
Parent Company: Hartford Health Care Corporation
Annual Sales: $377.6 million
Number of Employees: 5,700
Expertise Needed: Nursing, occupational therapy, physical therapy, physician assistant
Contact: Ms Judy Brady
       Professional Recruiter
       (203) 545-5555

HARVARD COMMUNITY HEALTH PLAN

10 BROOKLINE PLACE WEST
BROOKLINE, MASSACHUSETTS 02146-7215

Description: Provides health insurance and health-care services
Founded: 1968
Annual Sales: $828.7 million
Number of Employees: 6,000
Expertise Needed: Health insurance, customer service and support, marketing, information systems, finance, hospital administration, real estate, accounting, human resources, law
Contact: Ms Anne Smith
       Human Resource Director
       (617) 731-8292

HAUSMANN INDUSTRIES, INC.

130 UNION STREET
NORTHVALE, NEW JERSEY 07647

Description: Manufactures physical therapy equipment
Founded: 1958
Number of Employees: 110
Expertise Needed: Accounting, marketing, sales
Contact: Mr Warren Hausmann
       President
       (201) 767-0255

HAWAII MEDICAL SERVICE ASSOCIATION

818 KEEAUMOKU STREET
HONOLULU, HAWAII 96814-2365

Description: Provides health-care insurance services
Founded: 1938
Annual Sales: $853.9 million
Number of Employees: 1,200
Expertise Needed: Actuarial, accounting, finance, data processing
Contact: Ms Jennie Roberts
       Personnel Department
       (808) 944-2110

HAZELTON WASHINGTON

9200 LEESBURG PIKE
VIENNA, VIRGINIA 22182-1656

Description: Researches pharmaceuticals and chemicals
Parent Company: Corning Lab Services, Inc.
Annual Sales: $165.0 million
Number of Employees: 2,193
Expertise Needed: Biology, biostatistics, veterinary, chemistry, accounting, finance, business administration, laboratory technology, toxicology
Contact: Mr David Howard
       Manager of Human Resources
       (703) 893-5400

HCA HEALTH SERVICES OF KANSAS, INC.

550 NORTH HILLSIDE AVENUE
WICHITA, KANSAS 67214

Description: Public hospital
Parent Company: Hospital Corporation of America
Annual Sales: $399.5 million
Number of Employees: 3,082
Number of Managerial and Professional Employees Hired 1993: 350
Expertise Needed: Occupational therapy, physical therapy, pharmacy
Contact: Ms Janet Hamous
       Director of Human Resources
       (316) 688-2468

HCA HEALTH SERVICES OF VIRGINIA

9100 ARBORETUM PARKWAY
RICHMOND, VIRGINIA 23229-5205

Description: Public hospital
Parent Company: Hospital Corporation of America
Annual Sales: $290.4 million
Number of Employees: 1,800
Contact: Ms Maria Roseberry
       Healthcare Recruiter
       (804) 289-4510

HCF, INC.
2615 FORT AMANDA ROAD
LIMA, OHIO 45804-3730

Description: Corporate office of nursing home
Founded: 1969
Annual Sales: $69.0 million
Number of Employees: 2,400
Expertise Needed: Administration, accounting, nursing, marketing
Contact: Mr Chuck Okodrowski
Director of Human Resources
(419) 999-2010

HEALTH ALLIANCE PLAN OF MICHIGAN
2850 WEST GRAND BOULEVARD
DETROIT, MICHIGAN 48202-2643

Description: Provides health-care insurance services
Founded: 1973
Annual Sales: $630.7 million
Number of Employees: 1,400
Expertise Needed: Accounting, finance, underwriting, actuarial, data processing
Contact: Ms Lisa Facemyer
Human Resources Representative
(313) 872-8100

HEALTH CARE AND RETIREMENT CORPORATION OF AMERICA
1 SEAGATE
TOLEDO, OHIO 43604-1558

Description: Develops, owns, and operates health-care and retirement facilities
Annual Sales: $476.0 million
Number of Employees: 16,000
Expertise Needed: Business administration, accounting, finance, marketing, information systems
Contact: Mr Wade O'Brian
Vice President of Human Resources
(419) 247-5000

HEALTH CARE PLAN, INC.
900 GUARANTY BUILDING
BUFFALO, NEW YORK 14202

Description: Provides health-care insurance services
Founded: 1976
Annual Sales: $112.5 million
Number of Employees: 1,225
Number of Managerial and Professional Employees Hired 1993: 30
Expertise Needed: Actuarial, accounting, finance, ophthalmology, nursing, licensed practical nursing
Contact: Ms Ginger Parysek
Director of Human Resources
(716) 847-1480

HEALTH CARE SERVICE CORPORATION-BLUE CROSS & BLUE SHIELD
233 NORTH MICHIGAN AVENUE
CHICAGO, ILLINOIS 60601-5519

Description: Provides health-care insurance services
Founded: 1936
Assets: $3.1 billion
Number of Employees: 4,224
Expertise Needed: Sales, marketing, accounting, finance, actuarial
Contact: Human Resources Department
(312) 930-7500

HEALTH CARE SUPPLIERS, INC.
3925 WEST NORTHSIDE DRIVE
JACKSON, MISSISSIPPI 39209-2562

Description: Distributes medical and convalescent equipment
Parent Company: Medical Enterprises
Founded: 1976
Annual Sales: $31.9 million
Number of Employees: 640
Expertise Needed: Sales, marketing, distribution
Contact: Ms. Laurie Gurvin
Human Resources Manager
(601) 922-2528

HEALTH-CHEM CORPORATION
1212 AVENUE OF THE AMERICAS
NEW YORK, NEW YORK 10036

Description: Manufactures and distributes industrial and health-care synthetic fabrics
Founded: 1955
Number of Employees: 250
Expertise Needed: Biology, chemistry, business management, marketing, sales, management information systems
Contact: Ms Joyce Montalvo
Administrative Personnel Coordinator
(717) 764-1191

THE HEALTH GROUP
875 8TH STREET NORTHEAST
MASSILLON, OHIO 44646-8503

Description: Community hospital
Annual Sales: $50.7 million
Number of Employees: 1,260
Expertise Needed: Physical therapy, respiratory therapy, occupational therapy
Contact: Ms Ann Butler
Nurse Recruitment
(216) 832-8761

HEALTH IMAGES, INC.
8601 DUNWOODY PLACE
ATLANTA, GEORGIA 30350-2506

Description: Owns and operates diagnostic imaging
  centers
Annual Sales: $61.2 million
Number of Employees: 540
Expertise Needed: Marketing, accounting, radiological
  technology, sales
Contact: Ms Carol Tharilkel
        Manager of Human Resources
        (404) 587-5084

HEALTH MANAGEMENT ASSOCIATES, INC.
5811 PELICAN BAY BOULEVARD
NAPLES, FLORIDA 33963-2710

Description: Owns and operates general hospitals
Annual Sales: $278.0 million
Number of Employees: 4,500
Expertise Needed: Accounting, finance, data processing,
  law
Contact: Mr Fred Drow
        Director of Human Resources
        (813) 598-3131

HEALTH MIDWEST
2304 EAST MEYER BOULEVARD
KANSAS CITY, MISSOURI 64132-4104

Description: Provides hospital management and
  outreach clinical services
Annual Sales: $329.7 million
Number of Employees: 7,000
Expertise Needed: Dietetics, data processing, food
  services, hospital administration, medical records,
  pharmacy, registered nursing, licensed practical
  nursing
Contact: Ms Karen Lowe
        Human Resources Specialist
        (816) 276-9111

HEALTH NET
21600 OXNARD STREET
WOODLAND HILLS, CALIFORNIA 91367-4966

Description: Provides health-care insurance services
Annual Sales: $74.2 million
Number of Employees: 1,077
Expertise Needed: Accounting, finance, marketing,
  health care, sales, registered nursing, licensed
  practical nursing
Contact: Ms Ariella Ginoza
        Human Resources Representative
        (818) 719-6901

HEALTH-O-METER PRODUCTS, INC.
7400 WEST 100TH PLACE
BRIDGEVIEW, ILLINOIS 60455

Description: Designs and manufactures consumer,
  medical, office, and food service scales
Founded: 1919
Number of Employees: 300
Expertise Needed: Manufacturing engineering, electrical
  engineering, sales, marketing, accounting,
  management information systems
Contact: Mr Valentine Zilinskas
        Vice President of Human Resources
        (708) 598-9100

HEALTH PLAN OF NEVADA, INC.
2720 NORTH TENAYA WAY
LAS VEGAS, NEVADA 89128-0424

Description: Health maintenance organization
Parent Company: Sierra Health Services, Inc.
Annual Sales: $175.8 million
Number of Employees: 250
Expertise Needed: Health care, health insurance, claims
  adjustment/examination
Contact: Ms Carmel Fritz
        Manager of Employment
        (702) 242-7200

HEALTH PLUS OF NEW MEXICO, INC.
7500 JEFFERSON STREET NORTHEAST
ALBUQUERQUE, NEW MEXICO 87109-4335

Description: Health maintenance organization
Parent Company: Presbyterian Healthcare Services
Annual Sales: $46.9 million
Number of Employees: 105
Expertise Needed: Data processing, health insurance,
  actuarial
Contact: Human Resources Department
        (505) 823-0700

HEALTH RESOURCES NORTHWEST
HOSPITAL
1550 NORTH 115TH STREET
SEATTLE, WASHINGTON 98133-8401

Description: General and surgical hospital
Annual Sales: $104.1 million
Number of Employees: 1,896
Expertise Needed: Occupational therapy, physical
  therapy, nursing, radiology, administration
Contact: Ms Karlyn Byaham
        Acting Director of Human Resources
        (206) 364-0500

HEALTH SERVICES, INC.
3190 SOUTH BASCOM AVENUE
SAN JOSE, CALIFORNIA 95124-2568

Description: Provides hospital management services
Founded: 1976

Health Services, Inc. (continued)
Annual Sales: $26.0 million
Number of Employees: 720
Expertise Needed: Hospital administration, nursing, physical therapy, physicians
Contact: Mr Gary Collins
　　　　Vice President of Operations
　　　　(408) 369-0500

HEALTH SOUTH, INC.
3627 UNIVERSITY BOULEVARD SOUTH
JACKSONVILLE, FLORIDA 32216-4236

Description: General and surgical hospital
Annual Sales: $169.8 million
Number of Employees: 1,900
Expertise Needed: Accounting, finance, data processing, registered nursing, licensed practical nursing, certified nursing and nursing assistance
Contact: Ms Nancy Moredock
　　　　Director of Personnel
　　　　(904) 391-1200

HEALTH STAFFERS, INC.
5636 NORTH BROADWAY
CHICAGO, ILLINOIS 60660

Description: Provides temporary health-care personnel services
Number of Employees: 10
Expertise Needed: Health insurance
Contact: Ms Rose Houston
　　　　President
　　　　(312) 561-5400

HEALTHCARE AMERICA, INC.
912 CAPITOL OF TEXAS HIGHWAY SOUTH
AUSTIN, TEXAS 78746

Description: Provides health-care insurance services
Founded: 1979
Annual Sales: $193.7 million
Number of Employees: 2,340
Expertise Needed: Accounting
Contact: Mr. Jay Gemperle
　　　　Director of Human Resources
　　　　(512) 329-8829

HEALTHCARE COMPARE CORPORATION
750 RIVERPOINT DRIVE
WEST SACRAMENTO, CALIFORNIA 95605-1625

Description: Provides health-care utilization review and cost management services
Annual Sales: $30.0 million
Number of Employees: 400
Expertise Needed: Health care, sales, medical records, credit/credit analysis
Contact: Ms Lori Pasteur
　　　　Human Resources Representative
　　　　(916) 374-4600

HEALTHCARE CORPORATION
30 BURTON HILLS BOULEVARD
NASHVILLE, TENNESSEE 37215

Description: Owns and manages kidney dialysis clinics
Number of Employees: 200
Expertise Needed: Nursing, accounting, social work, management information systems
Contact: Ms Lynn Mangrum
　　　　Director of Human Resources
　　　　(615) 665-9900

HEALTHCARE REHABILITATION CENTER
1106 WEST DITTMAR ROAD
AUSTIN, TEXAS 78745-6328

Description: For-profit rehabilitation hospital
Parent Company: Healthcare International, Inc.
Annual Sales: $22.2 million
Number of Employees: 600
Expertise Needed: Physical therapy, occupational therapy, speech therapy, psychology
Contact: Ms Lisa Roper
　　　　Recruiter
　　　　(512) 444-4835

HEALTHCARE SERVICES GROUP, INC.
2643 HUNTINGDON PIKE
HUNTINGDON VALLEY, PENNSYLVANIA 19006-5109

Description: Provides management, administrative, and operating services to health-care facilities
Founded: 1976
Annual Sales: $82.9 million
Number of Employees: 5,000
Expertise Needed: Business management, data processing, accounting, finance, industrial hygiene, human resources
Contact: Human Resources Department
　　　　(215) 938-1661

HEALTHDYNE, INC.
1850 PARKWAY PLACE
MARIETTA, GEORGIA 30067-8237

Description: Provides products and services for home health care
Founded: 1970
Annual Sales: $247.4 million
Number of Employees: 3,319
Expertise Needed: Accounting, finance, data processing, law
Contact: Ms Dee Neabers
　　　　Manager of Employment
　　　　(404) 423-4500

HEALTHDYNE TECHNOLOGIES, INC.
1255 KENNESTONE CIRCLE
MARIETTA, GEORGIA 30066-6029

Description: Manufactures home care monitoring and respiratory equipment

Parent Company: Healthdyne, Inc.
Annual Sales: $28.5 million
Number of Employees: 340
Expertise Needed: Research and development, electrical engineering, mechanical engineering, manufacturing engineering, quality engineering, project management
Contact: Ms Claudia Snyder
Manager of Human Resources
(404) 499-1212

HEALTHINFUSION, INC.
5200 BLUE LAGOON DRIVE
MIAMI, FLORIDA 33126-7000

Description: Provides outpatient rehabilitation services
Annual Sales: $28.6 million
Number of Employees: 450
Expertise Needed: Nursing, pharmacy
Contact: Ms Susan Taylor
Director of Human Resources
(305) 267-1177

HEALTHPLUS OF MICHIGAN, INC.
G2050 SOUTH LINDEN ROAD
FLINT, MICHIGAN 48501-1700

Description: Provides health maintenance services
Founded: 1979
Annual Sales: $192.7 million
Number of Employees: 290
Expertise Needed: Nursing, licensed practical nursing, claims adjustment/examination, accounting, marketing, finance
Contact: Ms Kathy Kaza
Human Resources Specialist
(313) 230-2222

HEALTHPRO
1 RESEARCH DRIVE
WESTBORO, MASSACHUSETTS 01581

Description: Provides health-care cost management services
Founded: 1975
Number of Employees: 169
Expertise Needed: Case management, accounting, finance, analysis, clinical accounting, marketing, medical technology, clinical research, planning
Contact: Department of Human Resources
(508) 366-3100

HEALTHSOURCE, INC.
54 REGIONAL DRIVE
CONCORD, NEW HAMPSHIRE 03301-8507

Description: Provides managed care services
Annual Sales: $177.6 million
Number of Employees: 570

Expertise Needed: Nursing
Contact: Mr Walter Corinno
Human Resources Coordinator
(603) 225-5077

HEALTHSOUTH REHABILITATION CORPORATION
2 PERIMETER PARK SOUTH
BIRMINGHAM, ALABAMA 35243

Description: Provides outpatient rehabilitation services
Annual Sales: $407.0 million
Number of Employees: 7,000
Expertise Needed: Allied health, physical therapy, occupational therapy, speech therapy, exercise physiology
Contact: Mr Tod Burkhalter
Director of Clinical Employment
(205) 967-7116

HEALTHSOUTH REHABILITATION HOSPITAL OF GREATER PITTSBURGH
2380 MCGINLEY ROAD
MONROEVILLE, PENNSYLVANIA 15146-4416

Description: Rehabilitation hospital
Parent Company: Rehab Hospital Services Corporation
Number of Employees: 400
Expertise Needed: Physical therapy, occupational therapy, nursing, registered nursing, licensed practical nursing
Contact: Human Resources Department
(412) 856-2400

HEALTHTRUST, INC.
4525 HARDING ROAD
NASHVILLE, TENNESSEE 37205-2119

Description: Owns and manages hospitals
Annual Sales: $2.0 billion
Number of Employees: 19,500
Expertise Needed: Information systems, purchasing, hospital administration, finance, accounting
Contact: Ms Carolyn Schneider
Director of Recruitment and Development
(615) 383-4444

HEBREW REHABILITATION CENTER FOR THE AGED
120 CENTRE STREET
BOSTON, MASSACHUSETTS 02131-1011

Description: Not-for-profit chronic disease hospital
Founded: 1903
Annual Sales: $41.3 million
Number of Employees: 840
Expertise Needed: Registered nursing, physical therapy, respiratory therapy, occupational therapy, accounting, management information systems
Contact: Human Resources Department
(617) 325-8000

HELENA PLASTICS
632 IRWIN STREET
SAN RAFAEL, CALIFORNIA 94901

Description: Manufactures disposable plasticware for clinical hospital laboratories
Founded: 1959
Expertise Needed: Product design and development, plastics engineering, product design engineering, sales
Contact: Personnel Department
(510) 456-0100

HELENE FULD MEDICAL CENTER
750 BRUNSWICK AVENUE
TRENTON, NEW JERSEY 08638-4143

Description: Nonprofit hospital
Parent Company: Helene Fuld Health Care
Annual Sales: $92.5 million
Number of Employees: 1,200
Expertise Needed: Nursing, physical therapy, occupational therapy, accounting, anesthesiology, social work, mental health, speech therapy, laboratory technology
Contact: Ms Gail Miranda
Nursing Recruiter and Retention
(609) 394-6000

HELPING CARE, INC.
175 WEST JACKSON BOULEVARD
CHICAGO, ILLINOIS 60604-2601

Description: Provides home health-care services
Annual Sales: $40.7 million
Number of Employees: 2,550
Expertise Needed: Home health care
Contact: Ms Elizabeth Wirth
Registered Nurse and Training Coordinator
(312) 663-0833

HEMET VALLEY MEDICAL CENTER
1117 EAST DEVONSHIRE AVENUE
HEMET, CALIFORNIA 92543-3083

Description: General hospital
Founded: 1941
Annual Sales: $93.4 million
Number of Employees: 2,000
Expertise Needed: Registered nursing, licensed practical nursing, laboratory technology, medical technology, radiology
Contact: Ms Michelle Bird
Employment Manager
(909) 652-2811

HERBALIFE INTERNATIONAL, INC.
9800 SOUTH LA CIENEGA BOULEVARD
INGLEWOOD, CALIFORNIA 90301-4440

Description: Markets and sells nutritional products
Annual Sales: $214.4 million

Number of Employees: 500
Expertise Needed: Sales, accounting
Contact: Ms Linda Nadler
Recruiter
(310) 216-5169

HERITAGE ENTERPRISES, INC.
115 WEST JEFFERSON STREET
BLOOMINGTON, ILLINOIS 61701-3946

Description: Operates nursing homes
Annual Sales: $28.6 million
Number of Employees: 1,300
Number of Managerial and Professional Employees Hired 1993: 100
Expertise Needed: Nursing, licensed practical nursing, certified nursing and nursing assistance
Contact: Ms Connie Hoselton
Manager of Employment
(309) 828-4361

HERMANN HOSPITAL, INC.
6410 FANNIN STREET
HOUSTON, TEXAS 77030-1501

Description: General hospital
Founded: 1914
Annual Sales: $343.5 million
Number of Employees: 4,300
Expertise Needed: Nursing, licensed practical nursing, occupational therapy, physical therapy, radiology, medical technology, respiratory therapy
Contact: Ms Charlotte Carnagie
Manager of Professional Recruitment
(713) 704-4000

HHC, INC.
1420 DUTCH VALLEY ROAD
KNOXVILLE, TENNESSEE 37918-1424

Description: Home health-care agency
Parent Company: Housecall, Inc.
Annual Sales: $35.0 million
Number of Employees: 900
Expertise Needed: Physical therapy, occupational therapy, speech therapy, registered nursing, licensed practical nursing, social work
Contact: Ms Charlene Sparks
Director of Personnel
(615) 687-6230

DOW B. HICKAM PHARMACEUTICALS, INC.
10410 CORPORATE DRIVE
SUGARLAND, TEXAS 77487

Description: Manufactures and markets bandages and hospital supplies
Founded: 1961
Number of Employees: 120

Expertise Needed: Sales, chemistry, laboratory technology
Contact: Mr William Richardson
President
(713) 240-1000

HIGHLAND PARK HOSPITAL
718 GLENVIEW AVENUE
HIGHLAND PARK, ILLINOIS 60035-2432

Description: Private hospital
Parent Company: Lakeland Health Services, Inc.
Founded: 1916
Annual Sales: $81.4 million
Number of Employees: 1,200
Expertise Needed: Registered nursing, physical therapy
Contact: Mr John Vicik
Director of Human Resources
(708) 432-8000

HILLHAVEN CORPORATION
1148 BROADWAY
TACOMA, WASHINGTON 98402-3513

Description: Owns, leases, and operates long-term care centers and retirement communities
Founded: 1946
Annual Sales: $1.3 billion
Number of Employees: 40,800
Expertise Needed: Human resources, data processing, finance, accounting, physical therapy, occupational therapy, speech therapy, risk management, marketing
Contact: Ms Donna Proudfit
National Director of Recruitment and Employment
(206) 572-9901

HINSDALE HOSPITAL
120 NORTH OAK STREET
HINSDALE, ILLINOIS 60521-3829

Description: Church-operated general medical and surgical hospital
Founded: 1902
Annual Sales: $151.4 million
Number of Employees: 2,500
Expertise Needed: Registered nursing, physical therapy, occupational therapy
Contact: Personnel Department
(708) 856-9000

MARY HITCHCOCK MEMORIAL HOSPITAL
1 MEDICAL CENTER DRIVE
LEBANON, NEW HAMPSHIRE 03756-0001

Description: Public hospital specializing in trauma and primary care
Founded: 1889
Annual Sales: $207.3 million
Number of Employees: 2,650

Expertise Needed: Registered nursing, physical therapy, occupational therapy
Contact: Human Resources Department
(603) 650-5000

HMO AMERICA, INC.
540 NORTH LA SALLE
CHICAGO, ILLINOIS 60610-4217

Description: Health maintenance organization
Annual Sales: $218.3 million
Number of Employees: 339
Expertise Needed: Actuarial, underwriting, claims adjustment/examination, accounting
Contact: Ms Josie Bautista
Human Resources Manager
(312) 751-7500

HMO COLORADO, INC.
700 BROADWAY
DENVER, COLORADO 80203-3421

Description: Health maintenance organization
Parent Company: General Health Corporation
Annual Sales: $89.2 million
Number of Employees: 100
Expertise Needed: Registered nursing, licensed practical nursing, certified nursing and nursing assistance, physicians, law
Contact: Ms Shannon Anderson
Acting Director of Human Resources
(303) 831-2131

HMO MISSOURI, INC.
1831 CHESTNUT STREET
SAINT LOUIS, MISSOURI 63103-2231

Description: Health maintenance organization
Parent Company: Blue Cross & Blue Shield of Missouri
Annual Sales: $81.1 million
Number of Employees: 93
Expertise Needed: Actuarial, underwriting
Contact: Mr Jim Winter
Human Resources Representative for Employment and Placement
(314) 923-7700

HMSS, INC.
12450 GREENSPOINT DRIVE
HOUSTON, TEXAS 77060

Description: Provides home health-care services
Number of Employees: 600
Expertise Needed: IV nursing, pharmacy
Contact: Ms Pat Kapscia
Human Resources Manager
(713) 873-4677

HNU SYSTEMS, INC.
160 CHARLEMONT STREET
NEWTON, MASSACHUSETTS 02161

Description: Manufactures chemical monitoring systems
Founded: 1973
Number of Employees: 200
Number of Managerial and Professional Employees Hired 1993: 6
Expertise Needed: Electronics/electronics engineering, mechanical engineering, electrical engineering, industrial engineering
Contact: Department of Human Resources
(617) 964-6690

HOAG MEMORIAL HOSPITAL
301 NEWPORT BOULEVARD
NEWPORT BEACH, CALIFORNIA 92663-4120

Description: General medical and surgical hospital
Founded: 1944
Annual Sales: $188.4 million
Number of Employees: 2,500
Expertise Needed: Registered nursing, occupational therapy, respiratory therapy, physical therapy
Contact: Human Resources Department
(714) 645-8600

HOECHST-ROUSSEL PHARMACEUTICALS, INC.
ROUTE 202 & 206 NORTH
SOMERVILLE, NEW JERSEY 08876

Description: Pharmaceutical research company and prescription drug manufacturer
Founded: 1960
Number of Employees: 2,200
Expertise Needed: Chemistry, laboratory technology, biology
Contact: Mr John Clark
Vice President of Human Resources, Life Sciences Group
(908) 231-2000

HOFFMANN-LA ROCHE, INC.
340 KINGSLAND STREET
NUTLEY, NEW JERSEY 07110-1150

Description: Manufactures pharmaceutical products
Founded: 1905
Annual Sales: $2.3 billion
Number of Employees: 16,000
Expertise Needed: Accounting, finance, marketing, data processing, computer science, business administration, pharmacy, pharmaceutical, biochemistry, chemistry
Contact: Mr Alvin L Vinson
Director of Human Resources
(201) 235-5000

HOLLISTER, INC.
2000 HOLLISTER DRIVE
LIBERTYVILLE, ILLINOIS 60048-3746

Description: Manufactures disposable plastic products for the health-care and automotive industries
Founded: 1956
Annual Sales: $145.1 million
Number of Employees: 1,900
Expertise Needed: Mechanical engineering, design engineering, manufacturing engineering, accounting, sales, computer programming, computer science, chemistry
Contact: Mr James Karlovsky
Vice President of Human Resources
(708) 680-1000

HOLY CROSS HEALTH SYSTEM CORPORATION
3606 EAST JEFFERSON BOULEVARD
SOUTH BEND, INDIANA 46615-3036

Description: Provides health-care services
Founded: 1978
Annual Sales: $1.2 billion
Number of Employees: 18,360
Expertise Needed: Communications, accounting, finance, marketing, data processing
Contact: Mr Jeff Bernard
Director of Human Resources
(219) 233-8558

HOLY CROSS HOSPITAL OF SILVER SPRING
1500 FOREST GLEN ROAD
SILVER SPRING, MARYLAND 20910-1460

Description: Nonprofit private hospital
Parent Company: Holy Cross Health System Corporation
Founded: 1959
Annual Sales: $143.2 million
Number of Employees: 1,960
Expertise Needed: Occupational therapy, respiratory therapy, dialysis, cardiac care, management
Contact: Human Resources Department
(301) 905-1325

HOLY REDEEMER HOSPITAL AND MEDICAL CENTER
1648 HUNTINGDON PIKE
JENKINTOWN, PENNSYLVANIA 19046-8001

Description: Private general hospital
Parent Company: Holy Redeemer Health System
Annual Sales: $83.9 million
Number of Employees: 1,700
Expertise Needed: Physical therapy
Contact: Ms Linda Bivenour
Professional Recruiter
(215) 938-3128

HOME CARE AFFILIATES, INC.
9100 SHELBYVILLE ROAD
LOUISVILLE, KENTUCKY 40222-5153

Description: Provides home health-care services
Annual Sales: $42.9 million
Number of Employees: 1,500
Expertise Needed: Accounting, licensed practical nursing, registered nursing
Contact: Ms Patti Walker
    Assistant Vice President of Human Relations
    (502) 339-7025

HOME HEALTH CORPORATION OF AMERICA
2200 RENAISSANCE BOULEVARD
KING OF PRUSSIA, PENNSYLVANIA 19406-2755

Description: Provides home health-care services
Founded: 1978
Annual Sales: $22.6 million
Number of Employees: 750
Expertise Needed: Nursing, licensed practical nursing, accounting, finance, data processing, physical therapy, occupational therapy, social work, speech therapy, certified nursing and nursing assistance
Contact: Ms Joyce Fullington
    Personnel Administrator
    (215) 272-1717

HOME NURSING SERVICES, INC.
3725 AIRPORT BOULEVARD
MOBILE, ALABAMA 36608-1633

Description: Home health-care agency
Parent Company: SAAD Enterprises, Inc.
Annual Sales: $20.7 million
Number of Employees: 800
Expertise Needed: Registered nursing, licensed practical nursing, social service, physical therapy, speech therapy, occupational therapy
Contact: Ms Alice Bassenberg
    Director of Personnel
    (205) 343-9600

HOME X-RAY SERVICES OF AMERICA
2750 SOUTHWEST 37TH AVENUE
MIAMI, FLORIDA 33133

Description: Provides on-site X-ray services to nursing homes
Founded: 1962
Annual Sales: $25.0 million
Number of Employees: 250
Expertise Needed: X-ray technology, home health care, customer service and support
Contact: Mr Phil Edinger
    Vice President
    (800) 669-8642

HOMECARE MANAGEMENT, INC.
80 AIR PACK DRIVE
RONKONKOMA, NEW YORK 11779-7360

Description: Provides home infusion therapy, support, and specialized pharmaceutical services to organ transplant patients
Annual Sales: $26.4 million
Number of Employees: 85
Expertise Needed: Pharmacology, nursing, social work, sales, pharmaceutical technology
Contact: Employment Department
    (516) 981-0034

HOMEDCO GROUP, INC.
17650 NEWHOPE STREET
FOUNTAIN VALLEY, CALIFORNIA 92708-4220

Description: Provides home health-care services
Annual Sales: $303.4 million
Number of Employees: 5,000
Expertise Needed: Management information systems, finance, human resources, accounting, registered nursing, operations, respiratory therapy, pharmacy
Contact: Ms Sandy Northrutt
    Professional Staffing
    (714) 755-5600

HOOK-SUPERX, INC.
175 TRI COUNTY PARKWAY
CINCINNATI, OHIO 45246-3222

Description: Owns and operates retail pharmacies and eyewear stores
Founded: 1961
Annual Sales: $2.1 billion
Number of Employees: 18,000
Number of Managerial and Professional Employees Hired 1993: 10
Expertise Needed: Human resources, risk management, accounting, finance, management information systems, pharmacy
Contact: Mr John Kellner
    Human Resources Representative
    (513) 782-3000

HOOPER HOLMES, INC.
170 MOUNT AIRY ROAD
BASKING RIDGE, NEW JERSEY 07920-2021

Description: Provides health-care information services and medical personnel
Founded: 1899
Annual Sales: $154.8 million
Number of Employees: 10,500

Hooper Holmes, Inc. (continued)

Expertise Needed: Accounting, finance, marketing, management information systems

Contact for College Students and Recent Graduates:
Ms Jennifer Ferluga
Human Resources Specialist
(908) 766-5000

Contact for All Other Candidates:
Mr Richard D'Alesandro
Manager of Human Resources
(908) 766-5000

HORIZON HEALTH SYSTEM
26100 AMERICAN DRIVE
SOUTHFIELD, MICHIGAN 48034-6179

Description: Owns and operates hospitals and clinics
Annual Sales: $164.3 million
Number of Employees: 3,524
Expertise Needed: Accounting, finance
Contact: Ms Marian Deland
Personnel Coordinator
(313) 746-4300

HORIZON HEALTHCARE CORPORATION
6001 INDIAN SCHOOL ROAD NORTHEAST
ALBUQUERQUE, NEW MEXICO 87110-4139

Description: Owns and operates long-term care facilities
Annual Sales: $156.9 million
Number of Employees: 6,500
Expertise Needed: Administration, nursing, physical therapy
Contact: Ms Peggy Cave
Recruiter
(505) 881-4961

HOSPITAL AUTHORITY OF FLOYD COUNTY
304 TURNER MCCALL BOULEVARD
ROME, GEORGIA 30165-2734

Description: Public hospital
Founded: 1942
Annual Sales: $130.2 million
Number of Employees: 1,400
Expertise Needed: Physical therapy, pharmacy, registered nursing, licensed practical nursing
Contact for College Students and Recent Graduates:
Ms Faye Hicks
Personnel Coordinator
Contact for All Other Candidates:
Mr Hal Golden
Director of Personnel
(706) 295-5500

HOSPITAL AUTHORITY OF FULTON COUNTY
1000 JOHNSON FERRY ROAD NORTHEAST
ATLANTA, GEORGIA 30342-1606

Description: Nonprofit public hospital specializing in maternity and prenatal care
Founded: 1970
Annual Sales: $199.2 million
Number of Employees: 2,500
Expertise Needed: Registered nursing, physical therapy, respiratory therapy
Contact: Ms Martha Arnold
Employment Manager
(404) 851-8000

THE HOSPITAL CENTER AT ORANGE
188 SOUTH ESSEX AVENUE
ORANGE, NEW JERSEY 07051-3421

Description: Public hospital specializing in orthopedics
Parent Company: Orange Mountain Healthcare
Founded: 1874
Annual Sales: $86.4 million
Number of Employees: 1,300
Expertise Needed: Nursing, physical therapy, radiology, nuclear medicine, occupational therapy, accounting, management information systems
Contact: Ms Paula Nearier
Director of Human Resources
(201) 266-2265

HOSPITAL CORPORATION OF AMERICA
1 PARK PLAZA
NASHVILLE, TENNESSEE 37203-1121

Description: Owns and operates medical, surgical, and psychiatric hospitals
Founded: 1968
Annual Sales: $5.1 billion
Number of Employees: 66,000
Expertise Needed: Health care, information systems, medical records, physical therapy, management
Contact: Mr Terry Brock
Director of Staffing
(615) 327-9551

HOSPITAL FOR JOINT DISEASES
301 EAST 17TH STREET
NEW YORK, NEW YORK 10003-3804

Description: Orthopedic hospital
Founded: 1905
Annual Sales: $110.4 million
Number of Employees: 1,192
Expertise Needed: Physical therapy, occupational therapy, orthopedics, nursing
Contact: Ms Nora Donoher
Manager of Employment
(212) 460-0138

HOSPITAL OF THE GOOD SAMARITAN

616 SOUTH WITMER STREET
LOS ANGELES, CALIFORNIA 90017-2308

Description: Private nonprofit hospital specializing in tertiary care and open-heart surgery
Founded: 1887
Annual Sales: $174.9 million
Number of Employees: 1,800
Expertise Needed: Registered nursing, occupational therapy, physical therapy, pharmacology

Contact: Ms Randi Katz
Director of Recruiting
(213) 977-2300

HOSPITAL SISTERS HEALTH SYSTEM

SANGAMON TOWER APARTMENTS
SPRINGFIELD, ILLINOIS 62794-5262

Description: Owns and operates hospitals and medical centers
Founded: 1979
Annual Sales: $701.2 million
Number of Employees: 12,500
Number of Managerial and Professional Employees Hired 1993: 5
Expertise Needed: Finance, management information systems, accounting, auditing, computer programming

Contact for College Students and Recent Graduates:
Ms Billie Johnston
Manager of Personnel
(217) 522-6969

Contact for All Other Candidates:
Mr Charles Moe
Vice President of Human Resources
(217) 522-6969

HOSPITAL STAFFING SERVICES

6245 NORTH FEDERAL HIGHWAY
FORT LAUDERDALE, FLORIDA 33308

Description: Provides home health-care services
Annual Sales: $120.6 million
Number of Employees: 700
Expertise Needed: Nursing, occupational therapy, physical therapy

Contact: Human Resources Department
(305) 771-0500

THE HOUSE OF THE GOOD SAMARITAN

830 WASHINGTON STREET
WATERTOWN, NEW YORK 13601-4034

Description: Nonprofit, public acute-care hospital and nursing home
Founded: 1881
Annual Sales: $59.9 million
Number of Employees: 1,300

Expertise Needed: Nursing, licensed practical nursing, radiation technology, physical therapy, occupational therapy, social work, accounting, management information systems

Contact: Mr Tim Ryan
Director of Human Resources
(315) 785-4000

HOUSECALL, INC.

117 CENTRAL PARK DRIVE
KNOXVILLE, TENNESSEE 37922-1424

Description: Provides home health-care services
Annual Sales: $45.0 million
Number of Employees: 1,200
Expertise Needed: Nursing

Contact: Ms Dorothy Stiles
Director of Human Resources
(615) 687-6230

HOWARD COUNTY GENERAL HOSPITAL

5755 CEDAR LANE
COLUMBIA, MARYLAND 21044-2928

Description: Private hospital with a special-care nursery
Founded: 1969
Annual Sales: $70.0 million
Number of Employees: 1,225
Expertise Needed: Nursing, physical therapy, occupational therapy

Contact: Ms Kathy Anderson
Director of Human Resources
(410) 740-7815

HPI HEALTH CARE SERVICES, INC.

4500 ALEXANDER NORTHEAST
ALBUQUERQUE, NEW MEXICO 87107-3536

Description: Provides pharmacy management services to health-care institutions
Parent Company: Diagnostek, Inc.
Annual Sales: $78.1 million
Number of Employees: 1,100
Expertise Needed: Pharmacy, accounting, marketing, finance, management information systems

Contact: Ms Mary Dornellas
Manager of Human Resources
(505) 761-6100

HU-FRIEDY MANUFACTURING COMPANY, INC.

3232 NORTH ROCKWELL STREET
CHICAGO, ILLINOIS 60618-5935

Description: Manufactures dental surgical instruments
Founded: 1958
Annual Sales: $21.2 million
Number of Employees: 300

Hu-Friedy Manufacturing Company, Inc. (continued)

Expertise Needed: Design engineering, mechanical engineering, accounting, production

Contact: Mr Ed Khamis
Vice President of Human Resources
(312) 975-6100

HUDSON RESPIRATORY CARE, INC.
27711 DIAZ ROAD
TEMECULA, CALIFORNIA 92390-0740

Description: Manufactures and distributes respiratory therapy equipment
Founded: 1945
Expertise Needed: Administration, respiratory technology, respiratory therapy, home health care
Contact: Human Resources Manager
(908) 676-5611

HUMAN GENOME SCIENCES
9410 KEY WEST AVENUE
ROCKVILLE, MARYLAND 20850

Description: Biotechnology research company
Number of Employees: 170
Expertise Needed: Biology, chemistry
Contact: Ms Barbara Mitchell
Human Resources Director
(301) 309-8504

HUMANA, INC.
500 WEST MAIN STREET
LOUISVILLE, KENTUCKY 40202-2946

Description: Provides hospital management and health-care services
Founded: 1961
Annual Sales: $4.0 billion
Number of Employees: 65,000
Expertise Needed: Accounting, finance, actuarial, economics, sales, chemical engineering, mechanical engineering, industrial engineering, civil engineering
Contact: Ms Ann Spalding
Senior Recruiting Coordinator
(502) 580-1000

HURLEY MEDICAL CENTER
1 HURLEY PLAZA
FLINT, MICHIGAN 48503-5902

Description: General hospital
Founded: 1905
Annual Sales: $166.7 million
Number of Employees: 2,750

Expertise Needed: Social work, biomedical engineering, radiation technology, physical therapy, microwave engineering, nutrition, licensed practical nursing, nuclear medicine, anesthesiology

Contact: Mr Tyree Walker
Director of Employment
(313) 257-9140

HUTZEL HOSPITAL
4707 SAINT ANTOINE STREET
DETROIT, MICHIGAN 48201-1498

Description: General medical and surgical hospital
Parent Company: The Detroit Medical Center
Annual Sales: $154.1 million
Number of Employees: 2,100
Expertise Needed: Hospital administration, radiology, registered nursing, physical therapy, occupational therapy, licensed practical nursing, respiratory therapy
Contact: Ms Colleen Aiello
Manager of Employment
(313) 745-7015

HYBRITECH, INC.
11095 TORREYANA ROAD
SAN DIEGO, CALIFORNIA 92121-1104

Description: Manufactures medical diagnostic test kits
Annual Sales: $123.5 million
Number of Employees: 820
Expertise Needed: Biomedical, biomedical engineering, mechanical engineering, cardiopulmonary technology, cardiovascular technology, design engineering, computer science, electronics/ electronics engineering, product design and development
Contact: Human Resources Department
(619) 455-6700

HYCLONE LABORATORIES, INC.
1725 SOUTH HYCLONE ROAD
LOGAN, UTAH 84321

Description: Manufactures and markets biochemicals, chemicals, and pharmaceuticals
Founded: 1967
Number of Employees: 250
Number of Managerial and Professional Employees Hired 1993: 6
Expertise Needed: Mechanical engineering, laboratory technology, chemistry, biology, biochemistry
Contact: Mr Greg Cox
Director of Human Resources
(801) 753-4584

HYCOR BIOMEDICAL, INC.
18800 VON KARMAN AVENUE
IRVINE, CALIFORNIA 92715-1517

Description: Biomedical research firm and products manufacturer

Annual Sales: $27.4 million
Number of Employees: 250
Expertise Needed: Microbiology, biology, chemistry, chemical engineering
Contact: Ms Cheryl Graham
Human Resources Manager
(714) 440-2000

THE HYGIENIC CORPORATION
1245 HOME AVENUE
AKRON, OHIO 44310

Description: Manufactures dental disposables and medical supplies
Founded: 1930
Number of Employees: 250
Expertise Needed: Manufacturing engineering, design engineering, mechanical engineering, industrial engineering
Contact: Human Resources Department
(216) 633-8460

I CARE INDUSTRIES, INC.
4399 35TH STREET NORTH
SAINT PETERSBURG, FLORIDA 33714-3717

Description: Manufactures eyeglasses
Founded: 1968
Annual Sales: $16.2 million
Number of Employees: 300
Expertise Needed: Accounting, production, data processing
Contact: Personnel Department
(813) 327-5166

I-STAT
303 COLLEGE ROAD EAST
PRINCETON, NEW JERSEY 08540

Description: Provides patient care services and develops proprietary blood analysis products
Number of Employees: 300
Expertise Needed: Mechanical engineering, design engineering, accounting, automation, hardware engineering, software engineering/development, chemical engineering, chemistry, biochemistry, marketing
Contact: Human Resources Department
(609) 243-9300

ICI AMERICAS, INC.
3411 SILVERSIDE ROAD
WILMINGTON, DELAWARE 19810-4812

Description: Diversified company with operations in pharmaceuticals, paints, fibers, and financial services
Founded: 1912
Annual Sales: $5.2 billion
Number of Employees: 18,000

Expertise Needed: Chemical engineering, industrial engineering, marketing
Contact: Ms Nancy Bilson
Manager of Corporate Human Resources
(302) 887-3000

ICN PHARMACEUTICALS, INC.
3300 HYLAND AVENUE
COSTA MESA, CALIFORNIA 92626-1503

Description: Manufactures pharmaceuticals and medical diagnostic products and provides biotechnology research services
Founded: 1960
Annual Sales: $476.4 million
Number of Employees: 6,300
Expertise Needed: Pharmaceutical
Contact: Ms Christine Schumacher
Manager of Recruiting
(714) 545-0100

IDEC PHARMACEUTICALS CORPORATION
1101 TORREYANA ROAD
SAN DIEGO, CALIFORNIA 93121

Description: Develops antibodies for therapeutic applications
Founded: 1986
Number of Employees: 120
Expertise Needed: Manufacturing engineering, research and development
Contact: Mr Jeff White
Manager of Human Resources
(619) 458-0600

IDEXX LABORATORIES, INC.
1 IDEXX DRIVE
WESTBROOK, MAINE 04092-2040

Description: Develops and manufactures animal diagnostic test kits
Annual Sales: $57.7 million
Number of Employees: 350
Expertise Needed: Biology, chemistry, physics
Contact: Mr Matt Brush
Director of Human Resources
(207) 856-0300

IDX CORPORATION
1400 SHELBURNE ROAD
SOUTH BURLINGTON, VERMONT 05403-7754

Description: Designs and develops medical data processing systems and distributes computer hardware
Founded: 1969
Annual Sales: $75.5 million
Number of Employees: 674

IDX Corporation (continued)

Expertise Needed: Computer programming, program analysis

Contact: Ms Mary Paule-Bushey
Senior Human Resources Representative
(802) 862-1022

IGI, INC.
BUENA VISTA CORPORATE CENTER, LINCOLN
AND WHEAT ROADS
BUENA, NEW JERSEY 08310

Description: Manufactures and markets veterinary vaccines, health-care products, and pharmaceuticals
Founded: 1977
Number of Employees: 197
Expertise Needed: Chemistry, pharmacy
Contact: Ms Beverly Baxter
Personnel Manager
(609) 697-1441

IHC HOSPITALS, INC.
36 SOUTH STATE STREET
SALT LAKE CITY, UTAH 84111-1404

Description: Owns and operates hospitals and medical centers
Annual Sales: $843.3 million
Number of Employees: 13,656
Expertise Needed: Accounting, finance, marketing, law, data processing
Contact for College Students and Recent Graduates:
Ms Pam Alder
Human Resources Generalist
(801) 533-8282
Contact for All Other Candidates:
Ms Ruth Strong
Human Resources Generalist
(801) 533-8282

ILC TECHNOLOGY, INC.
399 JAVA DRIVE
SUNNYVALE, CALIFORNIA 94089

Description: Designs and develops medical lighting products
Founded: 1967
Number of Employees: 370
Expertise Needed: Manufacturing engineering, electrical engineering
Contact: Ms Margo Letesse
Human Resources Representative
(408) 745-7900

ILLINOIS MASONIC MEDICAL CENTER
836 WEST WELLINGTON AVENUE
CHICAGO, ILLINOIS 60657-5147

Description: Public nonprofit hospital specializing in trauma and open-heart surgery
Founded: 1909

Annual Sales: $222.5 million
Number of Employees: 3,000
Expertise Needed: Registered nursing, occupational therapy, physical therapy
Contact: Ms Ethyl Nunn
Manager of Employment
(312) 975-1600

IMAGEAMERICA, INC.
109 WESTPARK DRIVE 420
BRENTWOOD, TENNESSEE 37027-5032

Description: Provides outpatient services
Annual Sales: $70.0 million
Number of Employees: 445
Expertise Needed: Patient services, registered nursing, licensed practical nursing, health care
Contact: Human Resources Department
(615) 373-5400

IMATRON, INC.
389 OYSTER POINT BOULEVARD
SOUTH SAN FRANCISCO, CALIFORNIA 94080

Description: Designs and manufactures computer tomography products for medical diagnostic imaging
Founded: 1980
Number of Employees: 130
Expertise Needed: Manufacturing engineering, ultrasound technology
Contact: Ms Gina Caruso
Manager of Human Resources
(415) 583-9964

IMMANUEL HEALTHCARE SYSTEMS, INC.
6901 NORTH 72ND STREET
OMAHA, NEBRASKA 68122-1709

Description: Medical center
Founded: 1890
Annual Sales: $144.3 million
Number of Employees: 1,886
Expertise Needed: Registered nursing, licensed practical nursing, laboratory technology, medical technology, social work, respiratory therapy
Contact: Ms Nancy Fanders
Employment Manager
(402) 572-2121

IMMUCOR, INC.
P.O. BOX 5625
NORCROSS, GEORGIA 30091

Description: Manufactures and markets blood bank diagnostic and hospital laboratory reagents
Annual Sales: $27.3 million
Number of Employees: 120

Expertise Needed: Manufacturing engineering, electrical engineering, mechanical engineering

Contact: Ms Lauren Hayes
Human Resources Manager
(404) 441-2051

IMMULOGIC PHARMACEUTICAL CORPORATION

610 LINCOLN STREET
WALTHAM, MASSACHUSETTS 02154

Description: Develops products to treat allergic and autoimmune diseases
Annual Sales: $10.0 million
Number of Employees: 140
Expertise Needed: Research and development, chemical engineering, chemistry, biology

Contact: Ms Susan Black
Human Resources Coordinator
(617) 466-6000

IMMUNEX CORPORATION

51 UNIVERSITY STREET
SEATTLE, WASHINGTON 98101-2936

Description: Biomedical research firm
Parent Company: Lederle Parenterals, Inc.
Founded: 1981
Annual Sales: $43.0 million
Number of Employees: 572
Expertise Needed: Life sciences, accounting

Contact: Human Resources Department
(206) 587-0430

IMMUNOGEN, INC.

148 SIDNEY STREET
CAMBRIDGE, MASSACHUSETTS 02139

Description: Develops pharmaceuticals for cancer treatment
Founded: 1981
Annual Sales: $2.8 million
Expertise Needed: Biotechnology, biology, chemistry, biochemistry

Contact: Mr Jack Knox
Director of Human Resources
(617) 661-9312

IMPRA, INC.

1625 WEST 3RD STREET
TEMPE, ARIZONA 85281-2438

Description: Researches, develops, and produces cardiovascular surgery accessories
Founded: 1975
Annual Sales: $19.0 million
Number of Employees: 250
Expertise Needed: Accounting, finance, data processing, electrical engineering

Contact: Human Resources Department
(602) 894-9515

IN HOME HEALTH, INC.

601 LAKESHORE PARKWAY
MINNETONKA, MINNESOTA 55305-5214

Description: Provides in-home nursing care services
Founded: 1977
Annual Sales: $75.1 million
Number of Employees: 4,840
Expertise Needed: Accounting, nursing

Contact: Mr Mark Austin
Vice President of Administration
(612) 449-7500

INAMED CORPORATION

3800 HOWARD HUGHES PARKWAY
LAS VEGAS, NEVADA 89109-0925

Description: Develops and manufactures silicon implant products
Founded: 1961
Annual Sales: $42.3 million
Number of Employees: 489
Expertise Needed: Chemical engineering, pharmaceutical chemistry, medical technology, management information systems, accounting, finance, manufacturing engineering, electrical engineering, mechanical engineering

Contact: Ms Rose Herrera
Employment Manager
(702) 791-3388

INCSTAR CORPORATION

1990 INDUSTRIAL BOULEVARD SOUTH
STILLWATER, MINNESOTA 55082-6048

Description: Manufactures diagnostics test kits
Annual Sales: $46.0 million
Number of Employees: 350
Number of Managerial and Professional Employees Hired 1993: 10
Expertise Needed: Biochemistry, chemistry

Contact: Ms Pat O'Connor
Human Resources Representative
(612) 439-9710

INDEPENDENT HEALTH ASSOCIATION

511 FARBER LAKES DRIVE
WILLIAMSVILLE, NEW YORK 14221-5779

Description: Health maintenance organization
Founded: 1975
Annual Sales: $193.5 million
Number of Employees: 420
Expertise Needed: Health care, data processing, administration

Contact: Ms Joanne Reeb
Personnel Coordinator
(716) 631-3001

INDEPENDENCE BLUE CROSS
1901 MARKET STREET
PHILADELPHIA, PENNSYLVANIA 19103-1400

Description: Provides health-care insurance services
Founded: 1938
Annual Sales: $1.4 billion
Number of Employees: 2,400
Expertise Needed: Claims adjustment/examination, customer service and support, information systems

Contact: Mr Ronald Gilg
   Manager of Staffing
   (215) 241-3210

INDEPENDENCE REGIONAL HEALTH CENTER
1509 WEST TRUMAN ROAD
INDEPENDENCE, MISSOURI 64050-3436

Description: Public hospital
Founded: 1909
Annual Sales: $75.1 million
Number of Employees: 1,450
Expertise Needed: Nursing, physical therapy

Contact: Ms Teddy Jackson
   Director of Employment
   (816) 836-8100

INFOLAB, INC.
17400 HIGHWAY 61 NORTH
CLARKSDALE, MISSISSIPPI 38614

Description: Manufactures medical laboratory and diagnostic equipment
Founded: 1968
Annual Sales: $45.3 million
Number of Employees: 235
Expertise Needed: Sales

Contact: Human Resources Department
   (601) 627-2283

INFOMED
4365 ROUTE 1
PRINCETON, NEW JERSEY 08540

Description: Provides data processing services
Founded: 1969
Number of Employees: 200
Number of Managerial and Professional Employees Hired 1993: 60
Expertise Needed: Computer programming, network analysis, quality control, computer analysis

Contact: Ms Shari Reynold
   Human Resources Manager
   (609) 987-8181

INFRASONICS, INC.
3911 SORRENTO VALLEY BOULEVARD
SAN DIEGO, CALIFORNIA 92121

Description: Manufactures and markets respiratory care products

Number of Employees: 190
Expertise Needed: Biomedical engineering, chemistry

Contact: Ms Joyce Pedlow
   Manager of Human Resources
   (619) 450-9898

INGHAM MEDICAL CENTER CORPORATION
401 WEST GREENLAWN AVENUE
LANSING, MICHIGAN 48910-2819

Description: Public hospital
Founded: 1913
Annual Sales: $99.4 million
Number of Employees: 1,800
Expertise Needed: Nursing, physical therapy, occupational therapy

Contact: Ms Kris Garcia
   Nursing Recruiter
   (517) 334-2246

INNOVATIVE HEALTHCARE SYSTEMS
1900 INTERNATIONAL PARK DRIVE
BIRMINGHAM, ALABAMA 35243-4218

Description: Owns and operates psychiatric hospitals and mental health clinics
Annual Sales: $60.0 million
Number of Employees: 680
Expertise Needed: Accounting, finance, data processing, psychiatry, operations, marketing, social work

Contact: Mr David Hopper
   Personnel Director
   (205) 967-3455

INSTA-CARE PHARMACY SERVICES CORPORATION
8 HENSHAW STREET
WOBURN, MASSACHUSETTS 01801-4624

Description: Wholesale pharmacy company
Parent Company: Eckerd Corporation
Annual Sales: $271.1 million
Number of Employees: 900
Expertise Needed: Pharmacy

Contact: Mr Paul Colangelo
   Employment Manager
   (617) 935-2273

INSTROMEDIX, INC.
7431 NORTHEAST EVERGREEN PARKWAY
HILLSBORO, OREGON 97124

Description: Manufactures electromedical equipment
Founded: 1969
Number of Employees: 120
Expertise Needed: Design engineering, manufacturing engineering, mechanical engineering, electrical engineering

Contact: Mr Greg Semler
   Chief Executive Officer
   (505) 648-4576

INTEGRA LIFE SCIENCES CORPORATION

105 MORGAN LANE
PLAINSBORO, NEW JERSEY 08536

Description: Provides computer systems intergration and design services
Founded: 1990
Number of Employees: 100
Expertise Needed: Sales, mechanical engineering, electrical engineering
Contact: Ms Barbara Casis
Human Resources Manager
(609) 683-0900

INTEGRATED HEALTH SERVICES INC

10065 RED RUN BOULEVARD
OWINGS MILLS, MARYLAND 21117-4827

Description: Owns and operates subacute care facilities
Annual Sales: $195.3 million
Number of Employees: 5,050
Expertise Needed: Administration, accounting
Contact: Ms Jan Zdanis
Director of Administration
(410) 998-8400

INTEGRATED HEALTH SERVICES

5550 HARVEST HILL ROAD
DALLAS, TEXAS 75230

Description: Owns and operates skilled-care nursing facilities
Annual Sales: $32.8 million
Number of Employees: 1,020
Expertise Needed: Nursing management and administration
Contact: Ms Martha Royal
Regional Director of Human Resources
(214) 661-1862

INTERGROUP HEALTHCARE CORPORATION

1010 NORTH FINANCE CENTER DRIVE
TUCSON, ARIZONA 85710

Description: Provides managed care services
Annual Sales: $241.9 million
Number of Employees: 460
Expertise Needed: Health care, management, health insurance, claims adjustment/examination
Contact: Ms. Lori Haygood
Recruiter
(602) 721-1122

INTERIM HEALTHCARE DIVISION

2050 SPECTRUM BOULEVARD
FORT LAUDERDALE, FLORIDA 33309

Description: Provides temporary personnel placement services specializing in nurses and physical therapists
Founded: 1966
Annual Sales: $512.0 million

Number of Employees: 600
Expertise Needed: Licensed practical nursing, social work, accounting, law, information systems
Contact: Ms Ginny Chittem
Corporate Recruiter
(305) 938-7600

INTERMAGNETICS GENERAL CORPORATION

450 OLD NISKAYUNA
LATHAM, NEW YORK 12110

Description: Develops and manufactures products used in medical diagnostic imaging systems
Founded: 1971
Number of Employees: 450
Expertise Needed: Design engineering, manufacturing engineering, metallurgical engineering, cytotechnology
Contact: Ms Anna Prieto
Human Resources Director
(518) 782-1122

INTERMEDICS, INC.

4000 TECHNOLOGY ROAD
ANGLETON, TEXAS 77515-2523

Description: Manufactures surgical supplies and electromedical equipment
Parent Company: Sulzer Brothers, Inc.
Annual Sales: $400.0 million
Number of Employees: 3,020
Expertise Needed: Accounting, computer programming, marketing, finance, electrical engineering, mechanical engineering, biomedical engineering
Contact: Mr Robert Race
Senior Recruiter
(409) 848-4000

INTERMEDICS ORTHOPEDICS, INC.

1300 EAST ANDERSON LANE
AUSTIN, TEXAS 78752-1799

Description: Manufactures surgical and medical instruments and supplies
Parent Company: Intermedics, Inc.
Annual Sales: $100.0 million
Number of Employees: 600
Expertise Needed: Manufacturing engineering, mechanical engineering, quality engineering, marketing
Contact: Mr Jim Little
Employment Supervisor
(512) 835-1971

INTERMEDICS PACEMAKERS, INC.

4000 TECHNOLOGY ROAD
ANGLETON, TEXAS 77515-2523

Description: Manufactures cardiac rhythm management devices
Parent Company: Intermedics, Inc.

Intermedics Pacemakers, Inc. (continued)

Annual Sales: $190.0 million
Number of Employees: 1,400
Expertise Needed: Accounting, finance, data processing, electrical engineering, mechanical engineering, design engineering
Contact: Mr Steven Davis
Director of Human Resources
(409) 848-4000

INTERMOUNTAIN HEALTH CARE, INC.
36 SOUTH STATE STREET
SALT LAKE CITY, UTAH 84111-1453

Description: Owns and operates hospitals and health-care facilities
Founded: 1975
Annual Sales: $973.6 million
Number of Employees: 19,000
Expertise Needed: Accounting, systems engineering, computer programming, finance, economics, data processing, law
Contact: Ms Ruth Strong
Human Resources Generalist
(801) 530-3333

INTERNATIONAL MEDICATION SYSTEMS
17890 CASTLETON STREET
CITY OF INDUSTRY, CALIFORNIA 91748-1707

Description: Manufactures syringes
Annual Sales: $60.0 million
Number of Employees: 600
Expertise Needed: Chemistry, biology, microbiology, biomedical engineering, chemical engineering
Contact: Ms Debbie Klien
Supervisor of Recruiting
(818) 459-5297

INTERNATIONAL MUREX TECHNOLOGIES CORPORATION
3075 NORTHWOODS CIRCLE
NORCROSS, GEORGIA 30071

Description: Manufactures and markets medical diagnostic products
Number of Employees: 680
Expertise Needed: Design engineering, sales, marketing, accounting
Contact: Ms Nora Galloway
Human Resources Manager
(404) 662-0660

INTERNATIONAL TECHNIDYNE CORPORATION
8 OLSEN AVENUE
EDISON, NEW JERSEY 08820

Description: Manufactures blood coagulation testing equipment and related supplies
Founded: 1969

Number of Employees: 175
Expertise Needed: Manufacturing engineering, design engineering, electrical engineering, mechanical engineering, sales
Contact: Human Resources
(908) 548-6677

INTERSPEC, INC.
110 WEST BUTLER AVENUE
AMBLER, PENNSYLVANIA 19002-5795

Description: Manufactures and markets medical ultrasound systems
Founded: 1979
Annual Sales: $60.3 million
Number of Employees: 575
Expertise Needed: Design engineering, manufacturing engineering, software engineering/development, sales, marketing, accounting
Contact: Ms Paula Blumberg
Manager of Human Resources
(215) 540-9190

INTROSPECT HEALTHCARE CORPORATION
2797 NORTH INTROSPECT DRIVE
TUCSON, ARIZONA 85745-9454

Description: Psyciatric hospital
Parent Company: Diversification Association, Inc.
Founded: 1973
Annual Sales: $18.4 million
Number of Employees: 330
Number of Managerial and Professional Employees Hired 1993: 100
Expertise Needed: Psychology, psychiatry, nursing, social work
Contact: Ms Vicki DeGiso
Director of Personnel
(602) 792-6240

INVACARE CORPORATION
899 CLEVELAND STREET
ELYRIA, OHIO 44035-4107

Description: Manufactures and distributes home health-care equipment
Founded: 1971
Annual Sales: $263.2 million
Number of Employees: 2,455
Expertise Needed: Sales, purchasing, finance, marketing, accounting, mechanical engineering, electrical engineering
Contact: Ms Patti Stumpp
Employee Administrator
(216) 329-6000

ISIS PHARMACEUTICALS
2292 FARADAY AVENUE
CARLSBAD, CALIFORNIA 92008

Description: Develops and researches human therapeutic compounds

Annual Sales: $10.8 million
Number of Employees: 156
Expertise Needed: Research and development, chemistry, biology, biochemistry
Contact: Human Resources Department
(619) 931-9200

ISOLAB, INC.
3985 EASTERN ROAD
AKRON, OHIO 44321

Description: Manufactures diagnostic reagents and test kits and laboratory equipment
Founded: 1969
Number of Employees: 100
Expertise Needed: Manufacturing engineering, design engineering
Contact: Ms Jan Brownlee
(216) 825-4525

ISOMEDIX, INC.
11 APOLLO DRIVE
WHIPPANY, NEW JERSEY 07981

Description: Provides irradiation sterilization services
Founded: 1972
Number of Employees: 300
Expertise Needed: Accounting, marketing, sales
Contact: Human Resources Department
(201) 887-4700

IVAX CORPORATION
8800 NORTHWEST 36TH STREET
MIAMI, FLORIDA 33178-2433

Description: Researches, develops, and manufactures specialty chemicals, pharmaceuticals, and medical diagnostics
Annual Sales: $451.0 million
Number of Employees: 2,110
Expertise Needed: Chemical engineering, computer programming, accounting, sales
Contact: Ms Marcia Bucknor
Manager of Human Resources
(305) 590-2200

J.E. HANGER, INC. OF GEORGIA
5010 MCGINNIS FERRY ROAD
ALPHARETTA, GEORGIA 30202-3919

Description: Manufactures prosthetic devices
Founded: 1942
Annual Sales: $33.5 million
Number of Employees: 305
Expertise Needed: Accounting, finance, marketing, human resources
Contact: Ms Sue Katz
Director of Human Resources
(404) 667-9013

THE JACKSON LABORATORY
600 MAIN STREET
BAR HARBOR, MAINE 04609-1523

Description: Research laboratory and production facility
Founded: 1929
Annual Sales: $28.7 million
Number of Employees: 580
Expertise Needed: Production, medical technology, laboratory chemistry, technology research
Contact: Mr Harold Wheeler
Employment Manager
(207) 288-3371

JACKSON MADISON COUNTY GENERAL HOSPITAL
708 WEST FOREST AVENUE
JACKSON, TENNESSEE 38301-3901

Description: Nonprofit hospital specializing in behavioral problems
Founded: 1950
Annual Sales: $193.5 million
Number of Employees: 2,300
Expertise Needed: Registered nursing, occupational therapy, physical therapy
Contact: Ms Tracey Sadler
Professional Recruiter
(901) 423-3544

JAMAICA HOSPITAL, INC.
8900 VAN WYCK EXPRESSWAY
JAMAICA, NEW YORK 11418

Description: General hospital
Founded: 1892
Annual Sales: $140.3 million
Number of Employees: 1,600
Expertise Needed: Medical records, occupational therapy, dietetics, radiology
Contact: Ms Marguerite Verdi
Director of Human Resources
(718) 206-6000

JB DENTAL SUPPLY COMPANY
3515 EASTHAM DRIVE
CULVER CITY, CALIFORNIA 90232-2440

Description: Distributes dental equipment and supplies
Founded: 1973
Annual Sales: $26.8 million
Number of Employees: 240
Expertise Needed: Distribution, marketing, sales
Contact: Mr Dean Pasqualini
General Manager
(213) 935-7141

KEITH JEFFERS, INC.
OLD AIRPORT ROAD
WEST PLAINS, MISSOURI 65775

Description: Distributes veterinary equipment and
supplies
Founded: 1961
Annual Sales: $40.4 million
Number of Employees: 200
Expertise Needed: Accounting, finance, sales, marketing,
manufacturing engineering, mechanical
engineering, veterinary, chemical engineering,
medical laboratory technology
Contact: Ms Kathy Burke
Personnel Manager
(417) 256-3196

JEFFERSON-PILOT CORPORATION
100 NORTH GREENE STREET
GREENSBORO, NORTH CAROLINA 27401

Description: Provides life, health, accident, casualty, and
title insurance and reinsurance
Founded: 1903
Number of Employees: 5,000
Expertise Needed: Accounting, finance, marketing,
management information systems
Contact: Mr Alan Fields
Director of Human Resources
(910) 691-3000

THOMAS JEFFERSON UNIVERSITY
201 SOUTH 11TH STREET
PHILADELPHIA, PENNSYLVANIA 19107-5567

Description: Public hospital
Founded: 1824
Annual Sales: $639.8 million
Number of Employees: 8,000
Expertise Needed: Registered nursing, accounting,
finance, data processing, medical technology,
radiology, physician assistant, physical therapy,
occupational therapy, respiratory therapy
Contact: Ms Linda Mitchell
Manager of Employee Selection and
Placement
(215) 955-7700

JELRUS INTERNATIONAL
70 CANTIAGUE ROCK ROAD
HICKSVILLE, NEW YORK 11801

Description: Manufactures medical and dental
equipment
Founded: 1972
Number of Employees: 235
Expertise Needed: Mechanical engineering, electronics/
electronics engineering, computer programming,
laboratory technology
Contact: Ms Barbara Homburger
Personnel Administrator
(516) 942-0202

JERSEY CITY MEDICAL CENTER
50 BALDWIN AVENUE
JERSEY CITY, NEW JERSEY 07304

Description: Nonprofit hospital specializing in internal
medicine and surgery
Parent Company: Liberty Healthcare System, Inc.
Annual Sales: $145.1 million
Number of Employees: 2,200
Expertise Needed: Pharmaceutical technology
Contact: Mr Vincent Caidio
Assistant Director of Human Resources
(201) 915-2000

THE JEWETT REFRIGERATOR COMPANY
2 LETCHWORTH STREET
BUFFALO, NEW YORK 14213

Description: Manufacturers temperature-controlled
appliances for laboratories
Founded: 1849
Number of Employees: 100
Expertise Needed: Mechanical engineering, electrical
engineering, manufacturing engineering,
accounting, marketing, sales
Contact: Mr Martin Erdie
Human Resources Department
(716) 881-0030

JEWISH HOSPITAL, INC.
217 EAST CHESTNUT STREET
LOUISVILLE, KENTUCKY 40202-1821

Description: General hospital
Parent Company: Jewish Hospital Healthcare Services
Founded: 1903
Annual Sales: $170.9 million
Number of Employees: 2,054
Expertise Needed: Medical technology, radiation
technology, cardiology, physical therapy,
occupational therapy
Contact: Ms Judy Taylor
Employment Department
(502) 587-4011

JEWISH HOSPITALS, INC.
3200 BURNET AVENUE
CINCINNATI, OHIO 45229-3019

Description: Own general medical and surgical hospitals
Founded: 1854
Annual Sales: $158.3 million
Number of Employees: 2,350
Expertise Needed: Licensed practical nursing, registered
nursing, occupational therapy, physical therapy,
radiology, cardiopulmonary technology, certified
nursing and nursing assistance, cardiology, EKG
technology
Contact: Ms Theresa Murphy
Employment Coordinator
(513) 569-2021

JEWISH MEMORIAL HOSPITAL, INC.
59 TOWNSEND STREET
BOSTON, MASSACHUSETTS 02119-1318

Description: Private general hospital
Founded: 1929
Annual Sales: $34.1 million
Number of Employees: 552
Expertise Needed: Registered nursing, licensed practical nursing, social work
Contact: Ms Anne Borow
 Manager of Human Resources
 (617) 442-8760

JFK MEDICAL CENTER
98 JAMES STREET
EDISON, NEW JERSEY 08820-3902

Description: Private hospital
Parent Company: JFK Health Systems, Inc.
Annual Sales: $163.3 million
Number of Employees: 2,600
Expertise Needed: Occupational therapy, physical therapy, laboratory technology, medical technology, pharmacy
Contact: Ms Patricia Cook
 Lab and Medical Recruiter
 (908) 321-7875

JOHNS HOPKINS HEALTH SYSTEM CORPORATION
600 NORTH WOLFE STREET
BALTIMORE, MARYLAND 21205-2104

Description: Provides health-care services
Annual Sales: $658.5 million
Number of Employees: 5,598
Expertise Needed: Accounting, marketing, general nursing, health care, registered nursing
Contact: Ms Bonnie Alterwitz
 Director of Employment
 (410) 955-5000

JOHNS HOPKINS HOSPITAL, INC.
600 NORTH WOLFE STREET
BALTIMORE, MARYLAND 21205-2104

Description: Health-care provider of patient care diagnosis, treatment, and prevention services
Parent Company: Johns Hopkins Health System Corporation
Founded: 1890
Annual Sales: $469.3 million
Number of Employees: 5,357
Expertise Needed: Nursing, physical therapy, radiology, allied health
Contact: Ms Bonnie Alderwitz
 Director of Career Services
 (410) 955-6529

JOHNSON & JOHNSON
ONE JOHNSON & JOHNSON PLAZA
NEW BRUNSWICK, NEW JERSEY 08933

Description: Manufactures pharmaceuticals, surgical supplies, and health-care products
Founded: 1885
Annual Sales: $13.8 billion
Number of Employees: 84,900
Expertise Needed: Administration, finance, sales, marketing, law
Contact: Human Resources Department
 (908) 524-3258

JOHNSON & JOHNSON HEALTH MANAGEMENT
410 GEORGE STREET
NEW BRUNSWICK, NEW JERSEY 08901

Description: Provides health-care education and training services
Founded: 1986
Number of Employees: 250
Expertise Needed: Claims adjustment/examination, finance, marketing
Contact: Ms JoAnn Philweber
 Manager of Human Resources
 (908) 524-0400

JOHNSON & JOHNSON MEDICAL, INC.
2500 EAST ARBROOK BOULEVARD
ARLINGTON, TEXAS 76004-0130

Description: Manufactures disposable medical and surgical supplies and wound-care products
Parent Company: Johnson & Johnson
Founded: 1949
Annual Sales: $500.0 million
Number of Employees: 5,000
Expertise Needed: Accounting, information systems, mechanical engineering, industrial engineering, chemical engineering, technical engineering, electrical engineering, project engineering
Contact: Ms Sherry Brimley
 Employment Administrator
 (817) 465-3141

JOHNSON & JOHNSON PROFESSIONALS, INC.
41 PACELLA PARK DRIVE
RANDOLPH, MASSACHUSETTS 02368-1755

Description: Manufactures surgical instruments
Parent Company: Johnson & Johnson
Founded: 1964
Annual Sales: $75.7 million
Number of Employees: 900
Expertise Needed: Management information systems, mechanical engineering, electrical engineering
Contact: Ms Susan Piozzella
 Manager of Human Resources
 (617) 961-2300

JOHNSON CITY MEDICAL CENTER HOSPITAL

400 NORTH STATE OF FRANKLIN ROAD
JOHNSON CITY, TENNESSEE 37604-6035

Description: Public hospital specializing in acute care
Founded: 1945
Annual Sales: $138.4 million
Number of Employees: 1,990
Expertise Needed: Nursing, physical therapy, occupational therapy, speech pathology

Contact: Ms Jennine Vick
Manager of Recruitment and Employment
(615) 461-6111

ROBERT WOOD JOHNSON UNIVERSITY HOSPITAL

1 ROBERT WOOD JOHNSON PLACE
NEW BRUNSWICK, NEW JERSEY 08903-1928

Description: Nonprofit teaching hospital
Founded: 1884
Annual Sales: $212.3 million
Number of Employees: 2,410
Expertise Needed: Nursing, occupational therapy, physical therapy, licensed practical nursing

Contact: Ms Rose Bohlman
Supervisor of Employment
(908) 828-3000

JORDAN HEALTH SERVICES, INC.

PO BOX 889
MOUNT VERNON, TEXAS 75457

Description: Provides home health-care services
Annual Sales: $63.5 million
Number of Employees: 4,000
Expertise Needed: Finance, networking, licensed practical nursing

Contact: Human Resources Department
(903) 537-4588

JOSLIN DIABETES CENTER, INC.

1 JOSLIN PLACE
BOSTON, MASSACHUSETTS 02215-5397

Description: Diabetes control center
Founded: 1953
Annual Sales: $26.7 million
Number of Employees: 380
Expertise Needed: Diabetes, accounting, finance, data processing, biology, chemistry, physics

Contact: Ms Kathleen Clancy
Human Resources Specialist
(617) 732-2400

JSA HEALTHCARE CORPORATION

5565 STERRET PLACE
COLUMBIA, MARYLAND 21044-3422

Description: Provides management, physical examination, and testing services

Annual Sales: $30.0 million
Number of Employees: 785
Expertise Needed: Physicians

Contact: Ms Susan Mamakos
Physician Recruiter
(410) 964-2811

KAISER FOUNDATION HEALTH PLAN

1 KAISER PLAZA
OAKLAND, CALIFORNIA 94612-3610

Description: Provides health-care insurance and managed care services
Founded: 1955
Annual Sales: $23.0 billion
Number of Employees: 59,000
Expertise Needed: Nursing, radiology, pathology, anesthesiology, dialysis, emergency services, health care, intensive care, medical records

Contact: Human Resources Department
(510) 271-5833

KAISER FOUNDATION HEALTH PLAN OF COLORADO, INC.

10350 EAST DAKOTA AVENUE
DENVER, COLORADO 80231-1314

Description: Provides health-care services
Parent Company: Kaiser Foundation Health Plan
Founded: 1969
Annual Sales: $429.9 million
Number of Employees: 2,900
Expertise Needed: Optometry, ophthalmological engineering, physician assistant, registered nursing, licensed practical nursing, nursing, clinical services, physicians, radiology, sales

Contact: Ms Melanie Kaskaske
Director of Personnel Services
(303) 344-7660

KAISER FOUNDATION HEALTH PLAN OF TEXAS

12720 HILLCREST ROAD
DALLAS, TEXAS 75230

Description: Provides health-care services
Parent Company: Kaiser Foundation Health Plan
Annual Sales: $8.4 billion
Number of Employees: 1,065
Number of Managerial and Professional Employees Hired 1993: 270
Expertise Needed: Accounting, physical therapy, nursing, medical technology, radiation technology

Contact: Ms Linda Fonteneaux
Director of Human Resources Placement
(214) 458-5050

KAISER FOUNDATION HEALTH PLAN OF THE NORTHWEST
2701 NORTHWEST VAUGHN AVENUE
PORTLAND, OREGON 97210-5398

Description: Provides health-care insurance and managed care services
Parent Company: Kaiser Foundation Health Plan
Founded: 1945
Annual Sales: $2.7 billion
Number of Employees: 6,909
Expertise Needed: Management information systems, business administration, accounting, finance, data processing
Contact: Ms Mary Hinkley
Manager of Recruiting
(503) 721-4700

KAISER PERMANENTE, NORTHEAST DIVISION HEADQUARTERS
76 BATTERSON PARK ROAD
FARMINGTON, CONNECTICUT 06034-2571

Description: Provides health-care services
Parent Company: Kaiser Foundation Health Plan
Annual Sales: $67.2 million
Number of Employees: 300
Expertise Needed: Claims adjustment/examination, accounting
Contact: Ms Mary O'Connel
Director of Recruitment
(203) 678-6000

KAISER PERMANENTE, SOUTHEAST DIVISION HEADQUARTERS
3495 PIEDMONT ROAD NORTHEAST
ATLANTA, GEORGIA 30305

Description: Provides health-care services
Parent Company: Kaiser Foundation Health Plan
Annual Sales: $235.9 million
Number of Employees: 1,300
Number of Managerial and Professional Employees Hired 1993: 350
Expertise Needed: Accounting, law, licensed practical nursing, registered nursing, marketing, sales, medical technology, radiation technology, laboratory technology, hospital administration
Contact: Ms Jenny Wingard
Director of Employment
(404) 233-0555

KAISER PERMANENTE
1 KAISER PLAZA
OAKLAND, CALIFORNIA 94612-3610

Description: Provides health-care services
Founded: 1945
Annual Sales: $500.0 million
Number of Employees: 1,200

Expertise Needed: Administration, accounting, actuarial, management, health insurance, database management
Contact: Corporate Human Resources Department
(510) 271-6888

KEANE, INC.
10 CITY SQUARE
BOSTON, MASSACHUSETTS 02129-3714

Description: Designs, markets, and installs computer-based information systems
Founded: 1965
Annual Sales: $99.3 million
Number of Employees: 2,200
Number of Managerial and Professional Employees Hired 1993: 200
Expertise Needed: Accounting, finance, data processing, software engineering/development, consulting, computer programming
Contact: Mr Ken Mokler
Manager of Human Resources
(617) 241-9200

KELLOGG INDUSTRIES
159-163 WEST PEARL STREET
JACKSON, MICHIGAN 49201

Description: Manufacturers orthopedic soft goods
Parent Company: DePuy, Inc
Founded: 1907
Number of Employees: 125
Expertise Needed: Accounting, management information systems
Contact: Ms Shirley Johnson
Human Resources Department
(517) 782-0579

KELLY ASSISTED LIVING SERVICES
999 WEST BIG BEAVER ROAD
TROY, MICHIGAN 48084-4716

Description: Provides home health-care services
Parent Company: Kelly Services, Inc.
Founded: 1976
Annual Sales: $79.3 million
Number of Employees: 5,000
Expertise Needed: Customer service and support, management, finance, human resources, business, allied health, allied therapy, home health care, registered nursing, licensed practical nursing
Contact: Ms Krista Greiner
Recruiter
(313) 362-4444

THE KENDALL COMPANY
15 HAMPSHIRE STREET
MANSFIELD, MASSACHUSETTS 02048-1139

Description: Manufactures medical and health-care products and supplies
Founded: 1904

The Kendall Company (continued)

Annual Sales: $817.0 million
Number of Employees: 8,800
Number of Managerial and Professional Employees Hired 1993: 25
Expertise Needed: Marketing, data processing, health care, economics, finance, sales, accounting, auditing, engineering, chemistry
Contact: Mr Ken Smith
Manager of Employment
(508) 261-8000

KENMORE MERCY HOSPITAL, SISTERS OF MERCY

2950 ELMWOOD AVENUE
KENMORE, NEW YORK 14217-1304

Description: Acute-care residential facility
Parent Company: Mercy Health System of Western New York
Annual Sales: $35.5 million
Number of Employees: 1,300
Expertise Needed: Nursing, occupational therapy, physical therapy, X-ray technology, medical laboratory technology
Contact: Ms Mary Pat Garrett
Assistant Director of Personnel
(716) 879-6212

KENNEDY KRIEGER INSTITUTE, INC.

707 NORTH BROADWAY
BALTIMORE, MARYLAND 21205-1832

Description: Pediatric hospital
Annual Sales: $43.9 million
Number of Employees: 800
Expertise Needed: Registered nursing, licensed practical nursing, nursing, physical therapy, occupational therapy, speech therapy
Contact: Mr Michael Loughran
Director of Human Resources
(410) 550-9000

KENT COUNTY MEMORIAL HOSPITAL

455 TOLL GATE ROAD
WARWICK, RHODE ISLAND 02886-2759

Description: Public hospital
Founded: 1946
Annual Sales: $94.0 million
Number of Employees: 2,000
Expertise Needed: Registered nursing
Contact: Mr Anthony Solitro
Manager of Employment
(401) 737-7000

KEYSTONE HEALTH PLAN EAST, INC.

1901 MARKET STREET
PHILADELPHIA, PENNSYLVANIA 19103-1400

Description: Provides health-care insurance services

Parent Company: Medical Service Association of Pennsylvania
Annual Sales: $527.3 million
Number of Employees: 325
Expertise Needed: Claims adjustment/examination, accounting
Contact: Ms Kate Smith
Director of Personnel
(215) 241-2299

KIMBALL MEDICAL CENTER

600 RIVER AVENUE
LAKEWOOD, NEW JERSEY 08701-5237

Description: General hospital
Parent Company: Kimball Health Care Corporation
Annual Sales: $91.1 million
Number of Employees: 1,700
Expertise Needed: Radiology, cardiac care, pediatric care, oncology, maternity care
Contact: Ms Jean Moran
Professional Recruiter
(908) 363-1900

KIMBERLY-CLARK CORPORATION

2100 WINCHESTER ROAD
NEENAH, WISCONSIN 54956

Description: Manufactures paper and fiber products for consumer, health-care, and industrial use
Founded: 1872
Annual Sales: $7.0 billion
Number of Employees: 51,712
Expertise Needed: Research, operations, engineering, logistics, finance
Contact: Recruiting Department
(414) 721-6965

KING COUNTY MEDICAL BLUE SHIELD COMBINED SERVICES NORTHWEST

1800 9TH AVENUE
SEATTLE, WASHINGTON 98111-1322

Description: Provides health-care insurance services
Founded: 1933
Annual Sales: $1.0 billion
Number of Employees: 1,875
Expertise Needed: Actuarial, claims adjustment/examination
Contact: Mr Ray Olitt
Manager of Training and Development
(206) 464-3600

KING COUNTY PUBLIC HOSPITAL, VALLEY MEDICAL CENTER

400 SOUTH 43RD STREET
RENTON, WASHINGTON 98055

Description: Public hospital
Founded: 1948
Annual Sales: $117.9 million

Number of Employees: 1,927
Expertise Needed: Registered nursing, occupational therapy, physical therapy, pharmacology, respiratory therapy
Contact: Ms Michelle Bence
Nursing Recruiter
(206) 228-3450

KINNEY DRUGS, INC.
29 MAIN STREET
GOUVERNEUR, NEW YORK 13642

Description: Drug store chain
Founded: 1965
Annual Sales: $108.0 million
Number of Employees: 912
Expertise Needed: Pharmacy, management
Contact: Mr Ron Field
Director of Human Resources
(315) 287-1500

KNOLL PHARMACEUTICALS
30 NORTH JEFFERSON ROAD
WHIPPANY, NEW JERSEY 07981

Description: Pharmaceuticals company
Parent Company: BASF K&F Corporation
Founded: 1904
Annual Sales: $200.0 million
Number of Employees: 700
Expertise Needed: Chemistry, chemical engineering, marketing, sales
Contact: Mr Phillip Kluft
Director of Human Resources
(201) 887-8300

KNOWLES ELECTRONICS, INC.
1151 MAPLEWOOD DRIVE
ITASCA, ILLINOIS 60143-2058

Description: Manufactures miniature transducers for the hearing aid industry
Founded: 1954
Annual Sales: $60.0 million
Number of Employees: 701
Expertise Needed: Electronics/electronics engineering
Contact: Mr Robert Rasmussen
Director of Human Resources
(708) 250-5100

KV PHARMACEUTICAL COMPANY
2503 SOUTH HANLEY ROAD
SAINT LOUIS, MISSOURI 63144

Description: Develops and manufactures pharmaceuticals for the agricultural and health-care industries
Founded: 1942
Annual Sales: $43.5 million
Number of Employees: 330

Expertise Needed: Pharmaceutical science, operations, laboratory science, marketing, sales, pharmacy, accounting, finance
Contact: Ms Susan Wilson
Staffing Specialist
(314) 645-6600

L & F PRODUCTS, INC.
225 SUMMIT AVENUE
MONTVALE, NEW JERSEY 07645-1523

Description: Manufactures and distributes disinfectant products
Parent Company: Sterling Winthrop, Inc.
Founded: 1969
Annual Sales: $1.0 billion
Number of Employees: 3,300
Expertise Needed: Industrial engineering, computer programming, packaging engineering, accounting, management information systems, sales
Contact: Ms Marlene Fried
Manager of Recruitment and Human Resources
(201) 573-5700

LA GRANGE MEMORIAL HOSPITAL, INC.
5101 WILLOW SPRINGS ROAD
LA GRANGE, ILLINOIS 60525-2600

Description: Public community hospital
Founded: 1946
Annual Sales: $100.7 million
Number of Employees: 1,650
Expertise Needed: Registered nursing, nursing, respiratory therapy, nuclear medicine, laboratory technology
Contact: Ms Cathy Marquett
Nursing Recruiter
(708) 352-1200

LAB GLASS/LUREX DIVISION
1172 NORTHWEST BOULEVARD
VINELAND, NEW JERSEY 08360

Description: Manufactures specialty scientific glassware for research and development laboratories
Founded: 1937
Number of Employees: 100
Expertise Needed: Mechanical engineering, design engineering
Contact: Ms Cloud Volpe
Head of Engineering
(609) 691-3200

LAKELAND REGIONAL MEDICAL CENTER
1324 LAKELAND HILLS BOULEVARD
LAKELAND, FLORIDA 33805-4543

Description: General medical and surgical hospital
Founded: 1918
Annual Sales: $152.8 million
Number of Employees: 2,230

Lakeland Regional Medical Center (continued)

Expertise Needed: Licensed practical nursing, registered nursing

Contact: Employment Services
(813) 687-1100

LANCASTER LABORATORIES, INC.

2425 NEW HOLLAND PARK
LANCASTER, PENNSYLVANIA 17601-5946

Description: Commercial research laboratory and consulting firm
Founded: 1961
Annual Sales: $25.0 million
Number of Employees: 520
Expertise Needed: Chemistry, biology, analysis, biochemistry
Contact: Human Resources Department
(717) 656-2301

LASERSCOPE, INC.

3052 ORCHARD DRIVE
SAN JOSE, CALIFORNIA 95134-2011

Description: Designs and manufactures laser systems, related accessories, and disposable supplies
Founded: 1979
Annual Sales: $36.0 million
Number of Employees: 240
Expertise Needed: Design engineering, sales, marketing
Contact: Ms. Bonnie Jones
Vice President of Human Resources
(408) 943-0636

LAVERDIERES ENTERPRISES

BENTON AVENUE
WINSLOW, MAINE 04901

Description: Drug store chain
Annual Sales: $100.0 million
Number of Employees: 1,500
Expertise Needed: Retail, marketing, sales, pharmacy, accounting, finance
Contact: Mr Robert Bishop
Assistant Vice President of Human Resources
(207) 873-1151

LAWRENCE AND MEMORIAL HOSPITAL

365 MONTAUK AVENUE
NEW LONDON, CONNECTICUT 06320-4700

Description: General medical and surgical hospital
Annual Sales: $103.2 million
Number of Employees: 1,600
Expertise Needed: Physical therapy, physician assistant, occupational therapy, tax accounting
Contact: Ms Nancy Zembruski
Human Resources Representative
(203) 442-0711

LEE MEMORIAL HOSPITAL, INC.

2776 CLEVELAND AVENUE
FORT MYERS, FLORIDA 33901-5864

Description: Public hospital
Founded: 1916
Annual Sales: $190.3 million
Number of Employees: 2,700
Expertise Needed: Physical therapy, occupational therapy, pharmacy, nursing, CT scanning
Contact: Human Resources Department
(800) 334-5272

LEGACY HEALTH SYSTEM, INC.

1919 NORTHWEST LOVEJOY STREET
PORTLAND, OREGON 97209-1566

Description: Provides hospital, nursing, and personal care facility management services
Founded: 1971
Annual Sales: $27.8 million
Number of Employees: 5,280
Expertise Needed: Hospital administration, management, information systems, systems analysis, marketing
Contact: Mr Dennis Phister
Director of Human Resources
(503) 225-8740

LEHIGH VALLEY HOSPITAL, INC.

17TH AND CHEW STREET
ALLENTOWN, PENNSYLVANIA 18105

Description: Nonprofit hospital
Annual Sales: $285.9 million
Number of Employees: 5,000
Expertise Needed: Health care, nursing
Contact: Ms Susan Fitch
Nursing Recruitment
(215) 402-8000

LEMMON COMPANY

650 CATHILL ROAD
KULPSVILLE, PENNSYLVANIA 19443-1512

Description: Manufactures pharmaceutical products
Parent Company: TAG Pharmaceuticals, Inc.
Annual Sales: $105.0 million
Number of Employees: 400
Expertise Needed: Chemistry
Contact: Ms Marge Cauley
Director of Human Resources
(215) 723-5544

LENOX HILL HOSPITAL

100 EAST 77TH STREET
NEW YORK, NEW YORK 10021-1803

Description: General medical and surgical hospital
Founded: 1916
Annual Sales: $244.6 million
Number of Employees: 2,975

Expertise Needed: Dialysis, CAT/MRI technology, emergency services

Contact: Mr Alan Seiler
Assistant Director of Human Resources
(212) 434-2000

LEXINGTON MEDICAL CENTER
2720 SUNSET BOULEVARD
WEST COLUMBIA, SOUTH CAROLINA 29169-4810

Description: Nonprofit hospital
Parent Company: Lexington County Health Services District
Annual Sales: $107.1 million
Number of Employees: 1,600
Expertise Needed: Registered nursing

Contact: Ms B. Wynne
Manager of Personnel
(803) 791-2000

LIEBEL FLARSHEIM COMPANY
2111 EAST GALBRAITH ROAD
CINCINNATI, OHIO 45237-1624

Description: Manufactures X-ray equipment and accessories, and surgical devices
Annual Sales: $38.8 million
Number of Employees: 275
Number of Managerial and Professional Employees Hired 1993: 20
Expertise Needed: Marketing, sales, mechanical engineering, electronics/electronics engineering, electrical engineering, quality engineering, field engineering

Contact: Personnel Department
(513) 761-2700

LIFE CARE CENTERS OF AMERICA
3570 KEITH STREET NORTHWEST
CLEVELAND, TENNESSEE 37312-4309

Description: Operates long-term care facilities and retirement centers
Founded: 1975
Annual Sales: $414.3 million
Number of Employees: 18,000
Expertise Needed: Nursing, accounting, finance, data processing, computer programming

Contact: Mr Mark Gibson
Vice President of Professional Development
(615) 472-9585

LIFE FITNESS
10601 WEST BELMONT AVENUE
FRANKLIN PARK, ILLINOIS 60131-1545

Description: Markets exercise equipment
Annual Sales: $115.0 million
Number of Employees: 475

Expertise Needed: Engineering, manufacturing engineering, software engineering/development, computer science

Contact: Ms Christine Lockwood
Human Resources Assistant
(708) 451-3100

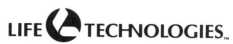

LIFE TECHNOLOGIES, INC.
8400 HELGERMAN COURT
GAITHERSBURG, MARYLAND 20884-9980

Description: Researches, develops, and manufactures products used in the biotechnology industry
Founded: 1983
Annual Sales: $204.9 million
Number of Employees: 1,400
Expertise Needed: Life science, molecular biology, biochemistry, biochemical engineering, chemical engineering

Contact: Ms J Clancy Kress
Manager of Staffing and College Relations
(301) 840-8000

CORPORATE PROFILE

The Company. LTI develops, manufactures, and markets more than 3,000 products for use in life sciences research and biomedical manufacturing. LTI has operations in 17 countries in Europe, North America, and the Asia-Pacific region, as well as distributors in Africa, the Middle East, and Latin America. LTI serves more than 20,000 customers around the world in universities, public and private research institutes, and the biotechnology and pharmaceutical manufacturing industries.

The Business. LTI products are used in the study of diseases, including AIDS, cancer, diabetes, and Alzheimer's and genetic disorders such as cystic fibrosis and Down Syndrome. LTI products are also used in genetic therapy research, as well as to develop improved techniques for bone marrow transplants, wound healing, and the treatment of burns. A further application is in the development of large-scale manufacturing of a wide range of gentically engineered health-care products, including vaccines, therapeutic drugs for cardiovascular and other diseases, and improved tests for infectious diseases such as hepatitis and AIDS.

Job Opportunities for Entry-Level and Experienced Personnel. Graduates with a PhD., M.S., or B.S. in any life science, biochemical engineering, or chemical engineering with a focus in biochemistry are encouraged to apply.

Student Requirements include a résumé, photocopy of transcripts, and a list of lab skills/techniques. Pertinent summer, co-op, or other related laboratory experience is required.

Company Locations. Opportunities are available at both the Maryland corporate headquarters and site of **BRL** products, and Grand Island, New York, site of **GIBCO** products.

Benefits. Offers unique benefits "FlexChoice" program providing core benefits for basic protection, and the ability to select optional benefits to fit individual needs. All employees are eligible to participate in LTI's incentive compensation plan, pension plan, 401K, and stock purchase plan.

Tuition reimbursement is an additional benefit also offered to all employees.

LIFELINK CORPORATION
331 SOUTH YORK ROAD
BENSENVILLE, ILLINOIS 60106-2673

Description: Operates nursing homes and retirement communities
Annual Sales: $24.4 million
Number of Employees: 690
Expertise Needed: Registered nursing, licensed practical nursing, certified nursing and nursing assistance, social service
Contact: Ms Kathy Schupbach
Director of Human Resources
(708) 766-3570

LIFESCAN, INC.
1000 GIBRALTER DRIVE
MILPITAS, CALIFORNIA 95035

Description: Manufactures blood glucose monitoring systems
Founded: 1985
Annual Sales: $125.0 million
Number of Employees: 700
Expertise Needed: Biomedical engineering, chemical analysis, dialysis, diabetes, electrical engineering, manufacturing engineering
Contact: Professional Staffing Department
(408) 263-9789

LIFESOURCE BLOOD SERVICES
1205 MILWAUKEE AVENUE
GLENVIEW, ILLINOIS 60025-2425

Description: Blood and bone marrow bank
Annual Sales: $27.7 million
Number of Employees: 450
Expertise Needed: Registered nursing, phlebotomy, medical laboratory technology
Contact: Ms Diane Beason
Employment Coordinator
(708) 298-9660

LINCARE, INC.
19337 US HIGHWAY 19 NORTH
CLEARWATER, FLORIDA 34618

Description: Provides home-based oxygen and therapy services
Annual Sales: $117.0 million
Number of Employees: 1,200
Expertise Needed: Accounting
Contact: Ms Sherry Lightfield
Manager of Human Resources
(813) 530-7700

JOHN C. LINCOLN HOSPITAL HEALTH CENTER
250 EAST DUNLAP AVENUE
PHOENIX, ARIZONA 85020

Description: Public hospital specializing in trauma
Founded: 1943
Annual Sales: $99.5 million
Number of Employees: 1,500
Number of Managerial and Professional Employees Hired 1993: 510
Expertise Needed: Registered nursing, physical therapy, occupational therapy
Contact: Ms Ann Essy
Employment Coordinator
(602) 870-6060

LINVATEC CORPORATION
11311 CONCEPT BOULEVARD
LARGO, FLORIDA 34643-4908

Description: Manufactures hospital and surgical equipment
Parent Company: Bristol-Myers Squibb Company
Annual Sales: $126.2 million
Number of Employees: 1,500
Expertise Needed: Mechanical engineering, electrical engineering, accounting, marketing, finance, computer programming
Contact: Ms Linda Abair
Human Resources Administrator
(813) 399-5106

LIVING CENTER OF AMERICA, INC.
15415 KATY FREEWAY
HOUSTON, TEXAS 77094-1899

Description: Owns and operates long-term health-care centers
Parent Company: ARA Group, Inc.
Annual Sales: $351.0 million
Number of Employees: 15,200
Number of Managerial and Professional Employees Hired 1993: 200

Expertise Needed: Accounting, marketing, information systems, computer programming, law, claims adjustment/examination, computer programming, program analysis

Contact: Ms Theresa Tucker
Director of Recruiting
(713) 578-4760

LOMA LINDA UNIVERSITY MEDICAL CENTER
11234 ANDERSON STREET
LOMA LINDA, CALIFORNIA 92354-2870

Description: Private hospital
Annual Sales: $318.2 million
Number of Employees: 4,352
Expertise Needed: Registered nursing, radiology, medical technology, physical therapy, occupational therapy, respiratory therapy

Contact: Mr Roger Miller
Manager of Employment
(909) 796-7311

LONG ISLAND COLLEGE HOSPITAL
340 HENRY STREET
BROOKLYN, NEW YORK 11201-5525

Description: General medical and surgical hospital
Parent Company: LICH Corporation
Annual Sales: $230.9 million
Number of Employees: 2,838
Expertise Needed: Nursing, hospital administration

Contact: Nurse Recruitment and Retention
(718) 756-1545

LONG'S DRUG STORES CORPORATION
141 NORTH CIVIC DRIVE
WALNUT CREEK, CALIFORNIA 94596-3815

Description: Drug store chain
Founded: 1938
Annual Sales: $2.5 billion
Number of Employees: 15,200

Contact: Ms Karen Cole
Supervisor of Employment
(510) 937-1170

LOOK, INC.
80 WASHINGTON STREET
NORWELL, MASSACHUSETTS 02061

Description: Manufactures medical sutures
Founded: 1936
Number of Employees: 130
Number of Managerial and Professional Employees Hired 1993: 20

Expertise Needed: Accounting, chemistry, biology, sales, mechanical engineering, management information systems

Contact: Mr Brian Gorley
Vice President of Operations
(617) 878-8220

LORAD CORPORATION
P.O. BOX 710
DANBURY, CONNECTICUT 06813-0710

Description: Manufactures diagnostic imaging equipment
Founded: 1983
Number of Employees: 210
Number of Managerial and Professional Employees Hired 1993: 45
Expertise Needed: Mechanical engineering, manufacturing engineering, electrical engineering

Contact: Ms Sharon Darnizo
Human Resources Supervisor
(203) 790-5544

LOURDES HOSPITAL, INC.
1530 LONE OAK ROAD
PADUCAH, KENTUCKY 42003-7901

Description: General medical and surgical hospital
Founded: 1962
Annual Sales: $108.2 million
Number of Employees: 1,446
Expertise Needed: Registered nursing, physical therapy

Contact: Department of Personnel
(502) 444-2444

LOVELACE MEDICAL FOUNDATION
2425 RIDGECREST DRIVE SOUTHEAST
ALBUQUERQUE, NEW MEXICO 87108-5129

Description: Medical research and educational foundation
Founded: 1947
Annual Sales: $25.2 million
Number of Employees: 332
Expertise Needed: Biology, physics, chemistry, technology

Contact: Ms Judy Coalson
Director of Human Resources
(505) 262-7155

LUBBOCK COUNTY HOSPITAL, UNIVERSITY MEDICAL CENTER
602 INDIANA AVENUE
LUBBOCK, TEXAS 79408-3364

Description: General hospital
Founded: 1967
Annual Sales: $116.4 million
Number of Employees: 1,750

Lubbock County Hospital, University Medical Center
(continued)

Expertise Needed: Nuclear medicine, emergency services, chemotherapy, real estate, physical therapy, occupational therapy

Contact: Ms Jennifer Gance
    Manager of Employment
    (806) 743-3355

LUMEX, INC.
100 SPENCE STREET
BAY SHORE, NEW YORK 11706

Description: Manufactures home health-care equipment
Founded: 1947
Number of Employees: 1,100
Expertise Needed: Structural engineering, engineering, finance, marketing, sales, manufacturing engineering, electrical engineering, mechanical engineering, accounting

Contact: Ms Sophie Cardon
    Director of Human Resources
    (516) 273-2200

THE LUMISCOPE COMPANY, INC.
400 RARITAN CENTER PARKWAY
EDISON, NEW JERSEY 08837

Description: Manufactures and distributes medical equipment and instruments
Founded: 1926
Number of Employees: 105
Expertise Needed: Accounting, engineering, management information systems

Contact: Human Resources Department
    (908) 225-5533

LUTHERAN GENERAL HEALTH CARE SYSTEM
1775 DEMPSTER STREET
PARK RIDGE, ILLINOIS 60068-1173

Description: Church-operated general medical and surgical hospitals
Founded: 1897
Annual Sales: $506.5 million
Number of Employees: 10,000
Expertise Needed: Social work, occupational therapy, nuclear technology, pharmacy, radiography, medical technology, registered nursing, speech pathology

Contact: Ms Robin Fell
    Director of Human Resources Placing, Recruitment, and Development
    (708) 696-8600

LUTHERAN MEDICAL CENTER, INC.
8300 WEST 38TH AVENUE
WHEAT RIDGE, COLORADO 80033-6005

Description: Private hospital
Founded: 1905

Annual Sales: $131.2 million
Number of Employees: 2,250
Expertise Needed: Nursing, allied health
Contact for College Students and Recent Graduates:
    Ms Sandy Cavonaugh
    Manager of Employment
    (303) 467-4200
Contact for All Other Candidates:
    Ms Lorrie Ham
    Nursing Recruiter
    (303) 420-9189

THE MACNEAL MEMORIAL HOSPITAL ASSOCIATION
3249 OAK PARK AVENUE
BERWYN, ILLINOIS 60402-3429

Description: Public hospital
Founded: 1919
Annual Sales: $125.5 million
Number of Employees: 1,700
Expertise Needed: Physical therapy, radiation technology, nursing, occupational therapy, accounting, finance, management information systems

Contact: Mr Jerry Lee
    Vice President of Human Resources
    (708) 795-9100

MAGEE WOMEN'S HOSPITAL
300 HALKET STREET
PITTSBURGH, PENNSYLVANIA 15213-3180

Description: Hospital specializing in women's care
Annual Sales: $126.9 million
Number of Employees: 1,900
Expertise Needed: Medical records, dietetics, food services, registered nursing

Contact: Human Resources Department
    (412) 641-1000

MAGNIVISION, INC.
5325 NORTHWEST 77TH AVENUE
MIAMI, FLORIDA 33166-4829

Description: Manufactures reading glasses
Parent Company: American Greetings Corporation
Founded: 1969
Annual Sales: $18.8 million
Number of Employees: 250
Expertise Needed: Accounting, marketing, sales, design engineering

Contact: Ms Ellen Rifkin
    Human Resources Manager
    (305) 477-4612

MAICO HEARING INSTRUMENTS, INC.
7375 BUSH LAKE ROAD
MINNEAPOLIS, MINNESOTA 55439

Description: Manufactures hearing aids
Founded: 1937

Number of Employees: 119
Expertise Needed: Mechanical engineering, electrical engineering, accounting, sales, marketing, management information systems, quality control
Contact: Ms Chris Chorzempa
Director of Human Resources
(612) 835-4400

MAIMONIDES MEDICAL CENTER, INC.
4802 10TH AVENUE
BROOKLYN, NEW YORK 11219-2916

Description: General hospital and medical center
Founded: 1947
Annual Sales: $284.1 million
Number of Employees: 3,900
Expertise Needed: Psychology, registered nursing, licensed practical nursing, physical therapy, occupational therapy
Contact: Ms Maryanne Sollecito
Recruiter
(718) 283-6000

MAINE MEDICAL CENTER
22 BRAMHALL STREET
PORTLAND, MAINE 04102-3175

Description: General medical and surgical hospital
Annual Sales: $204.4 million
Number of Employees: 3,800
Expertise Needed: Registered nursing, licensed practical nursing, operating room, intensive care, triage
Contact: Ms Holly MacEwan
Manager of Nursing Recruitment
(207) 871-0111

MALLINCKRODT, INC.
675 MCDONNELL BOULEVARD
HAZELWOOD, MISSOURI 63042-2301

Description: Manufactures medical equipment
Founded: 1867
Annual Sales: $1.2 billion
Number of Employees: 7,000
Expertise Needed: Manufacturing engineering, engineering, chemical engineering, chemistry, mechanical engineering, management information systems, industrial engineering
Contact: Ms Mary Monnet
Vice President of Human Resources
(314) 895-7367

MALLINCKRODT SPECIALTY CHEMICAL COMPANY
16305 SWINGLEY RIDGE ROAD
SAINT LOUIS, MISSOURI 63017-1777

Description: Manufactures drug-related and laboratory-related chemicals
Annual Sales: $395.3 million
Number of Employees: 2,000

Expertise Needed: Biology, biomedical engineering, biochemistry, accounting, chemistry, analog engineering
Contact: Ms Pam Thompson
Manager of Human Resources
(314) 530-2000

MANATEE MEMORIAL HOSPITAL
206 2ND STREET EAST
BRADENTON, FLORIDA 34208-1042

Description: Hospital
Founded: 1952
Annual Sales: $194.2 million
Number of Employees: 1,300
Expertise Needed: Registered nursing, certified nursing and nursing assistance, cardiology, pediatric care, oncology
Contact: Ms Andrea Pinnion
Director of Human Resources
(813) 746-5111

MANOR CARE, INC.
10750 COLUMBIA PIKE
SILVER SPRING, MARYLAND 20901-4427

Description: Owns and operates health-care facilities, hotels, and office buildings
Founded: 1968
Annual Sales: $1.0 billion
Number of Employees: 24,100
Number of Managerial and Professional Employees Hired 1993: 200
Expertise Needed: Finance, auditing, budgeting, computer programming, systems analysis, management information systems, accounting, administration
Contact: Ms Tracy Henshaw
Manager of Corporate Employment
(301) 681-9400

MANOR HEALTHCARE CORPORATION
10770 COLUMBIA PIKE
SILVER SPRING, MARYLAND 20901

Description: Provides nursing care and rehabilitation services
Number of Employees: 18,000
Expertise Needed: Marketing, sales, human resources, finance, nursing
Contact: Ms Susan Cardwell
Corporate Employment Manager
(301) 593-9600

MARCAL PAPER MILLS, INC.
1 MARKET STREET
ELMWOOD PARK, NEW JERSEY 07407

Description: Manufactures sanitary paper products
Founded: 1932
Number of Employees: 1,000

Marcal Paper Mills, Inc. (continued)

Expertise Needed: Engineering, marketing, sales, accounting

Contact: Mr James H Nelson
Director of Personnel
(201) 796-4000

MARCHON MARCOLIN EYEWEAR, INC.
35 HUB DRIVE
MELVILLE, NEW YORK 11747-3517

Description: Distributes eyeglass frames and sunglasses to optical retailers
Annual Sales: $120.0 million
Number of Employees: 250
Expertise Needed: Sales, marketing
Contact: Ms Tina Ombrellina
Personnel Supervisor
(516) 755-2020

MARIN GENERAL HOSPITAL
250 BON AIR ROAD
SAN RAFAEL, CALIFORNIA 94904-1702

Description: Public general hospital specializing in acute and trauma care
Annual Sales: $100.0 million
Number of Employees: 1,350
Expertise Needed: Registered nursing, physical therapy, pharmacy, speech pathology, social work, medical technology
Contact: Ms Rene Tomasello
Nursing Recruitment
(415) 925-7000

MARION MERRELL DOW, INC.
9300 WARD PARKWAY
KANSAS CITY, MISSOURI 64114-3321

Description: Produces prescription drugs and consumer health-care products
Parent Company: The Dow Chemical Company
Founded: 1952
Annual Sales: $3.3 billion
Number of Employees: 9,808
Expertise Needed: Pharmacy, packaging engineering, quality control, chemical engineering, mechanical engineering, industrial engineering, biology, physics
Contact: Mr Richard Bailey
Vice President of Human Resources
(816) 966-4000

MARION MERRELL DOW PHARMACEUTICALS
2110 EAST GALBRAITH ROAD
CINCINNATI, OHIO 45237-1625

Description: Produces prescription drugs and consumer health-care products
Parent Company: Marion Merrell Dow, Inc.
Annual Sales: $1.2 billion

Number of Employees: 6,500
Expertise Needed: Human resources, marketing, law, research and development, sales, operations, finance, information systems
Contact: Mr Richard Bailey
Vice President of Human Resources
(816) 966-4000

MARK CLARK PRODUCTS
3601 SOUTHWEST 29TH STREET
TOPEKA, KANSAS 66614-2074

Description: Manufactures patient identification bands, medical linens, and disposables
Founded: 1972
Annual Sales: $27.4 million
Number of Employees: 475
Expertise Needed: Manufacturing engineering, plastics engineering, product design and development
Contact: Personnel Department
(913) 273-3990

MARK STEVENS SERVICE MERCHANDISERS
1 CVS DRIVE
WOONSOCKET, RHODE ISLAND 02895-4239

Description: Drug store chain distributing health and beauty aides
Founded: 1969
Annual Sales: $1.9 billion
Number of Employees: 2,100
Contact: Mr Bob Botsford
Manager of Recruiting
(401) 765-1500

MARQUETTE ELECTRONICS, INC.
8200 WEST TOWER AVENUE
MILWAUKEE, WISCONSIN 53223-3219

Description: Manufactures monitoring and testing equipment
Founded: 1965
Annual Sales: $250.2 million
Number of Employees: 1,500
Number of Managerial and Professional Employees Hired 1993: 100
Expertise Needed: Mechanical engineering, accounting, clinical engineering, electronics/electronics engineering, computer-aided design, software engineering/development, hardware engineering
Contact: Mr Guy Hope
Manager of Personnel
(414) 355-5000

MARSAM PHARMACEUTICALS, INC.
24 OLNEY AVENUE
CHERRY HILL, NEW JERSEY 08003

Description: Manufactures and markets injectable generic prescription drug products
Annual Sales: $16.7 million
Number of Employees: 175

Number of Managerial and Professional Employees Hired 1993: 87

Expertise Needed: Accounting, marketing, sales, chemistry, research and development, quality control, management information systems

Contact: Ms Alice Mahoney
Administrative Assistant
(609) 424-5600

MARSHFIELD CLINIC
1000 NORTH OAK AVENUE
MARSHFIELD, WISCONSIN 54449-5703

Description: Multispecialty group practice
Founded: 1916
Annual Sales: $193.1 million
Number of Employees: 2,800
Expertise Needed: Physician assistant, nursing, general nursing, medical technology
Contact: Ms Renae Lein-Sheibley
Employment Manager
(715) 387-5511

MARTIN MEMORIAL MEDICAL CENTER
301 HOSPITAL AVENUE
STUART, FLORIDA 34994-2337

Description: General medical and surgical hospital
Annual Sales: $100.6 million
Number of Employees: 1,365
Expertise Needed: Nursing, radiation technology, occupational therapy, physical therapy
Contact: Ms Pauline Crahan
Employment Director
(407) 287-5200

MASSACHUSETTS GENERAL HOSPITAL CORPORATION
55 FRUIT STREET
BOSTON, MASSACHUSETTS 02114-2621

Description: General surgical hospital
Founded: 1811
Annual Sales: $692.0 million
Number of Employees: 10,000
Expertise Needed: Accounting, finance, marketing, data processing, auditing
Contact: Mr Steve Cancellieri
Manager of Employee Relations and Recruiting
(617) 726-2000

MASSACHUSETTS MUTUAL LIFE INSURANCE COMPANY
1295 STATE STREET
SPRINGFIELD, MASSACHUSETTS 01111

Description: Provides life, health, and disability insurance
Assets: $32.0 billion

Number of Employees: 9,000
Contact: Human Resources Department
(413) 788-8411

MAXICARE HEALTH PLANS, INC.
749 SOUTH BROADWAY STREET
LOS ANGELES, CALIFORNIA 90015

Description: Provides health-care insurance services
Annual Sales: $414.5 million
Number of Employees: 444
Expertise Needed: Marketing, customer service and support, actuarial, underwriting
Contact: Ms Heather Plumley
Vice President of Human Resources
(213) 765-2000

MAXUM HEALTH CORPORATION
14850 QUORUM DRIVE
DALLAS, TEXAS 75240-7012

Description: Provides mobile magnetic resonance imaging and other diagnostic services
Annual Sales: $45.1 million
Number of Employees: 386
Expertise Needed: Accounting, marketing, magnetic resonance imaging
Contact: Ms Pam Robertson
Supervisor of Payroll and Benefits
(214) 716-6200

MAXXIM MEDICAL
104 INDUSTRIAL BOULEVARD
SUGARLAND, TEXAS 77478-3128

Description: Medical and fitness equipment vendor
Annual Sales: $74.5 million
Number of Employees: 1,800
Expertise Needed: Accounting, finance, data processing, electrical engineering, mechanical engineering
Contact: Ms Donna Huestis
Director of Human Resources
(713) 240-2442

MAY'S DRUG STORES, INC.
6705 EAST 81ST STREET
TULSA, OKLAHOMA 74133-4158

Description: Operates retail drug stores
Founded: 1962
Annual Sales: $70.8 million
Number of Employees: 500
Expertise Needed: Pharmacy
Contact: Mr Jim Moomaw
Vice President of Operations
(918) 496-9646

MAYO FOUNDATION
200 1ST STREET SOUTHWEST
ROCHESTER, MINNESOTA 55905-0001

Description: Diagnostic medical center
Founded: 1863
Annual Sales: $1.5 billion
Number of Employees: 20,615
Expertise Needed: Chemistry, biology, microbiology, licensed practical nursing, registered nursing, nuclear medicine, medical technology
Contact: Mr Tony Enquist
    Personnel Representitive
    (507) 284-5391

MCGAW, INC.
2525 MCGAW AVENUE
IRVINE, CALIFORNIA 92714-5841

Description: Manufactures intravenous therapy and nutritional products
Founded: 1928
Annual Sales: $350.0 million
Number of Employees: 3,000
Expertise Needed: Project engineering, engineering management, computer engineering, biological sciences, research, marketing, sales, finance, laboratory technology, medical technology
Contact: Mr Robert Jacesko
    Manager of Human Resources
    (714) 660-2000

MCKESSON SERVICE MERCHANDISING
401 HIGHWAY 43 EAST
HARRISON, ARKANSAS 72602-8605

Description: Manufactures specialty foods, aspirin, and underwear
Parent Company: McKesson Corporation
Annual Sales: $575.0 million
Number of Employees: 3,000
Expertise Needed: Finance, sales, marketing, accounting, merchandising, purchasing, graphic arts, facilities management, computer programming
Contact: Ms Linda Eddings
    Employment Coordinator
    (501) 741-3402

MCLAREN REGIONAL MEDICAL CENTER
401 SOUTH BALLENGER HIGHWAY
FLINT, MICHIGAN 48532-3638

Description: Private, nonprofit facility specializing in rehabilitation
Annual Sales: $127.6 million
Number of Employees: 1,965
Expertise Needed: Occupational therapy, physical therapy, radiation therapy, speech pathology
Contact: Ms Roberta Shaw
    Human Resource Manager
    (810) 762-2463

MCLEOD REGIONAL MEDICAL CENTER
555 EAST CHEVES STREET
FLORENCE, SOUTH CAROLINA 29506-2617

Description: General hospital
Founded: 1906
Annual Sales: $151.7 million
Number of Employees: 2,005
Expertise Needed: Registered nursing, licensed practical nursing, medical technology, accounting, respiratory therapy, rehabilitation, anesthesiology
Contact: Ms Mariam Baldwin
    Director of Human Resources Recruitment
    (803) 667-2000

MCNEIL CONSUMER PRODUCTS
7050 CAMP HILL ROAD
FORT WASHINGTON, PENNSYLVANIA 19034

Description: Manufactures over-the-counter pharmaceuticals, and medications
Parent Company: Johnson & Johnson
Founded: 1959
Annual Sales: $230.4 million
Number of Employees: 1,800
Expertise Needed: Chemistry, research and development, finance, marketing, operations
Contact: Ms Jenny Pettis-Hassel
    Employment Manager
    (215) 233-7000

MDT CORPORATION
2300 WEST 205TH STREET
TORRANCE, CALIFORNIA 90501-1452

Description: Manufactures sterilization systems and medical equipment
Founded: 1971
Annual Sales: $119.2 million
Number of Employees: 1,140
Expertise Needed: Electrical engineering, mechanical engineering, finance, marketing, sales, accounting
Contact: Ms Shelly Knapp
    Employment Manager
    (716) 272-5050

MEAD JOHNSON & COMPANY
2400 WEST LLOYD EXPRESSWAY
EVANSVILLE, INDIANA 47721-0001

Description: Manufactures nutritional and pharmaceutical products
Parent Company: Bristol-Myers Squibb Company
Founded: 1967
Annual Sales: $1.5 billion
Number of Employees: 4,300
Expertise Needed: Sales, marketing, finance, accounting, engineering
Contact: Mr Pat Aquart
    Director of Staffing
    (812) 429-7150

MEADOWBROOK REHABILITATION GROUP

2200 POWELL STREET
EMERYVILLE, CALIFORNIA 94608-1809

Description: Physical rehabilitation center
Annual Sales: $28.7 million
Number of Employees: 555
Expertise Needed: Physical therapy, occupational therapy, speech therapy, registered nursing
Contact: Ms Alison Branstein
Director of Human Resources
(510) 420-0900

MED LABORATORY AUTOMATION, INC.

270 MARBLE AVENUE
PLEASANTVILLE, NEW YORK 10570

Description: Manufactures instrumentation products for clinical laboratories
Founded: 1963
Expertise Needed: Design engineering, mechanical engineering, electrical engineering, industrial engineering
Contact: Ms Sherry Borsesi
Human Resources Representative
(914) 747-3020

MED-X CORPORATION

3818 SOUTH 79TH EAST AVENUE
TULSA, OKLAHOMA 74170-0870

Description: Drug store chain
Founded: 1967
Annual Sales: $45.0 million
Number of Employees: 350
Expertise Needed: Pharmacy, sales, marketing
Contact: Mr John Conwell
Controller
(918) 628-1616

MEDAPHIS CORPORATION

2700 CUMBERLAND PARKWAY NORTHWEST
ATLANTA, GEORGIA 30339-3321

Description: Provides billing and accounting services to physicians and hospitals
Annual Sales: $97.4 million
Number of Employees: 3,100
Expertise Needed: Auditing, accounting
Contact: Human Resources Department
(404) 319-3300

MEDCENTERS HEALTHCARE, INC.

8100 34TH AVENUE SOUTH
MINNEAPOLIS, MINNESOTA 55425-1672

Description: Owns and operates health maintenance organizations and health-related companies
Parent Company: Health Partners, Inc.
Annual Sales: $352.3 million
Number of Employees: 4,000

Expertise Needed: Nursing, accounting, management information systems, management
Contact: Mr Robert Cooley
Human Resources Director
(612) 883-7600

MEDCO CONTAINMENT SERVICES, INC.

100 SUMMIT AVENUE
MONTVALE, NEW JERSEY 07645-1712

Description: Designs and manages prescription drug benefit plans
Parent Company: Merck & Company, Inc.
Founded: 1970
Annual Sales: $2.6 billion
Number of Employees: 9,250
Expertise Needed: Accounting, mechanical engineering, packaging engineering, design engineering, sales, computer programming, systems analysis, pharmacy
Contact: Mr David Lewis
Manager of Employment
(201) 358-3400

MEDEX, INC.

3637 LACON ROAD
HILLIARD, OHIO 43026-1202

Description: Designs and manufactures disposable hospital products
Founded: 1959
Annual Sales: $92.3 million
Number of Employees: 1,300
Expertise Needed: Mechanical engineering, design engineering, industrial engineering, accounting, law, sales, computer programming
Contact: Human Resources Department
(614) 876-2413

MEDI-CARE DATA SYSTEMS, INC.

223 STIGER STREET
HACKETTSTOWN, NEW JERSEY 07840

Description: Provides medical data processing services
Founded: 1969
Expertise Needed: Computer science, marketing, software engineering/development
Contact: Ms Jeannette Baker
Human Resources Department

MEDICAL AMERICA HEALTH SYSTEMS CORPORATION

1 WYOMING STREET
DAYTON, OHIO 45409-2722

Description: Provides health-care services
Annual Sales: $269.4 million
Number of Employees: 3,685

Expertise Needed: Physical therapy, occupational therapy, physician assistant, respiratory therapy, radiology

Contact: Ms Sandra Murphy
Manager of Human Resources
(513) 223-6192

MEDICAL ARTS LABORATORY, INC.

1111 NORTH LEE AVENUE, SUITE 100
OKLAHOMA CITY, OKLAHOMA 73103-2620

Description: Independent research laboratory
Founded: 1965
Annual Sales: $19.6 million
Number of Employees: 350
Expertise Needed: Medical laboratory technology, laboratory assistance, medical technology

Contact: Ms Cindy Goodwin
Recruiter
(405) 239-7111

MEDICAL CARE AMERICA, INC.

13455 NOEL ROAD
DALLAS, TEXAS 75240-6620

Description: Owns and operates outpatient surgical centers and provides home infusion therapy services
Annual Sales: $650.0 million
Number of Employees: 4,300
Expertise Needed: Licensed practical nursing

Contact: Benefits Department
(214) 701-2200

MEDICAL CENTER AT PRINCETON

253 WITHERSPOON STREET
PRINCETON, NEW JERSEY 08540-3213

Description: General hospital
Founded: 1929
Annual Sales: $91.4 million
Number of Employees: 1,800
Expertise Needed: Physical therapy, occupational therapy, laboratory technology, radiation technology

Contact: Ms Sharol Scialpi
Recruiter
(609) 497-4336

MEDICAL CENTER HOSPITAL

500 WEST 4TH STREET
ODESSA, TEXAS 79760-5059

Description: Public general hospital
Founded: 1949
Annual Sales: $109.9 million
Number of Employees: 1,556
Expertise Needed: X-ray technology, physical therapy, occupational therapy, speech therapy, radiation

technology, registered nursing, licensed practical nursing, certified nursing and nursing assistance

Contact: Ms Bernadette Fuentes
Allied Health Recruitment
(915) 333-7111

MEDICAL CENTER HOSPITAL OF VERMONT

111 COLCHESTER AVENUE
BURLINGTON, VERMONT 05401

Description: General medical and surgical hospital
Parent Company: Vermont Health Foundation, Inc.
Annual Sales: $155.1 million
Number of Employees: 2,414
Expertise Needed: Registered nursing, licensed practical nursing, occupational therapy, physical therapy, allied health, respiratory therapy, maternity care

Contact: Human Resources Department
(802) 656-2345

MEDICAL CENTER OF CENTRAL GEORGIA

777 HEMLOCK STREET
MACON, GEORGIA 31201-2102

Description: General hospital
Founded: 1895
Annual Sales: $208.2 million
Number of Employees: 3,371
Expertise Needed: Pharmacy, therapy, technology

Contact: Ms Donna Turner
Technical/Professional Recruiter
(912) 633-1334

MEDICAL CENTER OF CENTRAL MASSACHUSETTS

119 BELMONT STREET
WORCESTER, MASSACHUSETTS 01605-2903

Description: Nonprofit general hospital
Annual Sales: $172.2 million
Number of Employees: 3,300
Expertise Needed: Registered nursing, laboratory technology, radiation technology, medical technology, social work, physical therapy, occupational therapy, speech therapy, respiratory therapy

Contact: Ms Marita Thompson
Manager of Recruiting
(508) 793-6611

MEDICAL CENTER OF DELAWARE

501 WEST 14TH STREET
WILMINGTON, DELAWARE 19801-1013

Description: General hospital
Parent Company: MCD Foundation
Annual Sales: $369.7 million
Number of Employees: 5,613

Expertise Needed: Pharmacology, laboratory assistance, radiology, speech pathology, hearing, cardiac care, pediatric care

Contact: Mr Walt Szmidt
Director of Employment Services
(302) 428-2675

MEDICAL DATA ELECTRONICS, INC.
12720 WENTWORTH STREET
ARLITA, CALIFORNIA 91331-4329

Description: Manufactures and distributes medical monitoring devices
Founded: 1979
Annual Sales: $35.0 million
Number of Employees: 170
Expertise Needed: Electronics/electronics engineering, design engineering, marketing, accounting, product engineering

Contact: Ms Sherry Goldman
Director of Human Resources
(818) 768-6411

MEDICAL DISPOSABLES INBRAND
1165 HAYES INDUSTRIAL DRIVE
MARIETTA, GEORGIA 30062

Description: Manufactures sanitary paper products
Founded: 1975
Number of Employees: 400
Expertise Needed: Marketing, manufacturing, medical technology, accounting, customer service and support

Contact: Employment Department
(404) 422-3036

MEDICAL IMAGING CENTERS OF AMERICA
9444 FARNHAM STREET
SAN DIEGO, CALIFORNIA 92123-1309

Description: Provides medical imaging services to hospitals and physicians
Founded: 1981
Annual Sales: $84.6 million
Number of Employees: 492
Expertise Needed: Radiology, radiography, radiological technology

Contact: Ms Joan Robinson
Personnel Director
(619) 560-0110

MEDICAL INFORMATION TECHNOLOGY
MEDITECH CIRCLE
WESTWOOD, MASSACHUSETTS 02090

Description: Develops and sells computer software for hospitals
Founded: 1969
Annual Sales: $92.3 million
Number of Employees: 1,000

Expertise Needed: Marketing, software engineering/development, electrical engineering, data processing, accounting, finance

Contact: Ms Pamela Grant
Supervisor of Recruiting
(617) 821-3000

MEDICAL LABORATORY AUTOMATION, INC.
270 MARBLE AVENUE
PLEASANTVILLE, NEW YORK 10570-3411

Description: Manufactures instrumentation and specialty hospital products
Founded: 1963
Annual Sales: $50.5 million
Number of Employees: 365
Expertise Needed: Design engineering, mechanical engineering, electrical engineering, industrial engineering

Contact: Ms Sherry Borsesi
Human Resources Representative
(914) 747-3020

MEDICAL MANAGEMENT CONSULTANTS, INC.
8797 BEVERLY BOULEVARD
LOS ANGELES, CALIFORNIA 90048-1832

Description: Provides consulting services to hospitals
Annual Sales: $170.7 million
Number of Employees: 3,125
Expertise Needed: X-ray technology, laboratory technology, medical technology

Contact: Ms Jan Winter
Recruitment Consultant
(310) 659-3835

MEDICAL SERVICE BUREAU OF IDAHO
1602 21ST AVENUE
LEWISTON, IDAHO 83501-4061

Description: Provides medical, surgical, and dental health-care benefits
Founded: 1946
Annual Sales: $214.6 million
Number of Employees: 360
Expertise Needed: Accounting, claims processing/management, and administration, actuarial, law, finance

Contact: Ms Vickey Smith
Associate Director of Human Resources
(208) 746-2671

MEDIPLEX GROUP
5600 WYOMING BOULEVARD NORTHEAST
ALBUQUERUQE, NEW MEXICO 87109

Description: Provides surgical, inpatient, and outpatient health-care services
Founded: 1983
Number of Employees: 9,000

Mediplex Group (continued)

Expertise Needed: Nursing, physical therapy, respiratory therapy, speech pathology, languages

Contact: Mr Gary Stagher
Director of Corporate Recruiting
(505) 821-3355

MEDIQ IMAGING SERVICES, INC.

300 WILLOW STREET SOUTH
NORTH ANDOVER, MASSACHUSETTS 01845-5920

Description: Provides portable X-ray and electrocardiogram services
Parent Company: Mediq Corporation
Annual Sales: $17.4 million
Number of Employees: 170
Expertise Needed: Nuclear medicine, ultrasound technology, physicians

Contact: Mr James Clay
Human Resources Department
(508) 683-5901

MEDIQ, INC.

1 MEDIQ PLAZA
PENNSAUKEN, NEW JERSEY 08110-1439

Description: Provides health-care services
Founded: 1977
Annual Sales: $295.4 million
Number of Employees: 3,600
Expertise Needed: Occupational therapy, physical therapy, nursing

Contact: Ms Marianne Evans
Director of Human Resources
(609) 665-9300

MEDISENSE, INC.

266 2ND AVENUE
WALTHAM, MASSACHUSETTS 02154

Description: Manufactures home health-care equipment
Annual Sales: $95.0 million
Number of Employees: 750
Expertise Needed: Computer science, physics, chemistry, electronics/electronics engineering

Contact: Ms Carolyn White-Krueger
Employment Specialist
(617) 895-6195

MEDLAB, INC.

6600 SOUTHWEST HAMPTON STREET
PORTLAND, OREGON 97223

Description: Medical laboratory
Parent Company: Nichols Institute
Annual Sales: $23.3 million
Number of Employees: 485

Expertise Needed: Laboratory technology, chemical engineering, medical laboratory technology, data processing

Contact: Ms Jeanette Napoleon
Director of Human Resources
(503) 639-4500

MEDLINE INDUSTRIES, INC.

1 MEDLINE PLACE
MUNDELEIN, ILLINOIS 60060-4486

Description: Manufactures and distributes medical and surgical instruments and supplies, linens, and skin care products
Founded: 1966
Annual Sales: $385.7 million
Number of Employees: 2,000
Expertise Needed: Sales, finance, accounting, registered nursing

Contact: Ms Carna Keefe
Employment Manager
(708) 949-5500

MEDQUIST, INC.

20 CLEMENTON ROAD EAST
GIBBSBORO, NEW JERSEY 08026-1165

Description: Provides billing and collection services to hospitals and physicians
Annual Sales: $27.4 million
Number of Employees: 500
Expertise Needed: Accounting

Contact: Ms Laura Andersen
Director of Human Resources
(609) 782-0300

MEDRAD, INC.

271 KAPPA DRIVE
PITTSBURGH, PENNSYLVANIA 15238-2817

Description: Develops and manufactures medical imaging equipment and disposable medical products
Annual Sales: $67.4 million
Number of Employees: 725
Expertise Needed: Electrical engineering, mechanical engineering, industrial engineering, accounting, software engineering/development, quality control, research and development

Contact: Mr Martin Resick
Director of Human Resources
(412) 967-9700

THE MEDSTAT GROUP

777 EAST EISENHOWER PARKWAY
ANN ARBOR, MICHIGAN 48108

Description: Health-care information company
Founded: 1981
Number of Employees: 480
Number of Managerial and Professional Employees Hired 1993: 130

Expertise Needed: Business management, accounting, computer programming

Contact: Ms Helen Moyle
Vice President of Human Resources
(313) 996-1180

MEDTRONIC BIO-MEDICUS, INC.
9600 WEST 76TH STREET
EDEN PRAIRIE, MINNESOTA 55344-3718

Description: Manufactures surgical blood pumps and support systems
Parent Company: Medtronic, Inc.
Annual Sales: $27.9 million
Number of Employees: 280
Number of Managerial and Professional Employees Hired 1993: 3
Expertise Needed: Biomedical engineering, engineering, medical technology, analog engineering
Contact: Human Resources Department
(612) 944-7784

MEDTRONIC, INC.
7000 CENTRAL AVENUE NORTHEAST
MINNEAPOLIS, MINNESOTA 55432-3568

Description: Develops and manufactures biomedical devices for cardiovascular and neurological applications
Founded: 1949
Annual Sales: $1.3 billion
Number of Employees: 9,247
Expertise Needed: Finance, marketing, materials science, biomedical engineering, electrical engineering, chemical engineering, mechanical engineering, project engineering, software engineering/ development, biological sciences
Contact: Ms Diane Anderson
Employment Coordinator
(612) 574-4780

MEGA CARE, INC.
695 CHESTNUT STREET
UNION, NEW JERSEY 07083

Description: Provides acute-care services
Parent Company: Mega Source, Inc.
Annual Sales: $24.3 million
Number of Employees: 660
Expertise Needed: Registered nursing, licensed practical nursing, physical therapy, occupational therapy, speech therapy, accounting, administration, pharmacy
Contact: Ms Melinda Raggio
Employment Manager
(908) 851-7005

MELALEUCA, INC.
3910 SOUTH YELLOWSTONE HIGHWAY
IDAHO FALLS, IDAHO 83402-4342

Description: Manufactures drugs and sundries
Annual Sales: $200.1 million
Number of Employees: 500
Expertise Needed: Marketing, sales, customer service and support, manufacturing engineering
Contact: Human Resources Department
(208) 522-0700

MEMORIAL CITY GENERAL HOSPITAL CORPORATION
920 FROSTWOOD DRIVE
HOUSTON, TEXAS 77024-2412

Description: Public hospital specializing in acute care
Parent Company: Metro National Corporation
Founded: 1969
Annual Sales: $149.9 million
Number of Employees: 1,937
Expertise Needed: Nursing
Contact: Ms Mary Chomeau
Employment Representative
(713) 932-3000

MEMORIAL HOSPITAL AND MEDICAL CENTER
2200 WEST ILLINOIS AVENUE
MIDLAND, TEXAS 79701-6407

Description: General hospital
Founded: 1942
Annual Sales: $102.8 million
Number of Employees: 1,400
Expertise Needed: Radiation technology, physical therapy, occupational therapy
Contact: Ms Cathy Anwell
Assistant Director of Human Resources
(915) 685-1111

MEMORIAL HOSPITAL AT GULFPORT
4500 13TH STREET
GULFPORT, MISSISSIPPI 39502-2515

Description: Public general hospital
Founded: 1946
Annual Sales: $116.6 million
Number of Employees: 1,700
Expertise Needed: Registered nursing, physical therapy
Contact: Ms Lisa Benfield
Professional Recruitment
(601) 863-1441

MEMORIAL HOSPITAL OF SOUTH BEND
615 NORTH MICHIGAN STREET
SOUTH BEND, INDIANA 46601-1033

Description: Not-for-profit general medical and surgical hospital
Parent Company: Memorial Health System, Inc.

Memorial Hospital of South Bend (continued)

Annual Sales: $208.1 million
Number of Employees: 2,010
Expertise Needed: Allied health, physical therapy, occupational therapy, radiology, licensed practical nursing, registered nursing
Contact: Ms. Carol Ford
Recruiter for Allied Health
(219) 234-9041

MEMORIAL HOSPITAL SYSTEM

7600 BEACHNUT
HOUSTON, TEXAS 77074

Description: Not-for-profit general medical and surgical hospital and nursing home
Founded: 1971
Annual Sales: $316.5 million
Number of Employees: 3,200
Expertise Needed: Registered nursing, licensed practical nursing, occupational therapy, physical therapy
Contact: Ms Margaret Loper
Recruitment Coordinator
(713) 776-5000

MEMORIAL HOSPITALS ASSOCIATION

1700 COFFEE ROAD
MODESTO, CALIFORNIA 95355-2803

Description: Nonprofit hospital specializing in acute care
Founded: 1947
Annual Sales: $130.1 million
Number of Employees: 1,800
Expertise Needed: Registered nursing, radiology
Contact: Ms Toni Williams
Nursing Recruiter
(209) 526-4500

MEMORIAL MEDICAL CENTER

800 NORTH RUTLEDGE STREET
SPRINGFIELD, ILLINOIS 62781

Description: General medical and surgical hospital
Founded: 1897
Annual Sales: $184.5 million
Number of Employees: 2,800
Expertise Needed: Physical therapy, occupational therapy, laboratory technology
Contact: Ms Shirley Kirk
Director of Human Resources
(217) 788-3000

MEMORIAL MEDICAL CENTER OF JACKSONVILLE

3625 UNIVERSITY BOULEVARD SOUTH
JACKSONVILLE, FLORIDA 32216-4207

Description: Public hospital specializing in rehabilitation
Founded: 1964
Annual Sales: $136.6 million

Number of Employees: 1,729
Expertise Needed: Registered nursing, pharmacy, occupational therapy, physical therapy
Contact: Ms Nancy Murdock
Director of Personnel
(904) 399-6111

MEMORIAL MISSION HOSPITAL, INC.

509 BILTMORE AVENUE
ASHEVILLE, NORTH CAROLINA 28801-4690

Description: Nonprofit community hospital
Parent Company: Memorial Mission Medical Center
Founded: 1948
Annual Sales: $135.1 million
Number of Employees: 2,600
Expertise Needed: Nursing, laboratory assistance, respiratory care, rehabilitation
Contact: Ms Nancy Dexter
Personnel Director
(704) 255-4000

MEMORIAL SLOAN-KETTERING CANCER CENTER

1275 YORK AVENUE
NEW YORK, NEW YORK 10021

Description: Comprehensive cancer center engaged in biomedical research and patient care services
Founded: 1884
Number of Employees: 6,200
Expertise Needed: Management, customer service and support, information systems, molecular biology, biotechnology
Contact: Mr Edward L Kleinert
Administrator, College Relations
(212) 639-3479

For more information, see full corporate profile, pg. 208.

MENNINGER FOUNDATION, INC.

5800 SOUTHWEST 6TH AVENUE
TOPEKA, KANSAS 66606-9604

Description: Psychiatric hospital
Founded: 1919
Annual Sales: $63.6 million
Number of Employees: 1,150
Expertise Needed: Psychiatry, psychology, registered nursing, accounting, finance
Contact: Ms Sherry Harold
Employment Specialist
(913) 273-7500

MENTAL HEALTH MANAGEMENT, INC.

7601 LEWINSVILLE ROAD
MCLEAN, VIRGINIA 22102-2815

Description: Provides contract psychiatric care services to acute care hospitals
Parent Company: Mediq, Inc.
Annual Sales: $46.0 million
Number of Employees: 550
Expertise Needed: Psychiatry, clinical psychology, clinical services, social work
Contact: Mr Steve Short
　　　　Manager of Recruiting Services
　　　　(703) 749-4600

MERCK & COMPANY, INC.

1 MERCK DRIVE
WHITEHOUSE STATION, NEW JERSEY 08889

Description: Manufactures and markets pharmaceuticals, specialty chemicals, and animal health products
Founded: 1891
Annual Sales: $9.7 billion
Number of Employees: 38,400
Expertise Needed: Chemical engineering, biological sciences, biochemistry, life sciences, computer science, sales, marketing, statistics
Contact for College Students and Recent Graduates:
　　　　Ms Diane Dalinsky
　　　　Manager of College Relations
　　　　(908) 423-6221
Contact for All Other Candidates:
　　　　Human Resources Department
　　　　(908) 594-4000

MERCY CHILDREN'S HOSPITAL

2401 GILLHAM ROAD
KANSAS CITY, MISSOURI 64108-4619

Description: Pediatric hospital
Founded: 1897
Annual Sales: $106.6 million
Number of Employees: 2,000
Expertise Needed: Pediatric care, registered nursing, licensed practical nursing, anesthesiology, EKG technology, cardiology, accounting, operations
Contact: Ms Carol Medlin
　　　　Employment Interviewer
　　　　(816) 234-3143

MERCY HEALTH CENTER

4300 WEST MEMORIAL ROAD
OKLAHOMA CITY, OKLAHOMA 73120

Description: Nonprofit hospital
Founded: 1947
Annual Sales: $106.0 million
Number of Employees: 1,700

Expertise Needed: Registered nursing, respiratory therapy, occupational therapy, physical therapy
Contact: Ms Carol Grey
　　　　Professional Recruitment
　　　　(405) 755-1515

MERCY HEALTH SERVICES

34605 WEST 12 MILE ROAD
FARMINGTON HILLS, MICHIGAN 48331-3263

Description: Provides health-care services
Annual Sales: $1.6 billion
Number of Employees: 22,755
Expertise Needed: Accounting, finance, marketing, information systems
Contact: Ms Paula Huot
　　　　Director of Staffing
　　　　(810) 489-6000

MERCY HEALTH SERVICES, INC.

2001 VAIL AVENUE
CHARLOTTE, NORTH CAROLINA 28207-1219

Description: Nonprofit, private general hospital
Annual Sales: $99.2 million
Number of Employees: 1,375
Expertise Needed: Home health care, registered nursing, licensed practical nursing, physical therapy, occupational therapy, speech therapy, respiratory therapy, oncology, social work
Contact: Ms Marian Stamopolous
　　　　Human Resources Representative
　　　　(704) 379-5000

MERCY HEALTH SYSTEMS OF NEW YORK

515 ABBOTT ROAD
BUFFALO, NEW YORK 14220-1700

Description: Provides administrative management services for medical and surgical hospitals
Annual Sales: $118.2 million
Number of Employees: 3,503
Expertise Needed: Nursing, radiology, laboratory technology, physical therapy
Contact: Ms Melissa Bella
　　　　Employment Specialist
　　　　(716) 828-2750

MERCY HOSPITAL OF JANESVILLE, WISCONSIN

100 MINERAL POINT AVENUE
JANESVILLE, WISCONSIN 53545-2940

Description: General medical and surgical hospital
Founded: 1907
Annual Sales: $90.5 million
Number of Employees: 1,000

Mercy Hospital of Janesville, Wisconsin (continued)

Expertise Needed: Radiological technology, registered nursing, occupational therapy, respiratory therapy, physical therapy

Contact: Human Resources Department
(608) 756-6000

MERCY HOSPITAL & MEDICAL CENTER

STEVENSON EXPRESSWAY AT KING DRIVE
CHICAGO, ILLINOIS 60616

Description: Church-operated medical and surgical hospital
Founded: 1852
Annual Sales: $160.4 million
Number of Employees: 2,500
Expertise Needed: Registered nursing, physical therapy, occupational therapy, laboratory technology, radiology

Contact: Ms Mary Ann Sullivan
Employment Coordinator
(312) 567-2000

MERCY HOSPITAL, INC.

3663 SOUTH MIAMI AVENUE
MIAMI, FLORIDA 33133-4253

Description: General hospital
Founded: 1945
Annual Sales: $124.4 million
Number of Employees: 1,654
Expertise Needed: Occupational therapy, psychotherapy, chemotherapy, pathology, blood bank, operating room, administration supervision, radiation therapy

Contact: Mr Richard Sierra
Human Resources Generalist
(305) 854-4400

MERCY HOSPITAL OF LAREDO

1515 LOGAN AVENUE
LAREDO, TEXAS 78040-4617

Description: Public hospital
Annual Sales: $95.2 million
Number of Employees: 1,500
Expertise Needed: Registered nursing, occupational therapy, physical therapy

Contact: Mr Robert Chapa
Personnel Director
(210) 718-6222

THE MERCY HOSPITAL OF PITTSBURGH

1400 LOCUST STREET
PITTSBURGH, PENNSYLVANIA 15219-5166

Description: Nonprofit hospital specializing in trauma and cardiac care
Annual Sales: $199.8 million
Number of Employees: 2,500

Expertise Needed: Nursing, physical therapy, respiratory therapy, occupational therapy

Contact: Ms Judy Jim
Nursing Recruiter
(412) 232-8111

MERCY MEDICAL CENTER

1000 NORTH VILLAGE AVENUE
ROCKVILLE CENTRE, NEW YORK 11570-1000

Description: Church-operated medical and surgical hospital
Founded: 1913
Annual Sales: $126.1 million
Number of Employees: 1,800
Expertise Needed: Registered nursing

Contact: Mr John W Kafader
Vice President of Human Resources
(516) 255-0111

MERCY MEDICAL CENTER OF WILLISTON

1301 15TH AVENUE WEST
WILLISTON, NORTH DAKOTA 58801-3821

Description: Nonprofit private hospital
Founded: 1920
Annual Sales: $21.8 million
Number of Employees: 450
Expertise Needed: Registered nursing, licensed practical nursing, respiratory therapy, physical therapy, occupational therapy, anesthesiology nursing

Contact: Ms Janice Arnson
Director of Human Resources
(701) 774-7400

MERIDIA HEALTH SYSTEMS

6700 BETA DRIVE
CLEVELAND, OHIO 44143-2335

Description: Public hospital
Annual Sales: $101.4 million
Number of Employees: 1,200
Expertise Needed: Nursing, general surgery, surgical technology, physical therapy, occupational therapy

Contact: Professional Recruiter
(216) 446-8628

MERIS LABORATORIES, INC.

2890 ZANKER ROAD
SAN JOSE, CALIFORNIA 95134-2118

Description: Clinical laboratory
Annual Sales: $35.8 million
Number of Employees: 500
Expertise Needed: Phlebotomy, microbiology, medical laboratory technology

Contact: Ms Vicki Driver
Human Resources Manager
(408) 434-9200

MERIT MEDICAL SYSTEMS, INC.
79 WEST 4500
SALT LAKE CITY, UTAH 84107-2649

Description: Manufactures medical devices
Annual Sales: $18.4 million
Number of Employees: 325
Expertise Needed: Mechanical engineering, electrical
engineering, accounting, finance, data processing

Contact: Mr Brent Bowen
Manager of Human Resources
(801) 263-9300

MERITCARE MEDICAL GROUP
737 BROADWAY
FARGO, NORTH DAKOTA 58123

Description: Health-care clinic
Founded: 1919
Annual Sales: $120.1 million
Number of Employees: 1,600
Expertise Needed: Accounting, finance, data processing,
registered nursing, licensed practical nursing,
physicians

Contact: Ms Mona Lokken
Manager of Recruitment and Employment
(701) 234-2000

MET PATH LABORATORIES
5850 WEST CYPRESS STREET
TAMPA, FLORIDA 33607-1782

Description: Clinical laboratory
Parent Company: Damon Corporation
Annual Sales: $19.3 million
Number of Employees: 400
Expertise Needed: Laboratory technology

Contact: Ms Sandy Owen
Employment Manager
(813) 289-5400

METHODIST HOSPITAL
6500 EXCELSIOR BOULEVARD
ST. LOUIS PARK, MINNESOTA 55426-4702

Description: General medical and surgical hospital
Founded: 1892
Annual Sales: $143.7 million
Number of Employees: 2,423
Expertise Needed: Occupational therapy, physical
therapy, nursing

Contact: Ms Susan Salzman
Employment Representative
(612) 932-5000

THE METHODIST HOSPITAL
6565 FANNIN STREET
HOUSTON, TEXAS 77030-2707

Description: General hospital
Founded: 1923
Annual Sales: $482.7 million

Number of Employees: 6,
Expertise Needed: Nursing,
medical records, manage
occupational therapy, respi

Contact: Mr Fred Heskett
Manager of Human Resource
(713) 790-4295

METHODIST HOSPITAL FOUNDATION
2301 SOUTH BROAD STREET
PHILADELPHIA, PENNSYLVANIA 19148-3542

Description: Conducts medical research
Annual Sales: $80.5 million
Number of Employees: 1,150
Expertise Needed: Nursing, occupational therapy,
physical therapy

Contact: Ms Claudia Weinberg
Manager of Employment
(215) 952-9395

METHODIST HOSPITAL OF INDIANA
1701 SENATE BOULEVARD
INDIANAPOLIS, INDIANA 46206-1239

Description: Nonprofit hospital
Founded: 1899
Annual Sales: $500.0 million
Number of Employees: 7,100
Expertise Needed: Registered nursing, occupational
therapy, pharmacology, radiology, physical therapy

Contact: Ms Susie Burlich
Human Resources Consultant
(317) 929-8931

METHODIST HOSPITAL OF LUBBOCK, TEXAS
3615 19TH STREET
LUBBOCK, TEXAS 79410

Description: Public hospital
Founded: 1918
Annual Sales: $187.3 million
Number of Employees: 8,450
Expertise Needed: Nursing, physical therapy, radiology

Contact: Ms Susie Luker
Nursing Recruiter
(806) 792-1011

THE METHODIST HOSPITALS, INC.
600 GRANT STREET
GARY, INDIANA 46402-6001

Description: Public general hospital
Founded: 1941
Annual Sales: $213.9 million
Number of Employees: 3,005

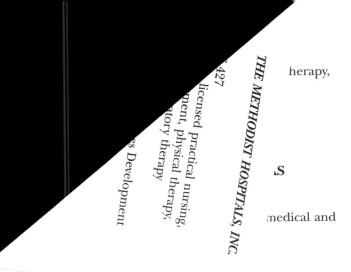

THE METHODIST HOSPITALS, INC.

...427

... licensed practical nursing,
... ment, physical therapy,
... tory therapy

...s Development

medical and

Number ...

Expertise Needed: Physician, ... apy,
occupational therapy, laboratory technology,
medical technology

Contact: Ms Joann Arias
Assistant Director of Human Relations
(214) 947-6510

METHODIST HOSPITALS OF MEMPHIS

1265 UNION AVENUE
MEMPHIS, TENNESSEE 38104-3415

Description: Private hospital
Founded: 1918
Annual Sales: $275.2 million
Number of Employees: 4,300
Expertise Needed: Physical therapy, registered nursing

Contact: Ms Mary Cavens
Director of Employment
(901) 726-7070

METHODIST MEDICAL CENTER OF OAK RIDGE

990 OAK RIDGE TURNPIKE
OAK RIDGE, TENNESSEE 37830-6976

Description: Public hospital providing general
health-care services
Founded: 1959
Annual Sales: $122.3 million
Number of Employees: 1,200
Expertise Needed: Registered nursing, physical therapy

Contact: Ms Rose Napier
Employment Manager
(615) 481-1124

METPATH, INC.

ONE MALCOLM AVENUE
TETERBORO, NEW JERSEY 07608-1011

Description: Provides medical and clinical laboratory
services
Parent Company: Corning, Inc.
Founded: 1967
Annual Sales: $1.8 billion
Number of Employees: 19,000

Expertise Needed: Customer service and support,
computer programming, laboratory assistance

Contact: Human Resources Administrator
(201) 393-5027

METPATH LABORATORIES

711 BINGHAM STREET
PITTSBURGH, PENNSYLVANIA 15203-1007

Description: Provides medical and clinical laboratory
services
Parent Company: Corning Lab Services, Inc.
Annual Sales: $107.2 million
Number of Employees: 2,000
Expertise Needed: Medical technology, biology,
chemistry, laboratory technology

Contact: Mr Edwin Koontz
Manager of Employment
(412) 488-7500

METPATH OF MICHIGAN

4444 GIDDINGS ROAD
AUBURN HILLS, MICHIGAN 48326-1533

Description: Provides medical and clinical laboratory
services
Parent Company: Corning Lab Services, Inc.
Annual Sales: $65.0 million
Number of Employees: 925
Expertise Needed: Medical technology, phlebotomy

Contact: Ms Cheryl Kaszuba
Manager of Employment
(810) 373-9120

METROHEALTH SYSTEM

2500 METROHEALTH DRIVE
CLEVELAND, OHIO 44109-1900

Description: Public general hospital
Founded: 1953
Annual Sales: $317.7 million
Number of Employees: 5,302
Expertise Needed: Registered nursing, physical therapy,
occupational therapy, pharmacology

Contact: Ms Kathy Bailor
Nursing Recruiter
(216) 459-3375

METROPOLITAN LIFE INSURANCE COMPANY

ONE MADISON AVENUE
NEW YORK, NEW YORK 10010-3603

Description: Provides life and health-care insurance
services
Founded: 1868
Assets: $118.0 billion
Number of Employees: 57,000

Expertise Needed: Health insurance, credit/credit analysis, computer programming, sales, law, advertising, marketing, actuarial, auditing

Contact: Mr Thomas O'Brien
Director of Recruiting and Staffing
(212) 578-2211

METTLER ELECTRONICS CORPORATION
1333 SOUTH CLAUDINA
ANAHEIM, CALIFORNIA 92805

Description: Manufactures therapeutic and ultrasonic equipment
Founded: 1957
Number of Employees: 100
Expertise Needed: Sales, electronics/electronics engineering

Contact: Human Resources
(714) 533-2221

MEYROWITZ OPTICIANS
520 5TH AVENUE
NEW YORK, NEW YORK 10036

Description: Owns and operates a chain of retail optical stores
Founded: 1875
Number of Employees: 50
Expertise Needed: Optometry, sales

Contact: Mr Mark Turturro
Recruiting
(212) 840-3880

MIAMI CHILDREN'S HOSPITAL
3100 SOUTHWEST 62ND AVENUE
MIAMI, FLORIDA 33155-3003

Description: Public hospital specializing in pediatrics
Founded: 1940
Annual Sales: $149.7 million
Number of Employees: 2,200
Expertise Needed: Registered nursing, physical therapy, occupational therapy, respiratory therapy

Contact for College Students and Recent Graduates:
Ms Karen Nesbitt
Nursing Recruiter
(305) 666-6511

Contact for All Other Candidates:
Ms Dorayne Rubaine
Director of Human Resources
(305) 666-6511

MIAMI JEWISH HOME HOSPITAL
5200 NORTHEAST 2ND AVENUE
MIAMI, FLORIDA 33137-2706

Description: Provides nursing home and acute-care rehabilitation services
Founded: 1945
Annual Sales: $40.1 million
Number of Employees: 1,200

Expertise Needed: Registered nursing, licensed practical nursing, physical therapy, occupational therapy, certified nursing and nursing assistance

Contact: Mr Laz Carrandi
Assistant Director of Employment
(305) 751-8626

MIAMI VALLEY HOSPITAL
1 WYOMING STREET
DAYTON, OHIO 45409-2722

Description: Nonprofit private hospital
Parent Company: Medical America Health Systems Corporation
Annual Sales: $192.0 million
Number of Employees: 3,400
Expertise Needed: Physical therapy, nursing

Contact: Ms Monica Stachler
Nursing Recruiter
(513) 223-6192

MICHIGAN MEDICAL CORPORATION
700 WARD DRIVE
SANTA BARBARA, CALIFORNIA 93111-2919

Description: Manufactures medical equipment and implants
Parent Company: Inamed Corporation
Annual Sales: $20.1 million
Number of Employees: 265
Expertise Needed: Electrical engineering, mechanical engineering, accounting, finance, data processing

Contact: Ms Jo Campos
Employment Services Assistant
(805) 683-6761

MICRO HEALTHSYSTEMS, INC.
414 EAGLE ROCK AVENUE
WEST ORANGE, NEW JERSEY 07052-4211

Description: Designs and develops financial and patient information management systems
Founded: 1970
Annual Sales: $23.6 million
Number of Employees: 250
Number of Managerial and Professional Employees Hired 1993: 90
Expertise Needed: Sales, software engineering/development, computer programming, finance, registered nursing

Contact: Mr. Dan Beards
Vice President of Human Resources
(201) 731-9252

MICROBIOLOGICAL ASSOCIATES, INC.
9900 BLACKWELL ROAD
ROCKVILLE, MARYLAND 20850

Description: Provides biological, genetic, and microbial testing services
Founded: 1947
Annual Sales: $240.0 million

Microbiological Associates, Inc. (continued)

Number of Employees: 200
Expertise Needed: Biomedical technology, microbiology, life sciences, laboratory science, laboratory technology
Contact: Ms Pam Erickson
       Employee Services Manager
       (301) 728-1000

MICROBIOLOGY REFERENCE LAB
10703 PROGRESS WAY
CYPRESS, CALIFORNIA 90630

Description: Provides infectious disease testing
Founded: 1977
Number of Employees: 150
Expertise Needed: Biochemistry, microbiology, laboratory technology, laboratory science
Contact: Ms Mary Ann Aadnesen
       Recruiter
       (619) 726-9418

MICROGENICS CORPORATION
2380 A BISSO LANE
CONCORD, CALIFORNIA 94520

Description: Provides commercial research services and manufactures diagnostic substances
Founded: 1981
Number of Employees: 225
Number of Managerial and Professional Employees Hired 1993: 25
Expertise Needed: Chemistry, laboratory technology, accounting, management information systems, marketing, sales
Contact: Ms Terry Hansen
       Director of Human Resources
       (510) 674-0667

MICROMERITICS INSTRUMENT CORPORATION
1 MICROMERITICS DRIVE
NORCROSS, GEORGIA 30093-1877

Description: Manufactures analytical instruments, measuring devices, and controlling devices
Founded: 1962
Number of Employees: 220
Expertise Needed: Software engineering/development, manufacturing engineering
Contact: Ms Lori Smith
       Human Resources Specialist
       (404) 662-3620

MICROPUMP CORPORATION
1402 NORTHEAST 136TH AVENUE
VANCOUVER, WASHINGTON 98684-8975

Description: Manufactures pumps and pumping equipment
Founded: 1960

Number of Employees: 135
Expertise Needed: Mechanical engineering, electronics/electronics engineering, project engineering, product engineering, sales, management
Contact: Ms Mindy Harter
       Human Resources Assistant
       (206) 253-2008

MICROTEK MEDICAL, INC.
512 LEHMBERG ROAD
COLUMBUS, MISSISSIPPI 39702

Description: Manufactures medical supplies and devices
Annual Sales: $25.8 million
Number of Employees: 500
Expertise Needed: Production management, accounting, anesthesiology, mechanical engineering, medical laboratory technology, marketing, sales, controlling, management, purchasing
Contact: Ms Nancy Betts
       Manager of Employment
       (601) 327-1863

MID ATLANTIC MEDICAL SERVICES
4 TAFT COURT
ROCKVILLE, MARYLAND 20850-5310

Description: Provides administrative management services
Annual Sales: $579.4 million
Number of Employees: 725
Expertise Needed: Actuarial, underwriting
Contact: Ms Julie Roth
       Manager of Human Resources
       (301) 762-8205

MIDAS REX PNEUMATIC TOOLS, INC.
2925 RACE STREET
FORT WORTH, TEXAS 76111

Description: Manufactures surgical instruments
Founded: 1964
Number of Employees: 100
Expertise Needed: Sales
Contact: Ms Kim Betts
       Executive Assistant
       (817) 831-4181

MIDDLESEX HOSPITAL
28 CRESCENT STREET
MIDDLETOWN, CONNECTICUT 06457-3650

Description: General medical and surgical hospital
Annual Sales: $103.5 million
Number of Employees: 1,320
Expertise Needed: Radiology, physicians, registered nursing, operating room, triage, gynecology, obstetrics
Contact: Human Resources Department
       (203) 347-9471

MIDMARK CORPORATION
60 VISTA DRIVE
VERSAILLES, OHIO 45380

Description: Manufactures medical furniture, lighting equipment, and sterilizers
Founded: 1960
Annual Sales: $50.0 million
Number of Employees: 500
Expertise Needed: Mechanical engineering, industrial engineering
Contact: Mr Jeff Farley
Manager of Human Resources
(513) 526-3662

MIDWEST DENTAL PRODUCTS CORPORATION
901 WEST OAKTON STREET
DES PLAINES, ILLINOIS 60018-1843

Description: Manufactures dental equipment and cleaning solutions
Parent Company: Dentsply International, Inc.
Annual Sales: $156.0 million
Number of Employees: 980
Expertise Needed: Manufacturing engineering, mechanical engineering, research and development
Contact: Ms Gloria McFadden
Vice President of Human Resources
(708) 640-4800

MIDWEST FOUNDATION
655 EDEN PARK DRIVE
CINCINNATI, OHIO 45202

Description: Provides health and medical insurance services
Founded: 1978
Annual Sales: $242.8 million
Number of Employees: 340
Expertise Needed: Claims adjustment/examination, actuarial, accounting
Contact: Ms Susan Osha
Human Resources Recruiter
(513) 784-5200

MILES, INC.
500 GRANT STREET
PITTSBURGH, PENNSYLVANIA 15219

Description: Develops, manufactures, and distributes pharmaceuticals, chemicals, and imaging products
Founded: 1973
Annual Sales: $6.5 billion
Number of Employees: 27,000
Expertise Needed: Marketing, accounting, sales, finance, pharmacy, biology, chemistry, physics, chemical engineering, mechanical engineering
Contact: Mr Mark Sappir
Director of Staffing
(412) 394-5500

MILLENNIUM PHARMACEUTICALS
640 MEMORIAL DRIVE
CAMBRIDGE, MASSACHUSETTS 02139

Description: Biopharmaceutical research company
Number of Employees: 80
Expertise Needed: Biology, chemistry, biochemistry
Contact: Mr Tony Zaritheny
Director of Scientific Recruiting
(617) 374-9480

MINE SAFETY APPLIANCES COMPANY
121 GAMMA DRIVE
PITTSBURGH, PENNSYLVANIA 15238-2919

Description: Develops and manufactures safety equipment
Founded: 1914
Annual Sales: $502.4 million
Number of Employees: 5,100
Number of Managerial and Professional Employees Hired 1993: 25
Expertise Needed: Research and development, finance, accounting, manufacturing engineering, electrical engineering, chemical engineering, industrial engineering
Contact: Mr Kenneth Krall
Manager of Personnel Development
(412) 967-3000

MINNEAPOLIS CHILDREN'S MEDICAL CENTER
2525 CHICAGO AVENUE SOUTH
MINNEAPOLIS, MINNESOTA 55404-4518

Description: Nonprofit children's hospital
Founded: 1953
Annual Sales: $92.2 million
Number of Employees: 1,800
Expertise Needed: Child therapy, health care, registered nursing, licensed practical nursing, radiology, physical therapy, nursing management and administration, speech therapy, respiratory therapy
Contact: Human Resources Department
(612) 863-6112

MINNESOTA MINING & MANUFACTURING COMPANY
3M CENTER
SAINT PAUL, MINNESOTA 55144-1000

Description: Manufactures adhesives, polymers, coatings, digital information and imaging products, and surgical supplies
Founded: 1902
Annual Sales: $13.9 billion
Number of Employees: 87,015

Minneapolis Children's Medical Center (continued)

Expertise Needed: Chemical engineering, mechanical engineering, electrical engineering, materials science, chemistry

Contact: Mr Marty Hanson
College Relations Director
(612) 723-1755

MINNTECH CORPORATION
14605 28TH AVENUE NORTH
MINNEAPOLIS, MINNESOTA 55447-4822

Description: Develops and manufactures dialysis treatment and cardiovascular surgery devices
Founded: 1974
Annual Sales: $44.3 million
Number of Employees: 285
Expertise Needed: Biochemistry, laboratory technology, medical technology, physicians, biomedical engineering, mechanical engineering, electronics/ electronics engineering

Contact: Mr. Gene Johnson
Director of Human Resources
(612) 553-3300

MIRIAM HOSPITAL, INC.
164 SUMMIT AVENUE
PROVIDENCE, RHODE ISLAND 02906-2800

Description: Public hospital specializing in open-heart surgery
Annual Sales: $98.6 million
Number of Employees: 1,700
Expertise Needed: Nursing

Contact: Ms Vi Colabella
Nursing Recruiter
(401) 331-8500

MISSOURI BAPTIST MEDICAL CENTER
3015 NORTH BALLAS ROAD
SAINT LOUIS, MISSOURI 63131-2317

Description: Private hospital with a heart center
Founded: 1889
Annual Sales: $123.7 million
Number of Employees: 2,100
Expertise Needed: Occupational therapy, medical laboratory technology, nursing

Contact: Ms Joan Kulterer
Employment Manager
(314) 432-1212

MOLECULAR BIOSYSTEMS, INC.
10030 BARNES CANYON ROAD
SAN DIEGO, CALIFORNIA 92121

Description: Manufactures analytical instruments and biological products
Founded: 1980
Number of Employees: 169

Expertise Needed: Ultrasound technology, mechanical engineering

Contact: Ms. Cynthia Mendez
Director of Human Resources
(619) 452-0681

MOLECULAR DEVICES CORPORATION
1311 ORLEANS DRIVE
SUNNYVALE, CALIFORNIA 94089

Description: Manufactures and markets laboratory analytical systems
Number of Employees: 130
Expertise Needed: Design engineering, mechanical engineering, accounting

Contact: Ms Jan Dahlin
Director of Human Resources
(408) 747-1700

MONMOUTH MEDICAL CENTER
300 2ND AVENUE
LONG BRANCH, NEW JERSEY 07740-6300

Description: General hospital
Parent Company: Mid Atlantic Health Group, Inc.
Founded: 1889
Annual Sales: $167.0 million
Number of Employees: 1,975
Expertise Needed: Clinical services, biology, X-ray technology, chemistry, oncology, pediatric care, rehabilitation, dialysis, cardiology

Contact: Ms Karen Methot
Health Recruiter
(908) 222-5200

MONTEFIORE MEDICAL CENTER
111 EAST 210TH STREET
BRONX, NEW YORK 10467-2401

Description: General hospital
Founded: 1884
Annual Sales: $853.3 million
Number of Employees: 9,500
Expertise Needed: Radiology, cardiology, physicians, oncology

Contact: Ms Maria Alport
Director of Human Resources
(718) 920-4321

MONTEFIORE UNIVERSITY HOSPITAL
3459 5TH AVENUE
PITTSBURGH, PENNSYLVANIA 15213-3241

Description: General medical and surgical hospital
Annual Sales: $199.2 million
Number of Employees: 1,600

Expertise Needed: Registered nursing, radiology, licensed practical nursing, physical therapy, occupational therapy, cardiology, pediatric therapy, pediatric care, laboratory technology, accounting

Contact: Human Resources Department
(412) 647-3290

MORRISTOWN MEMORIAL HOSPITAL

100 MADISON AVENUE
MORRISTOWN, NEW JERSEY 07962-1956

Description: General medical and surgical hospital
Annual Sales: $247.2 million
Number of Employees: 2,900
Expertise Needed: Registered nursing, physical therapy, occupational therapy

Contact: Ms Leslie Meyer
Nursing Manager
(201) 971-5000

MOTHER FRANCES HOSPITAL

800 EAST DAWSON STREET
TYLER, TEXAS 75701-2093

Description: Nonprofit hospital specializing in cardiac care
Founded: 1937
Annual Sales: $114.1 million
Number of Employees: 1,600
Expertise Needed: Nursing, medical laboratory technology, physical therapy, nursing management and administration

Contact: Ms Susan West
Nurse Recruiter
(903) 531-4472

MOUNT CARMEL HEALTH

793 WEST STATE STREET
COLUMBUS, OHIO 43222-1551

Description: Health-care facility
Founded: 1978
Annual Sales: $304.1 million
Number of Employees: 4,295
Expertise Needed: Nursing, allied health

Contact: Ms Sharon Mason
Health Recruiter
(614) 225-5000

MOUNT CLEMENS GENERAL HOSPITAL

1000 HARRINGTON STREET
MOUNT CLEMENS, MICHIGAN 48043-2920

Description: General and surgical hospital
Parent Company: MCG Telesis, Inc.
Annual Sales: $108.0 million
Number of Employees: 1,300

Expertise Needed: Physical therapy, occupational therapy, registered nursing, respiratory therapy

Contact: Ms Lenore Snow
Recruitment Specialist
(810) 792-4180

THE MOUNT SINAI MEDICAL CENTER

1 MOUNT SINAI DRIVE
CLEVELAND, OHIO 44106-4191

Description: Not-for-profit medical and surgical hospital
Founded: 1913
Annual Sales: $161.1 million
Number of Employees: 2,400
Expertise Needed: Registered nursing, radiology, nursing management and administration, coronary care, cardiology, licensed practical nursing, occupational therapy, physical therapy, accounting, data processing

Contact: Mr Steve Drogus
Vice President of Human Resources
(216) 421-4000

JOHN MUIR MEDICAL CENTER

1601 YGNACIO VALLEY ROAD
WALNUT CREEK, CALIFORNIA 94598-3122

Description: Not-for-profit medical and surgical hospital
Founded: 1958
Annual Sales: $149.1 million
Number of Employees: 2,200
Expertise Needed: Registered nursing, occupational therapy, physical therapy

Contact: Ms Kathy Maxwell
Nursing Recruiter
(510) 939-3000

MVP HEALTH PLAN

111 LIBERTY STREET
SCHENECTADY, NEW YORK 12305-1892

Description: Health maintenance organization
Annual Sales: $178.8 million
Number of Employees: 240
Expertise Needed: Health care, health insurance, claims adjustment/examination

Contact: Mr James Morrill
Director of Human Resources
(518) 370-4793

MYCOGEN CORPORATION

4980 CARROLL CANYON ROAD
SAN DIEGO, CALIFORNIA 92121

Description: Diversified agricultural biotechnology company
Founded: 1982
Number of Employees: 200

Mycogen Corporation (continued)

Expertise Needed: Chemical engineering, chemistry

Contact: Ms Naomi Whitacre
Director of Human Resources
(619) 453-8030

MYLAN LABORATORIES, INC.
781 CHESTNUT RIDGE ROAD
MORGANTOWN, WEST VIRGINIA 26505

Description: Manufactures pharmaceutical products
Founded: 1976
Annual Sales: $212.0 million
Number of Employees: 1,037
Expertise Needed: Laboratory technology, chemistry,
microbiology, pharmacy, accounting, life sciences

Contact: Mr Robert L Myers
Director of Human Resources
(304) 599-2595

MYRIAD GENETICS
421 WAKARA
SALT LAKE CITY, UTAH 84108

Description: Genetic research firm
Number of Employees: 45
Expertise Needed: Genetics

Contact: Ms Heather Burton
Personnel Administrator
(801) 582-3400

NAD, INC.
3135 QUARRY ROAD
TELFORD, PENNSYLVANIA 18969-1049

Description: Manufactures medical supplies
Founded: 1977
Annual Sales: $36.1 million
Number of Employees: 430
Expertise Needed: Biomedical, design engineering,
mechanical engineering, technology

Contact: Mr William Kysor
Employment Manager
(215) 723-9824

NALGE COMPANY
75 PANORAMA CREEK DRIVE
ROCHESTER, NEW YORK 14602-0365

Description: Manufactures plastic products
Founded: 1949
Number of Employees: 580
*Number of Managerial and Professional Employees Hired
1993:* 10
Expertise Needed: Plastics engineering, design
engineering, mechanical engineering, chemical
engineering, manufacturing engineering, product
management, sales, marketing

Contact: Mr Marty Wheeler
Manager of Employment and Compensation
(716) 586-8800

NAPLES COMMUNITY HOSPITAL, INC.
350 7TH STREET NORTH
NAPLES, FLORIDA 33940-5754

Description: Public hospital specializing in acute care
Founded: 1956
Annual Sales: $142.4 million
Number of Employees: 1,800
Expertise Needed: Nursing, allied health

Contact: Ms Dianne Janson
Allied Health Recruiter
(813) 262-3131

NATIONAL HEALTH CARE AFFILIATES
651 DELAWARE AVENUE
BUFFALO, NEW YORK 14202-1001

Description: Owns and operates skilled and
intermediate nursing care and residential care
facilities
Founded: 1977
Annual Sales: $50.2 million
Number of Employees: 2,300
Expertise Needed: Administration

Contact: Human Resources Department
(716) 881-4425

NATIONAL HEALTH LABS, INC.
4225 EXECUTIVE SQUARE
LA JOLLA, CALIFORNIA 92037-4849

Description: Owns and operates clinical laboratories
Founded: 1966
Annual Sales: $721.4 million
Number of Employees: 14,500
*Number of Managerial and Professional Employees Hired
1993:* 754
Expertise Needed: Accounting, finance, auditing,
marketing, computer programming, systems
integration, medical laboratory technology

Contact: Ms Kathie Livingston
Manager of Personnel
(619) 550-0600

NATIONAL HEALTHCORP
100 EAST VINE STREET
MURFREESBORO, TENNESSEE 37130-3734

Description: Owns, leases, and operates long-term
health-care facilities
Founded: 1971
Annual Sales: $216.4 million
Number of Employees: 10,543
Expertise Needed: Accounting, finance, data processing,
law, physical therapy, occupational therapy, speech
pathology

Contact: Mr Jim Keathley
Vice President of Corporate Affairs
(615) 890-2020

NATIONAL HEALTHTECH CORPORATION

10101 SLATER AVENUE STREET
FOUNTAIN VALLEY, CALIFORNIA 92708-4741

Description: Provides computer systems for hospitals and physicians
Founded: 1991
Annual Sales: $27.5 million
Number of Employees: 300
Expertise Needed: Information systems, management information systems, facilities management, project management, management
Contact: Ms Eileen Sepulveda
　　　　Director of Human Resources
　　　　(714) 963-0379

NATIONAL HMO (NEW YORK), INC.

850 BRONX RIVER ROAD
YONKERS, NEW YORK 10708

Description: Health maintenance organization
Number of Employees: 100
Expertise Needed: Accounting, finance, registered nursing, licensed practical nursing, physicians, marketing, data processing, health care, certified medical assistance, certified nursing and nursing assistance
Contact: Ms Maria DiVincenzo
　　　　Corporate Billing Director
　　　　(914) 776-2800

NATIONAL HOMECARE SYSTEMS, INC.

10 WEST KINZIE STREET
CHICAGO, ILLINOIS 60610

Description: Provides home health-care services
Founded: 1972
Annual Sales: $74.8 million
Number of Employees: 9,000
Expertise Needed: Registered nursing, accounting, administration
Contact: Ms Marlene Marley
　　　　Employment Manager
　　　　(312) 321-6244

NATIONAL INSTITUTIONAL PHARMACEUTICAL SERVICES

6001 INDIAN SCHOOL
ALBUQUERQUE, NEW MEXICO 87110-4139

Description: Provides pharmacy management services for nursing homes and hospitals
Parent Company: Horizon Healthcare Corporation
Annual Sales: $33.0 million
Number of Employees: 150
Expertise Needed: Nursing
Contact: Ms Peggy Cave
　　　　Recruiter
　　　　(505) 881-4961

NATIONAL MEDICAL CARE AND LIFE CHEM LABORATORIES SERVICES

22 PARIS AVENUE
ROCKLEIGH, NEW JERSEY 07647-2605

Description: Distributes and manufactures medical supplies
Parent Company: National Medical Care, Inc.
Annual Sales: $38.1 million
Number of Employees: 780
Expertise Needed: Engineering, accounting, business
Contact: Ms Glenna Antzak
　　　　Employment Manager
　　　　(201) 767-7700

NATIONAL MEDICAL CARE, HOME CARE DIVISION

1601 TRAPELO ROAD
WALTHAM, MASSACHUSETTS 02154

Description: Provides home health-care services specializing in home infusion therapy
Annual Sales: $60.9 million
Number of Employees: 1,200
Expertise Needed: Marketing, allied therapy, nursing, home health care
Contact: Human Resources Department
　　　　(800) 662-1237

NATIONAL MEDICAL CARE, INC.

1601 TRAPELO ROAD
WALTHAM, MASSACHUSETTS 02154

Description: Provides home health-care and nursing care services and distributes medical equipment
Parent Company: W. R. Grace & Company, Inc.
Founded: 1968
Annual Sales: $1.0 billion
Number of Employees: 14,000
Expertise Needed: Accounting, marketing, finance, computer programming, mechanical engineering, data processing, project engineering
Contact: Mr Tim Kerrigan
　　　　Manager of Employee Relations
　　　　(617) 466-9850

NATIONAL MEDICAL COMPUTER SERVICE

8928 TERMAN COURT
SAN DIEGO, CALIFORNIA 92121

Description: Develops and sells computer systems for hospitals and physicians
Founded: 1974
Number of Employees: 250
Expertise Needed: Software engineering/development, computer programming
Contact: Ms Denise Key
　　　　Human Resources Assistant
　　　　(619) 566-5800

NATIONAL MEDICAL ENTERPRISES

2700 COLORADO AVENUE
SANTA MONICA, CALIFORNIA 90404-3521

Description: Owns and operates hospitals and substance abuse treatment facilities
Founded: 1968
Annual Sales: $3.8 billion
Number of Employees: 50,423
Expertise Needed: Accounting, finance, marketing
Contact: Mr Alan Ewalt
Senior Vice President of Human Resources
(310) 998-8238

NATIONAL MEDICAL HOMECARE CORPORATION

1601 TRAPELO ROAD
WALTHAM, MASSACHUSETTS 02154-8237

Description: Provides home infusion therapy services
Parent Company: Healthdyne, Inc.
Annual Sales: $129.0 million
Number of Employees: 1,000
Expertise Needed: Home health care, nursing, nutrition, physical therapy
Contact: Human Resources Department
(617) 466-9850

NATIONAL SERVICE INDUSTRIES, INC.

1420 PEACHTREE STREET NORTHEAST
ATLANTA, GEORGIA 30309

Description: Manufactures textiles, lighting fixtures, and industrial chemicals
Founded: 1928
Expertise Needed: Sales, marketing
Contact: Human Resources Department
(404) 853-1000

NATIONAL VISION ASSOCIATES, LTD.

296 SOUTH CLAYTON STREET
LAWRENCEVILLE, GEORGIA 30245

Description: Operates leased vision centers
Number of Employees: 200
Expertise Needed: Accounting
Contact: Ms Lisa Schultz
Administrative Assistant
(404) 822-3600

NATURE'S BOUNTY, INC.

90 ORVILLE DRIVE
BOHEMIA, NEW YORK 11716

Description: Manufactures and markets vitamins and other nutritional supplements
Founded: 1971
Number of Employees: 1,000
Number of Managerial and Professional Employees Hired 1993: 6

Expertise Needed: Chemistry, biology, biochemistry
Contact: Personnel Department
(516) 567-9500

NATURE'S SUNSHINE PRODUCTS, INC.

75 EAST 1700 SOUTH
PROVO, UTAH 84606-7319

Description: Manufactures and distributes nutritional and personal care products
Founded: 1976
Annual Sales: $31.6 million
Number of Employees: 430
Expertise Needed: Mechanical engineering, electrical engineering, production engineering
Contact: Mr Dan Gelisen
Human Resources Director
(801) 342-4300

NDC FEDERAL SYSTEMS, INC.

1300 PICARD DRIVE
ROCKVILLE, MARYLAND 20850-4303

Description: Provides health-care practice management software
Number of Employees: 120
Expertise Needed: Software engineering/development, computer programming
Contact: Ms Lynn Schneider
Director of Human Resources
(201) 590-7700

NEDH CORPORATION

185 PILGRIM ROAD
BOSTON, MASSACHUSETTS 02215-5324

Description: General hospital
Founded: 1896
Annual Sales: $264.2 million
Number of Employees: 3,431
Expertise Needed: Cardiology, registered nursing, licensed practical nursing, oncology, dialysis
Contact: Ms Lisa Selleck
Recruiter
(617) 632-8137

NELLCOR, INC.

4280 HACIENDA DRIVE
PLEASANTON, CALIFORNIA 94588-3618

Description: Manufactures and markets blood oxygen monitoring equipment
Annual Sales: $218.2 million
Number of Employees: 1,720
Number of Managerial and Professional Employees Hired 1993: 150
Expertise Needed: Product design and development, software engineering/development, design

engineering, electrical engineering, marketing, finance, mechanical engineering, management information systems

Contact: Ms Victoria Campbell
      Manager of Employment
      (510) 463-4000

NEMOURS FOUNDATION
1650 PRUDENTIAL DRIVE
JACKSONVILLE, FLORIDA 32207-8147

Description: Health-care foundation for children
Founded: 1974
Annual Sales: $128.3 million
Number of Employees: 1,350
Expertise Needed: Physical therapy, registered nursing, licensed practical nursing, occupational therapy

Contact: Mr Gordon Joyner
      Director of Human Resources
      (904) 390-3647

NESLAB INSTRUMENTS, INC.
25 NIMBOE HILL ROAD
NEWINGTON, NEW HAMPSHIRE 03802-1178

Description: Manufactures refrigeration and heating equipment for laboratories
Founded: 1963
Number of Employees: 250
Expertise Needed: Manufacturing engineering, mechanical engineering

Contact: Ms Lori McHugh
      Manager of Human Resources
      (603) 436-9444

NEUMAN DISTRIBUTORS, INC.
175 RAILROAD AVENUE
RIDGEFIELD, NEW JERSEY 07657

Description: Distributes pharmaceutical goods
Parent Company: OCP International, Inc.
Annual Sales: $353.1 million
Number of Employees: 390
Expertise Needed: Accounting, sales, marketing, computer programming

Contact: Ms Barbara Toscano
      Director of Human Resources
      (201) 941-2000

NEUROMED, INC.
5000-A OAKES ROAD
FORT LAUDERDALE, FLORIDA 33314

Description: Develops and manufactures implantable neurosimulators
Expertise Needed: Engineering, electronics/electronics engineering, production, quality control

Contact: Human Resources Department
      (305) 587-3600

NEW BRITAIN GENERAL HOSPITAL
100 GRAND STREET
NEW BRITAIN, CONNECTICUT 06050

Description: Community hospital
Founded: 1893
Annual Sales: $122.0 million
Number of Employees: 2,548
Expertise Needed: Registered nursing, medical technology, EKG technology

Contact: Ms Kelly Scarrozzo
      Nursing Recruiter
      (203) 224-5011

NEW BRUNSWICK SCIENTIFIC COMPANY, INC.
44 TALMADGE ROAD
EDISON, NEW JERSEY 08818-4005

Description: Manufactures and markets biotechnology equipment, analytical instruments, and laboratory equipment
Founded: 1946
Expertise Needed: Design engineering, mechanical engineering, industrial engineering, accounting, sales, marketing

Contact: Human Resources Department
      (908) 287-1200

NEW HANOVER REGIONAL MEDICAL CENTER
2131 SOUTH 17TH STREET
WILMINGTON, NORTH CAROLINA 28402

Description: Public hospital
Founded: 1967
Annual Sales: $163.7 million
Number of Employees: 2,720
Expertise Needed: Registered nursing, occupational therapy, physical therapy

Contact: Ms Barbara Sturniolo
      Employment Manager
      (919) 343-7049

NEW YORK CITY HEALTH HOSPITALS CORPORATION
125 WORTH STREET
NEW YORK, NEW YORK 10013-4006

Description: Owns and operates hospitals
Founded: 1970
Annual Sales: $3.4 billion
Number of Employees: 47,000
Expertise Needed: Data processing, management information systems, accounting, finance, electrical engineering, marketing, mechanical engineering

Contact: Ms Gloria Velez
      Director of Human Resources
      (212) 730-3303

NEWARK BETH ISRAEL MEDICAL CENTER

201 LYONS AVENUE
NEWARK, NEW JERSEY 07112-2027

Description: General medical and surgical hospital
Annual Sales: $204.2 million
Number of Employees: 3,000
Expertise Needed: Social work, physical therapy, occupational therapy, obstetrics, gynecology, registered nursing, medical technology, laboratory technology

Contact: Ms Mary Kay Carter
Recruiter
(201) 926-7000

NEWPORT CORPORATION

1791 DEERE AVENUE
IRVINE, CALIFORNIA 92714-4814

Description: Manufactures laser-related and electro-optical laboratory equipment
Founded: 1938
Annual Sales: $87.8 million
Number of Employees: 748
Expertise Needed: Optics, electrical engineering, drafting, mechanical engineering

Contact: Ms Jan Denny
Manager of Human Resources
(714) 863-3144

NEWTON WELLESLEY HOSPITAL

2014 WASHINGTON STREET
NEWTON, MASSACHUSETTS 02162-1699

Description: General medical and surgical hospital
Founded: 1881
Annual Sales: $107.9 million
Number of Employees: 2,200
Expertise Needed: Registered nursing, nursing management and administration, emergency nursing, intensive care nursing, psychiatric nursing, certified nursing and nursing assistance, chemical dependency, occupational therapy, physical therapy

Contact: Human Resources Department
(617) 243-6000

NICHOLS INSTITUTE, INC.

1212 SOUTH EUCLID AVENUE
SIOUX FALLS, SOUTH DAKOTA 57105

Description: Clinical laboratory
Founded: 1988
Annual Sales: $21.2 million
Number of Employees: 440
Number of Managerial and Professional Employees Hired 1993: 10
Expertise Needed: Data processing, accounting, finance, medical technology

Contact: Mr Brian Bohn
Director of Human Resources
(605) 339-1212

NICHOLS INSTITUTE REFERENCE LABORATORIES

33608 ORTEGA HIGHWAY
SAN JUAN CAPISTRANO, CALIFORNIA 92675

Description: Clinical research laboratory
Parent Company: Nichols Institute
Founded: 1971
Annual Sales: $110.0 million
Number of Employees: 900
Expertise Needed: Laboratory assistance, medical laboratory technology, biology, chemistry, medical technology, marketing, sales, histology

Contact: Ms Debbie Conry
Human Resources Manager
(714) 728-4000

NICHOLS RESEARCH CORPORATION

4040 SOUTH MEMORIAL PARKWAY
HUNTSVILLE, ALABAMA 35802-1396

Description: Research and development laboratory
Founded: 1976
Annual Sales: $117.2 million
Number of Employees: 979
Expertise Needed: Electrical engineering, software engineering/development, computer programming

Contact: Ms Peggy Cerny
Employment Manager
(205) 883-1140

NME HOSPITALS, INC.

2700 COLORADO AVENUE
SANTA MONICA, CALIFORNIA 90404-3521

Description: Owns and operates hospitals and medical centers
Parent Company: National Medical Enterprises
Founded: 1968
Annual Sales: $2.1 billion
Number of Employees: 21,700
Expertise Needed: Accounting, finance, nursing, chemical engineering, electrical engineering, data processing

Contact: Ms Yvette Booker
Human Resources Administrator
(310) 988-8000

NME PROPERTIES, INC.

1145 BROADWAY PLAZA
TACOMA, WASHINGTON 98402-3513

Description: Leases health-care facilities
Parent Company: National Medical Enterprises
Founded: 1969
Annual Sales: $80.3 million
Number of Employees: 900
Expertise Needed: Accounting, marketing, finance, management information systems

Contact: Mr Alan Ewalt
Director of Human Resources
(206) 272-9203

NOR-LAKE, INC.
727 2ND STREET
HUDSON, WISCONSIN 54016

Description: Manufactures refrigeration equipment and laboratory incubators
Founded: 1947
Number of Employees: 200
Expertise Needed: Manufacturing engineering
Contact: Mr Paul Sederstrom
Personnel Manager
(715) 386-2323

NORDICTRACK, INC.
104 PEAVEY ROAD
CHASKA, MINNESOTA 55318-2324

Description: Manufactures exercise equipment
Parent Company: CML Group, Inc.
Annual Sales: $260.0 million
Number of Employees: 1,700
Expertise Needed: Accounting, finance, data processing, marketing, sales, manufacturing engineering, mechanical engineering, product design and development
Contact: Staffing Department
(612) 368-2500

NORRELL HEALTH CARE, INC.
3535 PIEDMONT ROAD NORTHEAST
ATLANTA, GEORGIA 30305

Description: Provides temporary and long-term health-care personnel services
Founded: 1981
Number of Employees: 500
Expertise Needed: Accounting, marketing, sales
Contact: Corporate Recruiter
(404) 240-3000

NORTEX DRUG DISTRIBUTORS, INC.
1021 NORTH CENTRAL EXPRESSWAY
PLANO, TEXAS 75075-8806

Description: Owns and operates drug stores
Founded: 1979
Annual Sales: $117.0 million
Number of Employees: 750
Expertise Needed: Management, sales, pharmaceutical
Contact: Mr Robert Anon
Operations Manager
(214) 424-2829

NORTH AMERICAN BIOLOGICALS, INC.
1111 PARK CENTER BOULEVARD
MIAMI, FLORIDA 33169

Description: Operates blood plasma centers
Annual Sales: $50.0 million
Number of Employees: 600

Expertise Needed: Chemistry, biology, laboratory technology
Contact: Ms Jan Cameron
Human Resources Assistant
(305) 625-5303

NORTH CAROLINA BAPTIST HOSPITAL
MEDICAL CENTER BOULEVARD
WINSTON SALEM, NORTH CAROLINA 27157-1185

Description: Provides health-care services
Founded: 1921
Annual Sales: $317.9 million
Number of Employees: 5,475
Expertise Needed: Nursing, pharmacy, radiation therapy, occupational therapy, physical therapy
Contact for College Students and Recent Graduates:
Ms Theresa Talbert
Nurse Recruiter
(910) 716-2933
Contact for All Other Candidates:
Ms Lisa Huffman
Corporate Recruiter
(910) 716-3367

NORTH CENTRAL HEALTH CARE FACILITY
1100 LAKEVIEW DRIVE
WAUSAU, WISCONSIN 54403-6778

Description: Psychiatric hospital and nursing home
Founded: 1974
Annual Sales: $30.7 million
Number of Employees: 875
Expertise Needed: Psychiatry, psychology, registered nursing, licensed practical nursing, physicians
Contact: Mr Michael Jelen
Human Resources Director
(715) 848-4600

NORTH MEMORIAL MEDICAL CENTER
3300 OAKDALE AVENUE NORTH
MINNEAPOLIS, MINNESOTA 55422-2926

Description: Nonprofit hospital, specializing in trauma
Founded: 1940
Annual Sales: $184.8 million
Number of Employees: 3,450
Expertise Needed: Registered nursing
Contact: Ms Lee Kern
Nursing Recruiter
(612) 520-5200

NORTH SHORE UNIVERSITY HOSPITAL
300 COMMUNITY DRIVE
MANHASSET, NEW YORK 11030-3801

Description: General hospital
Founded: 1946
Annual Sales: $398.9 million
Number of Employees: 4,720

North Shore University Hospital (continued)

Expertise Needed: Pediatric care, registered nursing, licensed practical nursing, laboratory technology

Contact: Ms Mary Ellen Beisner
Recruiter
(516) 562-4690

NORTH SUBURBAN CLINIC, LTD.
4801 CHURCH STREET
SKOKIE, ILLINOIS 60077-1362

Description: General health-care clinic
Founded: 1974
Annual Sales: $43.3 million
Number of Employees: 630
Expertise Needed: Registered nursing

Contact: Mr Mark Pieart
Director of Human Resources
(708) 674-9800

NORTHEAST GEORGIA HEALTH SERVICES
743 SPRING STREET EAST
GAINESVILLE, GEORGIA 30501

Description: Public hospital
Founded: 1951
Annual Sales: $122.0 million
Number of Employees: 2,000
Number of Managerial and Professional Employees Hired 1993: 200
Expertise Needed: Registered nursing, medical technology, physical therapy, nursing, occupational therapy

Contact: Mr Randy Johnson
Director of Human Resources
(404) 535-3500

NORTHERN HEALTH FACILITIES
105 WEST MICHIGAN STREET
MILWAUKEE, WISCONSIN 53203-2914

Description: Provides nursing home services
Parent Company: Unicare Health Facilities, Inc.
Annual Sales: $88.2 million
Number of Employees: 2,518
Expertise Needed: Registered nursing, physical therapy, home health care

Contact: Ms Io Schug
Director of Human Resources
(414) 271-9696

NORTHPORT HEALTH SERVICE, INC.
931 FAIRFAX PARK
TUSCALOOSA, ALABAMA 35406-2805

Description: Provides nursing home services
Annual Sales: $43.6 million
Number of Employees: 1,800

Expertise Needed: Home health care, registered nursing, licensed practical nursing, certified nursing and nursing assistance

Contact: Ms Debbie Elmore
Director of Human Resources
(205) 391-3600

NORTHWEST COMMUNITY HOSPITAL
800 WEST CENTRAL ROAD
ARLINGTON HEIGHTS, ILLINOIS 60005-2349

Description: Public hospital specializing in trauma and acute care
Founded: 1981
Annual Sales: $142.3 million
Number of Employees: 2,600
Expertise Needed: Registered nursing, physical therapy, medical technology, medical laboratory technology, accounting, occupational therapy

Contact for College Students and Recent Graduates:
Ms Donna Singer
Nursing Recruiter
(708) 259-1000

Contact for All Other Candidates:
Mr John Bauer
Manager of Employment
(708) 259-1000

NOVA MEDICAL SPECIALTIES, INC.
449 OAK SHADE ROAD
INDIAN MILLS, NEW JERSEY 08088

Description: Manufactures heart catheters
Founded: 1981
Number of Employees: 135
Expertise Needed: Nuclear engineering, mechanical engineering, accounting, quality engineering

Contact: Ms Katie Demko
Personnel Director
(609) 268-8080

NOVACARE, INC.
2570 BOULEVARD OF THE GENERALS
VALLEY FORGE, PENNSYLVANIA 19481

Description: Provides rehabilitation services and manufactures orthotics and prosthetics
Annual Sales: $539.1 million
Number of Employees: 7,750
Expertise Needed: Rehabilitation, nursing, physical therapy, occupational therapy, social work, psychology

Contact: Ms Elayne Patterson
Vice President of Human Resources Recruiting
(610) 992-7455

NU SKIN INTERNATIONAL
75 WEST CENTER STREET
PROVO, UTAH 84601-4479

Description: Manufactures skin-care and nutritional products
Founded: 1984
Annual Sales: $485.0 million
Number of Employees: 1,400
Expertise Needed: Marketing, sales, finance, accounting, data processing, law, nutrition, emergency services, biology, chemistry
Contact: Ms Liz Dalton
Director of Personnel and Human Resources
(801) 345-2500

NURSES PRN OF DENVER, INC.
9300 SOUTHWEST 87TH AVENUE
MIAMI, FLORIDA 33176-2413

Description: Provides temporary nursing personnel services
Founded: 1976
Annual Sales: $45.8 million
Number of Employees: 4,500
Expertise Needed: Registered nursing, licensed practical nursing, nursing management and administration, nursing, anesthesiology nursing, cardiovascular nursing, emergency nursing, intensive care nursing, maternity nursing
Contact: Human Resources Department
(305) 596-3331

NUTRAMAX PRODUCTS, INC.
9 BLACKBURN DRIVE
GLOUCESTER, MASSACHUSETTS 01930

Description: Manufactures health and personal care products
Number of Employees: 165
Expertise Needed: Accounting, sales
Contact: Human Resources Department
(508) 283-1800

NUVISION, INC.
2284 SOUTH BALLENGER HIGHWAY
FLINT, MICHIGAN 48501

Description: Owns and operates retail optical stores
Founded: 1952
Expertise Needed: Optometry, optics, sales, marketing, accounting
Contact: Mr Larry Warshaw
Executive Vice President of Retail Operations
(313) 767-0900

OAKWOOD HOSPITAL CORPORATION
1801 OAKWOOD BOULEVARD
DEABORN, MICHIGAN 48123-2500

Description: General hospital
Annual Sales: $265.1 million

Number of Employees: 4,200
Expertise Needed: Cardiac care, oncology, emergency services, hospital administration, pharmaceutical, geriatrics, communications
Contact: Human Resources
(313) 593-7000

OCCUPATIONAL HEALTH SERVICES
125 EAST SIR FRANCIS
LARKSPUR, CALIFORNIA 94939

Description: Mental health and substance abuse treatment center
Parent Company: Foundation Health Corporation
Annual Sales: $16.2 million
Number of Employees: 285
Expertise Needed: Rehabilitation, clinical services, social work, codependancy counseling, systems analysis
Contact: Ms Janet Paravanti-Holt
Director of Human Resources
(415) 461-8100

OCHSNER ALTON MEDICAL FOUNDATION
1516 JEFFERSON HIGHWAY
JEFFERSON, LOUISIANA 70121-2484

Description: General hospital
Founded: 1944
Annual Sales: $251.6 million
Number of Employees: 3,500
Expertise Needed: Registered nursing, licensed practical nursing, cardiopulmonary technology, oncology, pediatric care
Contact: Ms Barbara Johnson
Manager of Employment Staffing
(504) 838-3000

OCHSNER HEALTH PLAN
1 GALLERIA BOULEVARD
METAIRIE, LOUISIANA 70001-2082

Description: Health maintenance organization
Annual Sales: $112.7 million
Number of Employees: 110
Expertise Needed: Registered nursing, licensed practical nursing, accounting, claims adjustment/ examination, claims processing/management, and administration, case management
Contact: Ms Susan Senn
Human Resources Administrator
(504) 836-6600

OEC DIASONICS, INC.
384 WRIGHT BROTHERS DRIVE
SALT LAKE CITY, UTAH 84116

Description: Manufactures medical imaging equipment
Parent Company: OEC Medical Systems, Inc.
Founded: 1983
Annual Sales: $96.9 million
Number of Employees: 540

Expertise Needed: Mechanical engineering, design engineering, quality control, structural engineering, electrical engineering, software engineering/development, manufacturing engineering, test engineering

Contact: Mr Max Nezes
Director of Human Resources
(801) 328-9300

OHMEDA, INC.
110 ALLEN ROAD
LIBERTY CORNER, NEW JERSEY 07938-2097

Description: Produces respiratory therapy, anesthesia, and testing equipment
Parent Company: BOC Group, Inc.
Annual Sales: $800.0 million
Number of Employees: 2,000
Expertise Needed: Chemistry, mechanical engineering, manufacturing engineering

Contact: Mr William Decker
Manager of Human Resources
(908) 647-9200

OLSTEN KIMBERLY QUALITY CARE
1 MERRICK AVENUE
WESTBURY, NEW YORK 11590-6601

Description: Provides temporary health-care personnel services
Parent Company: Olsten Corporation
Annual Sales: $250.0 million
Number of Employees: 1,300
Expertise Needed: Occupational therapy, physical therapy, home health care, administration, registered nursing

Contact: Corporate Personnel Department
(516) 832-8200

OMEGA ENGINEERING, INC.
1 OMEGA DRIVE
STAMFORD, CONNECTICUT 06907

Description: Manufactures temperature measurement and control instrumentation
Founded: 1962
Number of Employees: 400
Expertise Needed: Electronics/electronics engineering, control engineering, mechanical engineering

Contact: Mr Ron Hemphill
Director of Human Resources
(203) 359-1660

OMEGA OPTICAL COMPANY, INC.
13515 NORTH STEMMONS FREEWAY
DALLAS, TEXAS 75234-5765

Description: Manufactures and distributes eyeglasses, contact lenses, and related accessories
Parent Company: Optical Radiation Corporation

Annual Sales: $85.0 million
Number of Employees: 1,052
Expertise Needed: Optics, mechanical engineering, design engineering, manufacturing engineering

Contact: Mr Victor Cortinas
Manager of Employment
(214) 241-4141

OMNICARE, INC.
2800 CHEMED CENTER
CINCINNATI, OHIO 45202-4728

Description: Provides pharmacy management services to hospitals and nursing homes
Annual Sales: $103.0 million
Number of Employees: 37
Expertise Needed: Accounting

Contact: Ms Janice Rice
Corporate Risk Manager
(513) 762-6666

ONCOGENE SCIENCE, INC.
106 CHARLES LINDBERGH BOULEVARD
UNIONDALE, NEW YORK 11553-3649

Description: Biopharmaceutical company that develops cancer and cardiovascular treatment products
Founded: 1983
Number of Employees: 200
Expertise Needed: Pharmacy, laboratory technology, chemistry

Contact: Ms Ann McDermott-Kane
Director of Human Resources
(516) 222-0023

OPTI-WORLD, INC.
1820 THE EXCHANGE NORTHWEST
ATLANTA, GEORGIA 30339-2018

Description: Owns and operates retail optical stores
Annual Sales: $55.0 million
Number of Employees: 1,300
Expertise Needed: Finance, sales, accounting, marketing

Contact: Mr Leslie Gaddis
Director of Management Information Systems
(404) 916-2020

OPTICAL RADIATION CORPORATION
1300 OPTICAL DRIVE
AZUSA, CALIFORNIA 91702-3251

Description: Designs and manufactures optical and electro-optical products
Founded: 1969
Annual Sales: $158.0 million
Number of Employees: 1,800
Expertise Needed: Electrical engineering, mechanical engineering, ophthalmology, accounting

Contact: Ms Joyce Dilley
Supervisor of Human Resources
(818) 969-3344

OPTOMETRIC EYECARE CENTERS
112 ZEBULON COURT
ROCKY MOUNT, NORTH CAROLINA 27804

Description: Owns and operates optometric retail stores
Founded: 1980
Number of Employees: 182
Number of Managerial and Professional Employees Hired 1993: 5
Expertise Needed: Warehousing, distribution, optics, optometry, accounting
Contact: Ms Alice Robbins
Payroll/Personnel Supervisor
(919) 937-6650

ORGANON, INC.
375 MOUNT PLEASANT AVENUE
WEST ORANGE, NEW JERSEY 07052-2724

Description: Manufactures anesthesia, obstetric, gynecologic, and reproductive pharmaceuticals
Parent Company: Akzona, Inc.
Founded: 1949
Annual Sales: $172.0 million
Number of Employees: 1,000
Expertise Needed: Sales, microbiology, quality control, analysis, pharmaceutical, chemical engineering
Contact: Ms Margan Mulvaney
Manager of Employee Relations
(201) 325-4500

ORTHO BIOTECH
700 ROUTE 202
RARITAN, NEW JERSEY 08869

Description: Manufactures pharmaceuticals used in the treatment of diseases
Parent Company: Johnson & Johnson
Founded: 1986
Number of Employees: 350
Expertise Needed: Biological sciences, biological engineering, biotechnology
Contact: Human Resources Department
(908) 704-5000

ORTHO DIAGNOSTIC SYSTEMS, INC.
1001 HIGHWAY 202
RARITAN, NEW JERSEY 08869

Description: Provides blood-related diagnostic services
Parent Company: Johnson & Johnson
Founded: 1973
Annual Sales: $500.0 million
Number of Employees: 1,600
Expertise Needed: Laboratory technology, biology, microbiology, chemistry
Contact: Ms Carol Peccarelli
Manager of Employment
(908) 218-8525

ORTHO PHARMACEUTICAL CORPORATION
ROUTE 202
RARITAN, NEW JERSEY 08869

Description: Manufactures pharmaceuticals and sanitary paper products
Parent Company: Johnson & Johnson
Founded: 1973
Annual Sales: $282.0 million
Number of Employees: 2,200
Expertise Needed: Marketing, sales, finance, accounting
Contact: Ms Lisa Libonati
Coordinator of Recruitment
(908) 218-6000

ORTHOMET, INC.
6301 CECILIA CIRCLE
MINNEAPOLIS, MINNESOTA 55439

Description: Manufactures and markets orthopedic products
Founded: 1974
Number of Employees: 128
Expertise Needed: Design engineering, manufacturing engineering, mechanical engineering
Contact: Mr Harlan Peterson
Director of Human Resources
(612) 944-6112

ORTHOPAEDIC HOSPITAL
2400 SOUTH FLOWER STREET
LOS ANGELES, CALIFORNIA 90007-2629

Description: Not-for-profit orthopedic hospital
Founded: 1923
Annual Sales: $30.7 million
Number of Employees: 500
Expertise Needed: Orthopedics, pharmacy, computer programming, computer science, personal computers, registered nursing, critical care nursing, medical technology, research
Contact: Human Resources Department
(213) 742-1154

OSF HEALTHCARE SYSTEM

800 NORTHEAST GLEN OAK AVENUE
PEORIA, ILLINOIS 61603-3255

Description: Provides health-care services for hospitals
Founded: 1875
Annual Sales: $455.2 million
Number of Employees: 7,266
Expertise Needed: Accounting, finance, auditing, data processing, computer programming
Contact: Mr Herbert Johnson
Director of Human Resources
(309) 691-1000

OSTEONICS CORPORATION

59 ROUTE 17 SOUTH
ALLENDALE, NEW JERSEY 07401-1614

Description: Manufactures orthopedic products
Parent Company: Stryker Corporation
Founded: 1979
Annual Sales: $45.7 million
Number of Employees: 600
Number of Managerial and Professional Employees Hired 1993: 5
Expertise Needed: Manufacturing engineering, orthopedics, mechanical engineering, product design and development, quality control, accounting, finance, marketing, sales
Contact: Ms Joanne Messler
Manager of Human Resources
(201) 825-4900

OUR LADY OF LOURDES MEDICAL CENTER

1600 HADDON AVENUE
CAMDEN, NEW JERSEY 08103-3101

Description: Private hospital, specializing in dialysis
Founded: 1950
Annual Sales: $125.2 million
Number of Employees: 2,250
Expertise Needed: Registered nursing, occupational therapy, medical technology, physical therapy
Contact: Mr Bob Thompson
Professional Recruiter
(609) 757-3500

OUR LADY OF THE LAKE REGIONAL MEDICAL CENTER

5000 HENNESSY BOULEVARD
BATON ROUGE, LOUISIANA 70808-4350

Description: Nonprofit, private hospital
Founded: 1920
Annual Sales: $222.3 million
Number of Employees: 3,000
Expertise Needed: Registered nursing, physical therapy
Contact: Ms Vicki Smith
Recruitment
(504) 765-6565

OVERLAKE HOSPITAL MEDICAL CENTER

1035 116TH AVENUE NORTHEAST
BELLEVUE, WASHINGTON 98004-4687

Description: Private hospital
Founded: 1952
Annual Sales: $100.6 million
Number of Employees: 1,760
Expertise Needed: Allied health, nursing
Contact: Ms Tracey Monteau
Nursing Coordinator
(206) 454-4011

OVERLOOK HOSPITAL ASSOCIATION

99 BEAUVOIR AVENUE
SUMMIT, NEW JERSEY 07901-3567

Description: General medical and surgical hospital
Annual Sales: $174.5 million
Number of Employees: 3,200
Expertise Needed: Respiratory therapy, occupational therapy, physical therapy, registered nursing, medical technology
Contact: Mr Ray Pagano
Director of Human Resources
(908) 522-2000

OWEN HEALTHCARE, INC.

9800 CENTRE PARKWAY
HOUSTON, TEXAS 77036-8279

Description: Provides home infusion, pharmacy, and materials management services to hospitals
Founded: 1970
Annual Sales: $238.7 million
Number of Employees: 2,300
Expertise Needed: Quality control, program analysis
Contact: Ms Deborah Thurman
Recruiter
(713) 777-8173

OXFORD HEALTH PLANS

OXFORD HEALTH PLANS, INC.

800 CONNECTICUT AVENUE
NORWALK, CONNECTICUT 06854

Description: Provides managed health-care services
Annual Sales: $311.0 million
Number of Employees: 1,000
Expertise Needed: Business, marketing, management, finance, operations, customer service and support, claims processing/management, and administration, sales, management information systems
Contact: Human Resources Department-PG

For more information, see full corporate profile, pg. 210.

PACIFIC MEDICAL CENTER AND CLINICS

1200 12TH AVENUE SOUTH
SEATTLE, WASHINGTON 98144-2733

Description: Owns and manages outpatient clinics
Founded: 1981
Annual Sales: $54.0 million
Number of Employees: 700
Expertise Needed: Physical therapy, occupational therapy, respiratory therapy, registered nursing
Contact: Ms Liz Ottaveli
     Human Resources Recruiter
     (206) 326-4000

PACIFIC PHYSICIAN SERVICES

1826 ORANGE TREE LANE
REDLANDS, CALIFORNIA 92374-4566

Description: Network of physician groups providing managed care services
Founded: 1983
Annual Sales: $131.2 million
Number of Employees: 1,000
Expertise Needed: Accounting, marketing, finance, management information systems
Contact: Human Resources Department
     (909) 825-4401

PACIFICARE OF CALIFORNIA

5701 KATELLA AVENUE
CYPRESS, CALIFORNIA 90630-5028

Description: Health maintenance organization
Founded: 1975
Annual Sales: $1.7 billion
Number of Employees: 1,300
Expertise Needed: Management, clinical nursing, social work, claims adjustment/examination, accounting, customer service and support, sales, marketing
Contact: Human Resources Department
     (800) 577-5627

PACIFICARE OF TEXAS, INC.

8200 HIGHWAY 10 WEST
SAN ANTONIO, TEXAS 78230-3878

Description: Health maintenance organization
Parent Company: Pacificare Health Systems
Annual Sales: $85.7 million
Number of Employees: 180
Expertise Needed: Allied health, clinical accounting, health insurance, finance, data processing, disability insurance
Contact: Ms Gloria King
     Human Resources Administrator
     (210) 524-9800

PACKAGING SERVICE CORPORATION

1100 WEST MARKET STREET
LOUISVILLE, KENTUCKY 40203

Description: Provides contract packaging services and manufactures surgical laser supplies and accessories
Number of Employees: 250
Expertise Needed: Marketing, sales
Contact: Ms Dawn Warren
     Human Resources Director
     (502) 625-7700

L. SALTER PACKARD CHILDREN'S HOSPITAL

725 WELCH ROAD
PALO ALTO, CALIFORNIA 94304-1601

Description: Non-profit pediatric hospital
Founded: 1919
Annual Sales: $183.7 million
Number of Employees: 1,200
Expertise Needed: Nursing
Contact: Mr Dave Thomas
     Recruiter
     (415) 497-8000

PACO PHARMACEUTICAL SERVICES, INC.

1200 PACO WAY
LAKEWOOD, NEW JERSEY 08701-5938

Description: Provides packaging services to pharmaceutical companies
Founded: 1925
Annual Sales: $72.0 million
Number of Employees: 1,354
Expertise Needed: Pharmaceutical, process engineering, marketing, product design and development, accounting, management information systems, microbiology, purchasing, quality control, project management
Contact: Mr Mark Traum
     Manager of Human Resources
     (908) 367-9000

PALL BIOMEDICAL PRODUCTS CORPORATION

77 CRESCENT BEACH ROAD
GLEN COVE, NEW YORK 11542-1323

Description: Manufactures filtration products for biomedical applications
Parent Company: Pall Corporation
Founded: 1975
Annual Sales: $25.1 million
Number of Employees: 300
Expertise Needed: Chemical engineering, mechanical engineering, accounting, management information systems, finance
Contact: Human Resources Department
     (516) 759-1900

PALL CORPORATION
2200 NORTHERN BOULEVARD
EAST HILLS, NEW YORK 11548

Description: Manufactures filtration products for medical applications
Founded: 1946
Annual Sales: $690.4 million
Number of Employees: 6,400
Expertise Needed: Accounting, finance, marketing, human resources, computer programming
Contact: Ms Jerri Schwalb
        Manager of Employment
        (516) 484-5400

PALL RAI, INC.
225 MARCUS BOULEVARD
HAUPPAUGE, NEW YORK 11788

Description: Manufactures filters for fluid processing
Parent Company: Pall Corporation
Founded: 1954
Number of Employees: 100
Expertise Needed: Manufacturing engineering, mechanical engineering
Contact: Ms Rita DeStefano
        Human Resources Manager
        (516) 273-0911

PALOMAR POMERADO HEALTH SYSTEM
15255 INNOVATION DRIVE
SAN DIEGO, CALIFORNIA 92128

Description: General hospital specializing in cardiac surgery and trauma
Founded: 1950
Annual Sales: $204.0 million
Number of Employees: 3,000
Expertise Needed: Emergency services, cardiology, networking, licensed practical nursing, psychology, laboratory technology, social work, medical technology, physical therapy
Contact: Ms Sally Chadwick
        Employment Coordinator
        (619) 739-3000

PANLABS, INC.
11804 NORTH CREEK PARKWAY SOUTH
BOTHELL, WASHINGTON 98011-8805

Description: Biotechnology and pharmaceutical research firm
Parent Company: Panlabs International, Inc.
Founded: 1983
Annual Sales: $17.3 million
Number of Employees: 340
Expertise Needed: Pharmacology, microbiology, chemistry, biology, molecular biology
Contact: Ms Jane Ramsey
        Manager of Human Resources
        (206) 487-8200

PAR-PHARMACEUTICAL
ONE RAM RIDGE ROAD
SPRING VALLEY, NEW YORK 10977

Description: Manufactures and markets generic drugs
Annual Sales: $52.5 million
Number of Employees: 430
Expertise Needed: Chemistry, pharmacy, research and development, sales, marketing
Contact: Ms Pamela Pekar
        Manager of Human Resources
        (914) 425-7100

PAREXEL INTERNATIONAL CORPORATION
195 WEST STREET
WALTHAM, MASSACHUSETTS 02154

Description: Pharmaceutical research company
Annual Sales: $700.0 million
Number of Employees: 700
Expertise Needed: Management, administration
Contact: Ms Cindy Robertson
        Manager of Human Resources
        (617) 487-9900

PARK HEALTHCARE COMPANY
4015 TRAVIS DRIVE
NASHVILLE, TENNESSEE 37211

Description: Owns and operates general and psychiatric hospitals and substance abuse treatment programs
Founded: 1983
Number of Employees: 300
Expertise Needed: Rehabilitation, counseling
Contact: Mr Robert Olsen
        Vice President and General Counsel
        (615) 833-1077

PARK NICOLLET MEDICAL CENTER
5000 WEST 39TH STREET
MINNEAPOLIS, MINNESOTA 55416-2620

Description: Medical center
Founded: 1950
Annual Sales: $164.8 million
Number of Employees: 2,270
Expertise Needed: Nursing, physicians, radiology
Contact: Ms Cindy Trussler
        Manager of Employee Relations
        (612) 927-3123

ⓅⒹ PARKE-DAVIS
People Who Care

PARKE-DAVIS, DIVISION OF WARNER-LAMBERT COMPANY
201 TABOR ROAD
MORRIS PLAINS, NEW JERSEY 07950

Description: Manufactures ethical pharmaceuticals
Founded: 1866

Annual Sales: $2.0 billion
Number of Employees: 4,700
Number of Managerial and Professional Employees Hired 1993: 275
Expertise Needed: Business, marketing, life sciences
Contact: Mr John L Woll
Director of Human Resources

CORPORATE PROFILE

Parke-Davis is a division of Warner-Lambert Company, one of the foremost producers of ethical pharmaceuticals in the world. The Parke-Davis tradition of caring reaches back 125 years to the days when the motto "Medicamenta Vera" was created. Parke-Davis created some of the finest quality standards in the pharmaceutical industry so that "true medicine" would always reach the patient. Over the years, Parke-Davis products and professionals have helped people worldwide lead longer, healthier, more productive lives.

The company's best efforts, however, are of little use without skilled communicators to explain their products and their uses to the medical community. This is the role of the Parke-Davis pharmaceutical sales representatives, located nationwide. These highly trained professionals are the prime link between Parke-Davis and the physicians who prescribe these medications to patients. Pharmacists also depend heavily on the information offered by their pharmaceutical sales representatives.

Each year, Parke-Davis asks a group of carefully selected graduates to consider becoming pharmaceutical sales representatives. Those who accept the invitation receive outstanding training, significant opportunity for professional growth, and excellent rewards for performance. As one of the People Who Care, a Parke-Davis professional can make a mark providing one of the world's most critical resources—better health care.

PARKVIEW MEMORIAL HOSPITAL
2200 RANDALLIA DRIVE
FORT WAYNE, INDIANA 46805-4638

Description: General medical and surgical hospital
Founded: 1920
Annual Sales: $178.6 million
Number of Employees: 3,407
Expertise Needed: Physical therapy
Contact: Ms. Christine Hursh
Manager of Employment
(219) 484-6636

PARTNERS HOME HEALTH, INC.
44 VANTAGE WAY
NASHVILLE, TENNESSEE 37228-1513

Description: Provides home health-care services
Annual Sales: $29.8 million
Number of Employees: 1,600

Expertise Needed: Accounting, finance, data processing
Contact: Ms Karen Dooley
Supervisor of Administration
(615) 256-8755

PASADENA RESEARCH CENTER
600 SOUTH LAKE AVENUE
PASADENA, CALIFORNIA 91106

Description: Manufactures and develops computer-aided molecular design software
Founded: 1984
Number of Employees: 100
Expertise Needed: Computer programming, software engineering/development
Contact: Human Resources Department
(818) 793-0151

PATHOLOGY LABORATORIES, LTD.
4200 MAMIE STREET
HATTIESBURG, MISSISSIPPI 39402-1733

Description: Clinical laboratory
Founded: 1956
Annual Sales: $17.1 million
Number of Employees: 368
Expertise Needed: Microbiology, biology, chemistry, laboratory technology, medical technology
Contact: Ms Gwen Kelly
Employment Manager
(601) 264-3856

PATHOLOGY MEDICAL LABORATORIES
10788 ROSELLE STREET
SAN DIEGO, CALIFORNIA 92121

Description: Provides laboratory testing services
Annual Sales: $20.5 million
Number of Employees: 375
Expertise Needed: Health insurance, phlebotomy
Contact: Ms Pam Witikko
Employment Manager
(619) 453-3141

PATIENT CARE, INC.
59 MAIN STREET
WEST ORANGE, NEW JERSEY 07052-5333

Description: Provides home health-care services
Founded: 1975
Annual Sales: $34.5 million
Number of Employees: 2,000
Expertise Needed: Nursing, licensed practical nursing, home health care, physical therapy, occupational therapy, speech therapy, accounting, management information systems, human resources
Contact: Ms Roberta Potaki
Manager of Personnel
(201) 325-3005

PATTERSON DENTAL COMPANY
1100 EAST 80TH STREET
MINNEAPOLIS, MINNESOTA 55420-1426

Description: Distributes dental products and equipment
Annual Sales: $277.1 million
Number of Employees: 1,478
Expertise Needed: Accounting, finance, customer service and support, sales
Contact: Ms Mary Martins
Director of Human Resources
(612) 854-2881

PAYLESS DRUG STORES
9275 SOUTHWEST PEYTON LANE
WILSONVILLE, OREGON 97070

Description: Drug store chain
Parent Company: Thrifty Corporation
Founded: 1939
Annual Sales: $547.0 million
Number of Employees: 19,000
Expertise Needed: Business management, accounting, marketing, finance, management information systems
Contact: Ms Jeannette Stone
Senior Vice President of Human Resources
(503) 682-4100

PEARLE, INC.
2534 ROYAL LANE
DALLAS, TEXAS 75229-3417

Description: Owns and operates retail optical stores
Annual Sales: $497.4 million
Number of Employees: 5,000
Expertise Needed: Sales, marketing, research, accounting, computer programming
Contact: Mr Malcom Greenslader
Vice President of Human Resources
(214) 277-5000

PEL-FREEZ BIOLOGICALS
219 NORTH ARKANSAS STREET
ROGERS, ARKANSAS 72756

Description: Manufactures and markets immunological compounds used for biomedical research and medical diagnosis
Founded: 1953
Number of Employees: 150
Expertise Needed: Laboratory technology
Contact: Ms Regina Stowe
Administrative Assistant to the President
(501) 636-4361

PENDLETON MEMORIAL METHODIST HOSPITAL
5620 READ BOULEVARD
NEW ORLEANS, LOUISIANA 70127-3106

Description: Private general hospital
Founded: 1961
Annual Sales: $94.7 million
Number of Employees: 1,067
Expertise Needed: Nursing, physical therapy, radiology
Contact: Ms Judy Quinn
Nurse Recruitment
(304) 244-5127

PERDUE FREDERICK COMPANY
700 UNION BOULEVARD
TOTOWA, NEW JERSEY 07512-2210

Description: Manufactures and distributes pharmaceuticals
Parent Company: Pharmaceutical Research Association
Founded: 1976
Annual Sales: $30.0 million
Number of Employees: 240
Expertise Needed: Pharmaceutical, pharmacology, pharmacy
Contact: Ms Danielle Nelson
Senior Vice President of Human Resources
(203) 853-0123

PERMANENTE MEDICAL GROUP, INC.
1950 FRANKLIN STREET
OAKLAND, CALIFORNIA 94612-5103

Description: Provides health-care services
Founded: 1945
Annual Sales: $2.0 billion
Number of Employees: 16,000
Expertise Needed: Management information systems, data processing, computer science, human resources, accounting, finance, marketing
Contact: Ms Nadine Wilbanks
Director of Personnel
(510) 987-2787

PERRIGO COMPANY
117 WATER STREET
ALLEGAN, MICHIGAN 49010-1371

Description: Manufactures over-the-counter pharmaceuticals, personal care products, and vitamins
Founded: 1887
Annual Sales: $409.8 million
Number of Employees: 2,012
Expertise Needed: Chemistry, production, marketing, mechanical engineering
Contact: Mr Mark Werre
Employment Specialist
(616) 673-8451

PFIZER, INC.
235 EAST 42ND STREET
NEW YORK, NEW YORK 10017-5703

Description: Develops and manufactures
pharmaceuticals, biochemicals, and medical devices
Founded: 1849
Annual Sales: $7.2 billion
Number of Employees: 40,700
*Number of Managerial and Professional Employees Hired
1993:* 115
Expertise Needed: Sales, chemistry, computer science,
marketing, biology
Contact: Ms Faye Williams
Associate Manager of University Relations
(212) 573-2323

PHAMIS, INC.
401 2ND AVENUE
SEATTLE, WASHINGTON 98104-2862

Description: Develops software for health-care facilities
Founded: 1981
Annual Sales: $22.0 million
Number of Employees: 165
Expertise Needed: Software engineering/development,
computer programming, program analysis
Contact: Ms. Kathy Dellplain
Director of Human Resources
(206) 622-9558

PHAR-MOR, INC.
20 FEDERAL PLAZA WEST
YOUNGSTOWN, OHIO 44501-1423

Description: Discount drug store chain
Annual Sales: $2.0 billion
Number of Employees: 19,800
Expertise Needed: Accounting, marketing, computer
programming, retail
Contact: Mr Greg Eckert
Director of Human Resources
(216) 746-6641

PHARMACHEM LABORATORIES
1505 O'BRIEN DRIVE
MENLO PARK, CALIFORNIA 94025-1435

Description: Drug testing laboratory
Annual Sales: $29.0 million
Number of Employees: 255
Expertise Needed: Chemistry, biological sciences,
laboratory assistance, analysis
Contact: Ms Debbie Sallen
Employment Manager
(415) 328-6200

PHARMACIA BIOTECH, INC.
800 CENTENNIAL AVENUE
PISCATAWAY, NEW JERSEY 08854-391

Description: Manufactures intravenous
fine chemicals
Parent Company: Procordia U.S., Inc.
Annual Sales: $250.0 million
Number of Employees: 700
Expertise Needed: Biomedical engineering, biochemistry,
instrumentation, medical laboratory technology
Contact: Ms Donna M Ross
Vice President of Human Resources
(908) 457-8000

PHARMACIA DELTEC, INC.
1265 GREY FOX ROAD
SAINT PAUL, MINNESOTA 55112-6967

Description: Develops and manufactures drug delivery
devices used for controlled infusion therapy
Parent Company: Pharmacia Biotech, Inc.
Annual Sales: $57.6 million
Number of Employees: 686
Expertise Needed: Manufacturing engineering,
mechanical engineering, electrical engineering
Contact: Ms Libby Shusterich
Staffing Manager
(612) 633-2556

PHARMACO LSR INTERNATIONAL, INC.
4009 BANISTER LANE
AUSTIN, TEXAS 78704-6853

Description: Contract biomedical research company
Parent Company: Applied Bioscience International
Annual Sales: $115.8 million
Number of Employees: 1,693
Expertise Needed: Pharmacology, nursing, biology, sales,
statistics
Contact: Ms Alyssa Pymdus
Manager of Employment
(512) 447-2663

PHARMACY MANAGEMENT SERVICES, INC.
3611 QUEEN PALM DRIVE
TAMPA, FLORIDA 33619

Description: Provides medical cost containment and
workers' compensation services
Founded: 1972
Annual Sales: $106.1 million
Number of Employees: 985
Expertise Needed: Customer service and support,
information systems, sales
Contact: Ms Barbara Younginer
Supervisor of Recruiting
(813) 626-7788

...AKINETICS LABORATORIES, INC.
...EST FAYETTE STREET
...TIMORE, MARYLAND 21201

Description: Provides pharmaceutical testing services
Founded: 1976
Number of Employees: 150
Expertise Needed: Laboratory technology, chemistry
Contact: Mr Joseph Goebbels
Director of Human Resources
(410) 385-4500

PHARMAVITE CORPORATION
15451 SAN FERNANDO MISSION BOULEVARD
MISSION HILLS, CALIFORNIA 91345

Description: Manufactures nutritional supplements and health and beauty products
Parent Company: Otsuka America, Inc.
Founded: 1989
Annual Sales: $82.0 million
Number of Employees: 642
Expertise Needed: Chemistry, chemical engineering, accounting, marketing
Contact: Ms Yolanda Mesa
Human Resources Representative
(818) 837-3633

PHOENIX MEDICAL TECHNOLOGY, INC.
ROUTE 521 WEST
ANDREWS, SOUTH CAROLINA 29510

Description: Manufactures and markets disposable medical products
Expertise Needed: Plastics engineering, design engineering
Contact: Mr Roger Hughes
Personnel Director
(803) 221-5100

PHOENIX PRODUCTS COMPANY, INC.
6161 NORTH 64TH STREET
MILWAUKEE, WISCONSIN 53218

Description: Manufactures sterile packaging materials
Founded: 1892
Expertise Needed: Packaging engineering, manufacturing engineering, electrical engineering
Contact: Ms Lisa Ziebell
Director of Human Resources
(414) 438-1200

PHONIC EAR, INC.
3880 CYPRESS DRIVE
PETALUMA, CALIFORNIA 94954-7600

Description: Manufactures assistive technology products for persons with speech and hearing impairments
Founded: 1963
Number of Employees: 170

Expertise Needed: Electronics/electronics engineering, mechanical engineering
Contact: Human Resources Department
(707) 769-1110

PHP HEALTHCARE CORPORATION
1140 COMMERCE PARK DRIVE
RESTON, VIRGINIA 22091-1811

Description: Provides managed care services
Founded: 1976
Annual Sales: $126.1 million
Number of Employees: 2,800
Expertise Needed: Accounting
Contact: Mr John Bukur
Vice President of Human Resources
(703) 758-3600

PHYSICIAN SALES & SERVICE, INC.
7800 BELFORT PARKWAY
JACKSONVILLE, FLORIDA 32256

Description: Distributes medical equipment and supplies
Founded: 1983
Number of Employees: 1,030
Number of Managerial and Professional Employees Hired 1993: 200
Expertise Needed: Sales
Contact: Ms Jean Collins
Director of Personnel
(904) 281-0011

PHYSICIANS CLINICAL LABORATORY
3301 C STREET 100 EAST
SACRAMENTO, CALIFORNIA 95816

Description: Clinical laboratory
Annual Sales: $40.7 million
Number of Employees: 900
Expertise Needed: Laboratory technology, phlebotomy, laboratory assistance
Contact: Human Resources Department
(916) 444-3500

PHYSICIANS HEALTH PLAN CORPORATION
3650 OLENTANGY RIVER ROAD
COLUMBUS, OHIO 43214-3454

Description: Provides health insurance and health-care services
Parent Company: UHC Management Company, Inc.
Annual Sales: $133.4 million
Number of Employees: 350
Expertise Needed: Accounting, finance, data processing, licensed practical nursing
Contact: Ms Jackie Abbott
Director of Human Resources
(614) 442-7100

PHYSICIANS MUTUAL INSURANCE COMPANY

2600 DODGE STREET
OMAHA, NEBRASKA 68131

Description: Provides health-care insurance services
Founded: 1902
Annual Sales: $477.7 million
Number of Employees: 1,410
Expertise Needed: Accounting, computer programming, systems analysis
Contact: Ms Lise Gjelsten
Assistant Vice President of Human Resources
(402) 633-1000

PICKER INTERNATIONAL, INC.

595 MINER ROAD
HIGHLAND HEIGHTS, OHIO 44143-2131

Description: Manufactures medical diagnostic equipment
Parent Company: GEC, Inc.
Founded: 1930
Annual Sales: $946.4 million
Number of Employees: 4,700
Expertise Needed: Marketing, finance, sales, accounting, nuclear engineering, electrical engineering, mechanical engineering, software engineering/development
Contact: Mr Steve Bogas
Technical Recruiter
(216) 473-3000

PIERCE COUNTY MEDICAL BUREAU

1501 MARKET STREET
TACOMA, WASHINGTON 98402-3333

Description: Provides health-care insurance services
Founded: 1917
Annual Sales: $200.0 million
Number of Employees: 365
Expertise Needed: Sales, marketing, computer programming, claims adjustment/examination
Contact: Human Resources Department
(206) 597-7047

PILGRIM HEALTH CARE, INC.

10 ACCORD EXECUTIVE DRIVE
NORWELL, MASSACHUSETTS 02061-1613

Description: Health maintenance organization
Founded: 1980
Annual Sales: $483.0 million
Number of Employees: 585
Expertise Needed: Computer programming, medical records
Contact: Human Resources Department
(617) 871-3950

PILLING-WECK

420 DELAWARE DRIVE
FORT WASHINGTON, PENNSYLVANIA 19034

Description: Manufactures surgical and medical instruments
Founded: 1814
Number of Employees: 300
Expertise Needed: Manufacturing engineering, industrial engineering
Contact: Ms Sandy Shook
Manager of Human Resources
(215) 643-2600

PILOT SOFTWARE, INC.

1 CANAL PARK
CAMBRIDGE, MASSACHUSETTS 02141

Description: Develops and sells computer software
Founded: 1983
Annual Sales: $50.0 million
Number of Employees: 350
Expertise Needed: Accounting, finance, software engineering/development, data processing, computer programming
Contact: Mr Ron Greenberg
Director of Human Resources
(617) 374-9400

PIONEER HEALTHCARE, INC.

36 COMMERCE WAY
WOBURN, MASSACHUSETTS 01801

Description: Owns and operates substance abuse treatment facilities
Founded: 1979
Number of Employees: 250
Expertise Needed: Accounting
Contact: Department of Human Resources
(617) 938-8888

PISCOR, INC.

16818 VIA DEL CAMPO COURT
SAN DIEGO, CALIFORNIA 92127-1714

Description: Provides equipment, and supplies to hospitals for open-heart surgical procedures
Founded: 1968
Annual Sales: $73.2 million
Number of Employees: 510
Expertise Needed: Medical technology
Contact: Ms Trish Lindgren
Recruiting Coordinator
(619) 485-5599

PITT COUNTY MEMORIAL HOSPITAL

200 STANTONSBURG ROAD
GREENVILLE, NORTH CAROLINA 27834

Description: Public hospital
Founded: 1953
Annual Sales: $238.9 million

Pitt County Memorial Hospital (continued)

Number of Employees: 3,700
Expertise Needed: Nursing, physical therapy, occupational therapy, law
Contact: Ms Connie Owens
Allied Health Recruiter
(910) 551-4100

PLANTATION BOTANICALS, INC.

1401 COUNTY ROAD 830
FELDA, FLORIDA 33930

Description: Manufactures medicinal products
Founded: 1964
Annual Sales: $59.6 million
Number of Employees: 470
Expertise Needed: Accounting, finance, data processing
Contact: Mr Marlin Hoffman
Chairman of the Board
(813) 675-2984

PLASTICS ONE, INC.

6591 MERRIMAN ROAD, SOUTHWEST
ROANOKE, VIRGINIA 24018

Description: Manufactures miniaturized connectors and electrodes for biomedical use
Founded: 1949
Number of Employees: 135
Number of Managerial and Professional Employees Hired 1993: 3
Expertise Needed: Manufacturing engineering, design engineering
Contact: Ms Debbie Honaker
Personnel Manager
(703) 772-7950

PML MICROBIOLOGICALS

9595 SOUTHWEST TUALATIN-SHERWOOD ROAD
TUALATIN, OREGON 97062

Description: Manufactures biochemicals, blood products, reagents, and test kits
Founded: 1967
Number of Employees: 140
Contact: Human Resources Department
(503) 692-1030

PMT CORPORATION

1500 PARK ROAD
CHANHASSEN, MINNESOTA 55317

Description: Manufactures and markets surgical instruments, patient monitoring equipment, and electrodes
Founded: 1979
Number of Employees: 100
Expertise Needed: Manufacturing engineering, mechanical engineering, design engineering
Contact: Human Resources Director
(612) 470-0866

POLAR WARE COMPANY

2806 NORTH 15TH STREET
SHEBOYGAN, WISCONSIN 53081

Description: Manufactures stainless steel equipment used for patient care and food service applications
Founded: 1907
Expertise Needed: Manufacturing engineering, mechanical engineering
Contact: Mr Richard Whiting
Personnel Director
(414) 458-3561

POLYCLINIC MEDICAL CENTER OF HARRISBURG

2601 NORTH 3RD STREET
HARRISBURG, PENNSYLVANIA 17110-2004

Description: Public hospital
Founded: 1909
Annual Sales: $139.2 million
Number of Employees: 2,200
Expertise Needed: Registered nursing, physical therapy, occupational therapy, respiratory therapy
Contact: Mr Bruce McIntosh
Employee Relations Specialist
(717) 782-2336

POLYMER TECHNOLOGY CORPORATION

100 RESEARCH DRIVE
WILMINGTON, MASSACHUSETTS 01887

Description: Manufactures ophthalmic goods and surgical devices
Founded: 1976
Number of Employees: 500
Expertise Needed: Marketing, advertising, mechanical engineering, industrial engineering, optics
Contact: Mr Kris Gregson
Manager of Human Resources
(508) 658-6111

POMONA VALLEY HOSPITAL MEDICAL CENTER

1798 NORTH GAREY AVENUE
POMONA, CALIFORNIA 91767-2918

Description: Nonprofit, public hospital
Founded: 1909
Annual Sales: $155.6 million
Number of Employees: 2,209
Expertise Needed: Registered nursing
Contact: Ms Mary Leahy
Human Resources Director
(714) 865-9500

POPPER & SONS, INC.

300 DENTON AVENUE
NEW HYDE PARK, NEW YORK 11040

Description: Manufactures needles and syringes, thermometers, and medical supplies

Founded: 1922
Expertise Needed: Biomedical engineering, biomedical technology, manufacturing
Contact: Ms Hilda Hoffman
Human Resources Manager
(516) 248-0300

PORTER INSTRUMENT COMPANY, INC.
245 TOWNSHIP LINE ROAD
HATFIELD, PENNSYLVANIA 19440

Description: Manufactures dental gas flowmeters, oxygen equipment, and sterilizers
Founded: 1968
Number of Employees: 180
Expertise Needed: Mechanical engineering, sales
Contact: Ms Millie Gabriel
Personnel Administrator
(215) 723-4000

J. T. POSEY COMPANY
5635 NORTH PECK ROAD
ARCADIA, CALIFORNIA 91006

Description: Manufactures patient care and restraint devices
Founded: 1937
Number of Employees: 150
Number of Managerial and Professional Employees Hired 1993: 5
Expertise Needed: Administration, customer service and support, marketing
Contact: Human Resources Department
(818) 443-3143

POUDRE VALLEY HOSPITAL
1024 SOUTH LEMAY AVENUE
FORT COLLINS, COLORADO 80524

Description: General medical and surgical hospital
Founded: 1962
Annual Sales: $106.2 million
Number of Employees: 1,800
Expertise Needed: Physical therapy, occupational therapy
Contact: Mr Chris Lujan
Employment Representative
(303) 482-4111

PREFERRED CARE
259 MONROE AVENUE
ROCHESTER, NEW YORK 14607-3632

Description: Health maintenance organization
Founded: 1977
Annual Sales: $215.0 million
Number of Employees: 230
Expertise Needed: Allied health, benefits management, actuarial, accounting, finance, data processing
Contact: Ms Cindy Wilson
Human Resources Representative
(716) 325-3920

PREFERRED HEALTH CARE, LTD.
15 RIVER ROAD
WILTON, CONNECTICUT 06897-4025

Description: Provides mental health and substance abuse treatment services
Annual Sales: $54.5 million
Number of Employees: 1,260
Expertise Needed: Psychology, nursing
Contact: Ms Debbie Grundle
Human Resources Manager
(203) 762-0993

PREMIER ANESTHESIA, INC.
1100 ASHWOOD PARKWAY SOUTH
ATLANTA, GEORGIA 30338-4768

Description: Provides anesthesiology staff to hospitals
Annual Sales: $58.8 million
Number of Employees: 320
Expertise Needed: Anesthesiology
Contact: Mr Bruce Powell
Director of Corporate Recruiting
(404) 668-9330

PREMIER DENTAL PRODUCTS COMPANY
1710 ROMANO DRIVE
NORRISTOWN, PENNSYLVANIA 19404

Description: Distributes surgical instruments, dental supplies, tubes, and catheters
Founded: 1913
Number of Employees: 140
Expertise Needed: Distribution, sales, marketing
Contact: Ms Barbara Rizzo
Director of Administration
(215) 277-3800

PREMIUM PLASTICS, INC.
465 WEST CERMAK ROAD
CHICAGO, ILLINOIS 60616

Description: Manufactures medical supplies
Founded: 1945
Number of Employees: 275
Number of Managerial and Professional Employees Hired 1993: 4
Expertise Needed: Computer programming
Contact: Ms Mary Barden
Human Resources Manager
(312) 225-8700

PRESBYTERIAN HEALTHCARE SERVICES
4775 INDIAN SCHOOL ROAD NORTHEAST
ALBUQUERQUE, NEW MEXICO 87110-3927

Description: General hospital
Founded: 1908
Annual Sales: $325.5 million
Number of Employees: 5,780

Expertise Needed: Nursing, occupational therapy, physical therapy

Contact: Ms Patti Galliher
Director of Employee Relations
(505) 260-6300

PRESBYTERIAN HEALTHCARE SYSTEM

8220 WALNUT HILL LANE
DALLAS, TEXAS 75231-9203

Description: Owns and operates general medical and surgical hospitals
Founded: 1976
Annual Sales: $284.0 million
Number of Employees: 4,500
Expertise Needed: Nursing, physical therapy, occupational therapy, respiratory therapy, medical technology, accounting, marketing, information systems, radiation technology

Contact: Ms Jan Blue
Director of Recruiting
(214) 345-7864

PRESBYTERIAN HOMES, INC.

1217 SLATE HILL ROAD
CAMP HILL, PENNSYLVANIA 17011-8012

Description: Nursing home
Founded: 1927
Annual Sales: $40.1 million
Number of Employees: 1,340
Expertise Needed: Registered nursing, licensed practical nursing

Contact: Ms Mary Ann Adamczyk
Vice President of Human Resources
(717) 737-9700

PRESBYTERIAN HOSPITAL

200 HAWTHORNE LANE
CHARLOTTE, NORTH CAROLINA 28204-2515

Description: Private hospital
Annual Sales: $247.7 million
Number of Employees: 3,000
Expertise Needed: Nursing, radiology, respiratory therapy, anesthesiology

Contact: Ms Marsie Cranford
Nursing Recruiter
(704) 384-4000

PRESBYTERIAN HOSPITAL OF DALLAS

8200 WALNUT HILL LANE
DALLAS, TEXAS 75231-4402

Description: General hospital
Founded: 1976
Annual Sales: $253.1 million
Number of Employees: 4,000

Expertise Needed: Physical therapy, occupational therapy, social work, medical technology, nursing, cardiac care, respiratory therapy, accounting, respiratory therapy, computer programming

Contact: Ms Marilyn Ambrose
Nurse Recruiter
(214) 345-7864

PRESBYTERIAN MANORS, INC.

6525 EAST MAINSGATE ROAD
WICHITA, KANSAS 67226-1062

Description: Continuing care facility for retirement communities
Founded: 1948
Annual Sales: $36.5 million
Number of Employees: 1,300
Expertise Needed: Nursing, administration

Contact: Ms Sally Ross
Vice President of Human Resources
(316) 685-1100

PRESENTATION SISTERS, INC.

800 EAST 21ST STREET
SIOUX FALLS, SOUTH DAKOTA 57105

Description: Private hospital
Annual Sales: $119.7 million
Number of Employees: 2,100
Expertise Needed: Physical therapy, occupational therapy, anesthesiology, respiratory therapy, medical technology, radiation technology, pharmacy, registered nursing

Contact: Ms Trish Trandahl
Director of Human Resources
(605) 339-8000

PRIMARK CORPORATION

8251 GREENSBORO DRIVE
MCLEAN, VIRGINIA 22102-3809

Description: Diversified company with interests in financial services, medical claims processing, transportation, and aircraft
Annual Sales: $309.7 million
Number of Employees: 3,339
Expertise Needed: Accounting, administration, human resources, data processing

Contact: Ms Helena O'Sullivan
Personnel Generalist
(703) 790-7600

PRIME MEDICAL SERVICES, INC.

1301 CAPITAL OF TEXAS HIGHWAY
AUSTIN, TEXAS 78746

Description: Provides management services for medical centers, hospitals, and outpatient facilities
Number of Employees: 150

Expertise Needed: Sales, administration
Contact: Ms Cheryl McCloud
      Chief Financial Officer
      (512) 328-2892

PRIMECARE HEALTH PLAN, INC.

1233 NORTH MAYFAIR ROAD
MILWAUKEE, WISCONSIN 53226-3255

Description: Health maintenance organization
Parent Company: UHC Management Company, Inc.
Annual Sales: $177.9 million
Number of Employees: 250
Expertise Needed: Nursing, case management,
   administration, computer programming,
   management information systems, program analysis
Contact: Human Resources Department
      (414) 453-9070

PRINCIPAL HEALTH CARE, INC.

1801 ROCKVILLE PIKE
ROCKVILLE, MARYLAND 20852-1632

Description: Health maintenance organization and
   preferred provider organization
Parent Company: Principal Mutual Life Insurance
   Company
Annual Sales: $235.1 million
Number of Employees: 800
Expertise Needed: Accounting, finance, computer
   science, actuarial, underwriting, nursing
   management and administration
Contact: Mr James Gillette
      Director of Human Resources
      (301) 881-1033

PRIVATE FORMULATIONS, INC.

460 PLAINFIELD AVENUE
EDISON, NEW JERSEY 08818

Description: Manufactures over-the-counter,
   non-prescription pharmaceuticals
Founded: 1963
Number of Employees: 220
Expertise Needed: Pharmacy, chemistry, biology
Contact: Ms Erma Gonzales
      Human Resources Manager
      (908) 985-7100

PRIVATE HEALTHCARE SYSTEMS, LTD.

20 MAGUIRE ROAD
LEXINGTON, MASSACHUSETTS 02173-3110

Description: Provides health-care management services
Annual Sales: $65.3 million
Number of Employees: 1,036
Expertise Needed: Business, business administration,
   accounting, health care
Contact: Employment Department
      (617) 863-1886

PROCTER & GAMBLE PHARMACEUTICALS

ONE PROCTER & GAMBLE PLAZA
CINCINNATI, OHIO 45202

Description: Manufactures ethical pharmaceuticals and
   respiratory care products
Founded: 1837
Annual Sales: $220.3 million
Number of Employees: 103,500
Expertise Needed: Accounting, marketing, finance,
   management information systems, sales, chemical
   engineering
Contact: Mr Benjamin L. Bethell
      Executive Vice President of Human Resources
      (513) 983-1100

PROCTOR COMMUNITY HOSPITAL

5409 NORTH KNOXVILLE AVENUE
PEORIA, ILLINOIS 61614-5016

Description: Community hospital
Parent Company: Proctor Health Care, Inc.
Annual Sales: $62.1 million
Number of Employees: 1,140
Expertise Needed: Nursing
Contact: Ms Nicki Baldi
      Employment Manager
      (309) 691-1000

PROCURANT CORPORATION

657 NORTH BROADWAY
ESCONDIDO, CALIFORNIA 92025-1801

Description: Manufactures surgical equipment and
   supplies
Annual Sales: $41.9 million
Number of Employees: 550
Expertise Needed: Manufacturing engineering,
   mechanical engineering
Contact: Mr Bert Theodore
      Director of Human Resources
      (619) 452-7106

PROFESSIONAL CARE PRODUCTS, INC.

1766 LA COSTA MEADOWS DRIVE
SAN MARCOS, CALIFORNIA 92069

Description: Manufactures orthopedic soft goods
   including anatomical and specialty braces
Founded: 1977
Number of Employees: 136
Expertise Needed: Manufacturing engineering,
   mechanical engineering
Contact: Ms Darcy Sondag
      Human Resources Assistant
      (619) 744-9410

PROFESSIONAL DENTAL TECHNOLOGIES

633 LAWRENCE STREET
BATESVILLE, ARKANSAS 72501

Description: Develops and manufactures dental
equipment and instruments
*Number of Managerial and Professional Employees Hired
1993:* 5
Expertise Needed: Manufacturing engineering,
mechanical engineering, industrial hygiene
Contact: Ms Ernestine Doucet
Personnel Director
(501) 698-2300

PROMEGA CORPORATION

2800 WOODS HOLLOW
MADISON, WISCONSIN 53711-5300

Description: Manufactures biochemical systems and
provides genetic engineering and biomedical
research services
Founded: 1978
Annual Sales: $35.0 million
Number of Employees: 310
Expertise Needed: Scientific research, production
engineering, finance, management information
systems, accounting, product design and
development, product engineering
Contact: Mr Timothy Seifriz
Employment Coordinator
(608) 274-4330

PROPPER MANUFACTURING COMPANY, INC.

36-04 SKILLMAN AVENUE
LONG ISLAND CITY, NEW YORK 11101

Description: Manufactures surgical and medical
instruments
Founded: 1935
Number of Employees: 160
Expertise Needed: Manufacturing engineering, design
engineering
Contact: Ms Maxine Kaplan
Personnel Director
(718) 392-6650

PROTOCOL SYSTEMS, INC.

8500 SOUTHWEST CREEKSIDE PLACE
BEAVERTON, OREGON 97005-7107

Description: Manufactures surgical and medical
instruments and electromedical equipment
Founded: 1986
Number of Employees: 211
Expertise Needed: Manufacturing engineering,
mechanical engineering, electrical engineering
Contact: Ms Trudy Wiedemann
Director of Human Resources
(503) 526-8500

PROVIDENCE HOSPITAL

16001 WEST 9 MILE ROAD
SOUTHFIELD, MICHIGAN 48075-4818

Description: Nonprofit hospital
Founded: 1923
Annual Sales: $230.7 million
Number of Employees: 3,621
Expertise Needed: Nursing, physical therapy,
occupational therapy
Contact: Ms Anne Boerkoel
Nursing Recruitment
(313) 424-3000

PRUDENTIAL INSURANCE OF AMERICA, INC.

751 BROAD STREET
NEWARK, NEW JERSEY 07102-3777

Description: Provides life, health, and other insurance
services
Founded: 1875
Assets: $218.4 billion
Number of Employees: 100,000
Expertise Needed: Computer programming, accounting,
finance
Contact: Ms Joan Ellen
Director of Human Resources
(201) 802-3917

PUREPAC, INC.

200 ELMORA AVENUE
ELIZABETH, NEW JERSEY 07202-1106

Description: Develops, manufactures, and markets
generic drugs
Parent Company: Faulding Holdings, Inc.
Annual Sales: $64.5 million
Number of Employees: 302
Expertise Needed: Accounting, chemistry
Contact: Mr. Douglass DiSalle
Vice President of Human Resources
(908) 527-9100

PURITAN-BENNETT CORPORATION

9401 INDIAN CREEK PARKWAY
SHAWNEE MISSION, KANSAS 66210

Description: Develops and manufactures respiratory
products and products for the aviation industry
Founded: 1913
Annual Sales: $256.1 million
Number of Employees: 2,400
*Number of Managerial and Professional Employees Hired
1993:* 6
Expertise Needed: Data processing, accounting,
marketing, sales, mechanical engineering, electrical
engineering, medical technology, electronics/

electronics engineering, manufacturing engineering, product design and development

Contact: Mr Fran Stowell
Manager of Training and Development
(913) 338-7454

PHOEBE PUTNEY MEMORIAL HOSPITAL

417 WEST 3RD AVENUE
ALBANY, GEORGIA 31701-1943

Description: Nonprofit hospital
Founded: 1897
Annual Sales: $192.0 million
Number of Employees: 1,950
Expertise Needed: Nursing, occupational therapy, physical therapy

Contact: Ms Joyce Ann Widner
Nursing Recruiter
(912) 883-1800

PYMAH CORPORATION

500 202 NORTH
FLEMINGTON, NEW JERSEY 08822

Description: Manufactures blood pressure measuring equipment, sterile packaging materials, and sterilization equipment and supplies
Founded: 1969
Number of Employees: 300
Expertise Needed: Manufacturing engineering, mechanical engineering, design engineering

Contact: Ms Debbie Katz
Manager of Personnel
(908) 788-4000

QUAL-MED, INC.

225 NORTH MAIN STREET
PUEBLO, COLORADO 81003-3234

Description: Provides managed care services
Annual Sales: $283.4 million
Number of Employees: 1,000
Expertise Needed: Actuarial, finance, data processing, disability insurance

Contact: Ms Sharon Maguire
Director of Human Resources
(709) 542-0500

QUAL-MED PLANS FOR HEALTH

155 GRAND AVENUE
OAKLAND, CALIFORNIA 94612-3763

Description: Health maintenance organization
Parent Company: Qual-Med, Inc.
Annual Sales: $301.2 million
Number of Employees: 380
Expertise Needed: Actuarial, accounting, business, claims adjustment/examination, customer service and support, sales

Contact: Human Resources Department
(510) 465-9600

QUALITONE DIVISION

4931 WEST 35TH STREET
MINNEAPOLIS, MINNESOTA 55416

Description: Manufactures surgical appliances and supplies
Founded: 1954
Number of Employees: 175
Expertise Needed: Manufacturing engineering, audio engineering

Contact: Ms Cleo Debing
Human Resources Manager
(612) 927-7161

QUALITY HEALTH CARE FACILITIES

1901 1ST AVENUE
NEBRASKA CITY, NEBRASKA 68410-2110

Description: Owns and operates health-care facilities
Founded: 1974
Annual Sales: $17.0 million
Number of Employees: 1,100
Expertise Needed: Nursing, physical therapy, administration

Contact: Mr John Buckles
Director of Human Resources
(402) 873-7791

QUALITY SYSTEMS, INC.

4000 LEGATO ROAD
FAIRFAX, VIRGINIA 22033-4055

Description: Provides medical data processing services
Parent Company: Vitro Corporation
Annual Sales: $17.5 million
Number of Employees: 340
Expertise Needed: Network management systems, computer programming, database management, systems engineering, software engineering/ development, network analysis, personal computers

Contact: Ms Lori Fravel
Quality Systems, Inc
(703) 352-9200

QUANTUM HEALTH RESOURCES, INC.

790 THE CITY DRIVE SOUTH
ORANGE, CALIFORNIA 92668-4941

Description: Provides home health-care services
Annual Sales: $118.3 million
Number of Employees: 663
Expertise Needed: Home health care, licensed practical nursing, physical therapy, occupational therapy, registered nursing

Contact: Ms Jan Brodowski
Employment Coordinator
(714) 750-1610

QUICKIE DESIGNS, INC.
2842 BUSINESS PARK AVENUE
FRESNO, CALIFORNIA 93727

Description: Manufactures wheelchairs
Parent Company: Sunrise Medical, Inc.
Annual Sales: $70.0 million
Number of Employees: 550
Expertise Needed: Design engineering, management information systems, accounting
Contact: Mr Dave Lauger
　　　　Director of Human Resources
　　　　(209) 292-2171

QUIDEL CORPORATION
10165 MCKELLAR COURT
SAN DIEGO, CALIFORNIA 92121-4201

Description: Develops and manufactures diagnostic test kits
Annual Sales: $28.8 million
Number of Employees: 260
Expertise Needed: Accounting, finance, marketing, sales, biology, mechanical engineering, electrical engineering
Contact: Mr Daryll Getzlaff
　　　　Vice President of Human Resources
　　　　(619) 552-1100

QUINTON INSTRUMENT COMPANY
2121 TERRY AVENUE
SEATTLE, WASHINGTON 98121-2791

Description: Manufactures surgical appliances and supplies
Founded: 1960
Number of Employees: 600
Expertise Needed: Manufacturing engineering, mechanical engineering, software engineering/development, electrical engineering, quality engineering
Contact: Ms Joyce Oldenburg
　　　　Employment Administrator
　　　　(206) 223-7373

RACAL HEALTH AND SAFETY, INC.
7305 EXECUTIVE WAY
FREDERICK, MARYLAND 21701

Description: Manufactures surgical equipment and supplies
Founded: 1976
Number of Employees: 150
Expertise Needed: Manufacturing engineering, mechanical engineering
Contact: Ms Linda Freeman
　　　　Human Resources Manager
　　　　(301) 695-8200

RADIOMETER AMERICA, INC.
811 SHARON DRIVE
CLEVELAND, OHIO 44145-1522

Description: Markets and distributes medical, analytical, and microbiology products
Founded: 1977
Annual Sales: $55.0 million
Number of Employees: 280
Expertise Needed: Biochemistry, chemistry, accounting, finance, data processing
Contact: Mr Dennis Cada
　　　　Director of Human Resources
　　　　(216) 871-8900

RAPID CITY REGIONAL HOSPITAL
353 FAIRMONT BOULEVARD
RAPID CITY, SOUTH DAKOTA 57701-7375

Description: Public hospital
Annual Sales: $116.5 million
Number of Employees: 1,675
Expertise Needed: Registered nursing, physical therapy, histology, radiology, laboratory technology
Contact: Ms Kelly Horton
　　　　Recruiter
　　　　(605) 341-1000

RAPIDES REGIONAL MEDICAL CENTER
211 4TH STREET
ALEXANDRIA, LOUISIANA 71301-8452

Description: General hospital
Founded: 1970
Annual Sales: $108.9 million
Number of Employees: 1,661
Expertise Needed: Medical technology, nuclear medicine, biological sciences, radiology
Contact: Mr. Allen Crane
　　　　Director of Personnel
　　　　(318) 473-3150

THE READING HOSPITAL AND MEDICAL CENTER
6TH AND SPRUCE STREETS
WEST READING, PENNSYLVANIA 19611

Description: General medical and surgical hospital
Founded: 1867
Annual Sales: $164.1 million
Number of Employees: 3,500
Expertise Needed: Health care, physical therapy, occupational therapy, rehabilitation, nursing
Contact: Ms Beth Clabria
　　　　Professional Nursing Recruiter

RED LINE HEALTHCARE CORPORATION
8121 10TH AVENUE NORTH
GOLDEN VALLEY, MINNESOTA 55427-4401

Description: Distributes medical equipment, furniture, drugs, and supplies

Annual Sales: $210.3 million

Number of Employees: 730

Expertise Needed: Computer programming, business management

Contact: Ms Theresa Rayner
Recruiter
(612) 545-5757

REGENCY HEALTH SERVICES, INC.
2742 DOW AVENUE
TUSTIN, CALIFORNIA 42680-2621

Description: Owns and manages long-term health-care facilities

Annual Sales: $115.4 million

Number of Employees: 3,200

Contact: Ms Dianne Krosner
Assistant Director of Human Resources
(714) 544-4443

REHABCARE CORPORATION
7733 FORSYTH BOULEVARD
SAINT LOUIS, MISSOURI 63105-1817

Description: Develops and manages physical rehabilitation programs

Annual Sales: $48.4 million

Number of Employees: 850

Expertise Needed: Occupational therapy, physical therapy, speech therapy, social work

Contact: Ms Ellen Jeffrey
Personnel Specialist
(314) 863-7422

REHABILITY CORPORATION
111 WESTWOOD PLACE
BRENTWOOD, TENNESSEE 37024-2549

Description: Provides outpatient rehabilitation services

Founded: 1985

Annual Sales: $24.4 million

Number of Employees: 800

Expertise Needed: Rehabilitation, nursing, physical therapy, occupational therapy

Contact: Manager of Human Resources
(615) 377-2937

REHABWORKS, INC.
521 SOUTH GREENWOOD AVENUE
CLEARWATER, FLORIDA 34616-5607

Description: Manages physical, occupational, and speech therapy facilities for hospitals and clinics

Parent Company: Continental Medical Systems

Founded: 1978

Annual Sales: $60.0 million

Number of Employees: 1,500

Expertise Needed: Speech therapy, physical therapy, occupational therapy

Contact: Mr Jay Healy
Director of Field Support Department
(813) 441-8954

RELIANCE MEDICAL PRODUCTS, INC.
3535 KINGS MILLS ROAD
MASON, OHIO 45040

Description: Designs and manufactures patient and instrument positioning systems

Founded: 1898

Number of Employees: 140

Expertise Needed: Manufacturing engineering, electrical engineering, mechanical engineering, design engineering

Contact: Mr Roy Grandstaff
Director of Employee Resources
(513) 398-3937

RELIFE, INC.
813 SHADES CREEK PARKWAY
BIRMINGHAM, ALABAMA 35209-6827

Description: Operates inpatient facilities and provides rehabilitation services

Annual Sales: $45.0 million

Number of Employees: 1,500

Expertise Needed: Registered nursing, occupational therapy, physical therapy, certified nursing and nursing assistance, accounting, finance, human resources, management information systems

Contact: Human Resources Department
(205) 870-8099

RENAISSANCE EYEWEAR, INC.
50 SOUTH AVENUE WEST
CRANFORD, NEW JERSEY 07016

Description: Manufactures ophthalmic goods

Founded: 1959

Annual Sales: $25.0 million

Number of Employees: 225

Expertise Needed: Optometry, accounting, sales, information systems

Contact: Personnel
(908) 709-0110

RESEARCH TRIANGLE INSTITUTE
3040 CORNWALLIS ROAD
RESEARCH TRIANGLE PARK, NORTH CAROLINA 27709-5206

Description: Research institute

Founded: 1958

Annual Sales: $118.0 million

Number of Employees: 1,552

Research Triangle Institute (continued)

Expertise Needed: Electrical engineering, mechanical engineering, industrial engineering, civil engineering, biology, chemistry, physics, social work, statistics

Contact for College Students and Recent Graduates:
> Mr Reed Manus
> Manager of Communications
> (919) 541-6200

Contact for All Other Candidates:
> Mr Jack Collins
> Manager of Recruiting
> (919) 541-6200

RESOURCES HOUSING AMERICA, INC.
3060 PEACHTREE ROAD NORTHWEST
ATLANTA, GEORGIA 30305-2228

Description: Owns and operates nursing homes
Annual Sales: $180.0 million
Number of Employees: 4,000
Expertise Needed: Accounting
Contact: Ms Diane Smith
> Office Manager
> (404) 364-2900

RESPIRONICS, INC.
1001 MURRY RIDGE DRIVE
MURRYSVILLE, PENNSYLVANIA 15668-8517

Description: Designs and manufactures respiratory products for home, hospital, and emergency use
Founded: 1976
Annual Sales: $69.3 million
Number of Employees: 1,200
Expertise Needed: Mechanical engineering, electrical engineering, accounting, finance, data processing, business administration, sales, design engineering, marketing
Contact: Mr Michael Ziemianski
> Director of Human Resources
> (412) 733-0200

RESPONSE TECHNOLOGIES, INC.
1775 MORIAH WOODS BOULEVARD
MEMPHIS, TENNESSEE 38117

Description: Outpatient cancer center
Number of Employees: 115
Expertise Needed: Radiology, laboratory technology
Contact: Ms Cindy Dill
> Human Resources Director
> (901) 683-0212

REVCO DISCOUNT DRUG CENTERS, INC.
1925 ENTERPRISE PARKWAY
TWINSBURG, OHIO 44087-2207

Description: Discount drug store chain
Parent Company: D. S. Revco, Inc.
Annual Sales: $204.6 million

Number of Employees: 2,309
Expertise Needed: Accounting, management information systems
Contact: Ms Marsha Ericson
> Manager of Employment Services
> (216) 425-9811

REX HOSPITAL
4420 LAKE BOONE TRAIL
RALEIGH, NORTH CAROLINA 27607-7505

Description: Private, nonprofit hospital
Founded: 1937
Annual Sales: $139.1 million
Number of Employees: 2,900
Expertise Needed: Nursing, occupational therapy
Contact: Ms Lynn Wilson
> Nurse Recruiter
> (919) 783-3100

RHONE MERIEUX, INC.
115 TRANS TECH DRIVE
ATHENS, GEORGIA 30601-1649

Description: Manufactures animal pharmaceuticals
Annual Sales: $46.0 million
Number of Employees: 535
Expertise Needed: Veterinary, laboratory technology, chemistry, microbiology, biochemistry
Contact: Ms Mary Jane Holcomb
> Personnel Manager
> (706) 548-9292

RHONE-POULENC RORER, INC.
500 ARCOLA ROAD
COLLEGEVILLE, PENNSYLVANIA 19426

Description: Develops and produces pharmaceutical products
Founded: 1968
Annual Sales: $4.0 billion
Number of Employees: 22,000
Expertise Needed: Marketing, industrial engineering, pharmacy, research and development, laboratory technology, sales
Contact: Human Resources Department
> (610) 454-8000

RHONE-POULENC RORER PHARMACEUTICALS
500 VIRGINIA DRIVE
FORT WASHINGTON, PENNSYLVANIA 19034

Description: Manufactures and markets prescription drugs
Parent Company: Rhone-Poulenc Rorer, Inc.
Annual Sales: $307.7 million
Number of Employees: 2,400
Number of Managerial and Professional Employees Hired 1993: 10

Expertise Needed: Biology, chemistry, chemical engineering, project management, electrical engineering, packaging engineering, pharmaceutical

Contact: Ms Susan Tierney
    Human Resources Coordinator
    (215) 628-6000

RHSC SALT LAKE CITY, INC.
8074 SOUTH 1300 EAST
SANDY, UTAH 84094-0743

Description: Physical rehabilitation center
Annual Sales: $27.8 million
Number of Employees: 250
Expertise Needed: Registered nursing, speech therapy, respiratory therapy, occupational therapy, physical therapy

Contact: Ms Peggy Hanover
    Human Resources Manager
    (801) 561-3400

RICHARD-ALLAN MEDICAL INDUSTRIES
8850 M-89
RICHLAND, MICHIGAN 49083

Description: Manufactures and markets medical supplies
Founded: 1953
Number of Employees: 200
Expertise Needed: Manufacturing engineering, mechanical engineering, design engineering, sales

Contact: Ms Kathy Zito
    Human Resources Specialist
    (616) 629-5811

RICHARDSON ELECTRONICS, LTD.
40W267 KESLINGER ROAD
LAFOX, ILLINOIS 60147

Description: Manufactures and distributes electronic components for medical imaging equipment
Founded: 1947
Number of Employees: 655
Expertise Needed: Manufacturing engineering, mechanical engineering, design engineering

Contact: Mr Joseph Grill
    Vice President of Human Resources
    (708) 208-2200

RICHLAND MEMORIAL HOSPITAL
5 RICHLAND MEDICAL PARK
COLUMBIA, SOUTH CAROLINA 29203-6805

Description: General hospital
Founded: 1890
Annual Sales: $268.3 million
Number of Employees: 3,612

Expertise Needed: Cardiac care, pediatrics, oncology, licensed practical nursing, physical therapy, occupational therapy

Contact: Mr James Gallieshaw
    Director of Employment and Nurse Recruitment
    (803) 765-7000

RIDGEWOOD BUSHWICK SENIOR CITIZEN HOMECARE COUNCIL
280 WYCKOFF AVENUE
BROOKLYN, NEW YORK 11237

Description: Home health-care agency
Founded: 1976
Annual Sales: $23.9 million
Number of Employees: 1,400
Expertise Needed: Registered nursing, licensed practical nursing

Contact: Personnel
    (718) 821-0254

RITE AID CORPORATION
30 HUNTER LANE
CAMP HILL, PENNSYLVANIA 17011

Description: Drug store chain
Founded: 1927
Annual Sales: $3.7 billion
Number of Employees: 30,490
Expertise Needed: Graphic arts, advertising, computer programming, finance

Contact: Mr Robert Souder
    Senior Vice President of Personnel
    (717) 975-2633

RIVENDELL OF AMERICA, INC.
3401 WEST END AVENUE
NASHVILLE, TENNESSEE 37203-1070

Description: Psychiatric hospitals
Parent Company: Vendell Healthcare, Inc.
Annual Sales: $62.2 million
Number of Employees: 1,050
Expertise Needed: Nursing, accounting, social work, psychology

Contact: Mr David Lassiter
    Vice President of Human Resources
    (615) 383-0376

RIVERSIDE HEALTH SYSTEM
500 J CLYDE MORRIS BOULEVARD
NEWPORT NEWS, VIRGINIA 23601-4442

Description: Nonprofit teaching hospital
Annual Sales: $254.6 million
Number of Employees: 5,200

Riverside Health System (continued)

Expertise Needed: Nursing, physical therapy, occupational therapy

Contact: Mr Raymond Schmidt
Director of Human Resources
(804) 875-7500

RIVERVIEW MEDICAL CENTER
1 RIVERVIEW PLAZA
RED BANK, NEW JERSEY 07701

Description: Public hospital
Parent Company: Riverview Health Care Services Corporation
Annual Sales: $125.0 million
Number of Employees: 2,000
Expertise Needed: Nursing

Contact: Ms Louise Horowitz
Employment Manager
(908) 741-2700

RJR DRUG DISTRIBUTORS, INC.
4944 SHELBYVILLE ROAD
LOUISVILLE, KENTUCKY 40207-3306

Description: Operates a drug store chain
Annual Sales: $27.7 million
Number of Employees: 210
Expertise Needed: Sales, management, retail, pharmacy

Contact: Department of Employment
(502) 893-7674

ROAD RESCUE, INC.
1133 RANKIN STREET
SAINT PAUL, MINNESOTA 55116

Description: Manufactures motor vehicle and truck bodies and medical and hospital equipment
Founded: 1976
Number of Employees: 130
Expertise Needed: Manufacturing engineering, mechanical engineering, electrical engineering

Contact: Human Resources Department
(612) 699-5588

ROBERTS OXYGEN COMPANY, INC.
7640 STANDISH PLACE
ROCKVILLE, MARYLAND 20855-2207

Description: Provides oxygen therapy equipment
Founded: 1966
Annual Sales: $30.0 million
Number of Employees: 225
Expertise Needed: Home health care, emergency services, respiratory therapy, sales

Contact: Human Resources Department
(301) 294-1950

ROBERTS PHARMACEUTICAL CORPORATION
4 INDUSTRIAL WAY WEST
EATONTOWN, NEW YORK 07724

Description: Researches and developes pharmaceuticals
Founded: 1983
Number of Employees: 325
Expertise Needed: Marketing, sales

Contact: Mr Tod McGovern
Director of Human Resources
(908) 389-1182

A.H. ROBINS COMPANY, INC.
1407 CUMMINGS DRIVE
RICHMOND, VIRGINIA 23220

Description: Pharmaceuticals company
Founded: 1866
Number of Employees: 1,400
Expertise Needed: Chemistry, chemical engineering, accounting

Contact: Manager of Recruitment
(804) 257-2000

ROCHE BIOMEDICAL LABORATORIES, INC.
1447 YORK COURT
BURLINGTON, NORTH CAROLINA 27215-3361

Description: Provides clinical testing services
Parent Company: Hoffmann-La Roche, Inc.
Annual Sales: $398.3 million
Number of Employees: 8,400
Expertise Needed: Biology, chemistry, microbiology, medical technology

Contact: Ms Patricia Noell
Personnel Administrator
(919) 584-5171

ROCHE PROFESSIONAL SERVICES CENTERS, INC.
140 EAST RIDGEWOOD AVENUE
PARAMUS, NEW JERSEY 07652-4025

Description: Provides home health-care services
Parent Company: Hoffmann-La Roche, Inc.
Founded: 1972
Annual Sales: $46.0 million
Number of Employees: 275
Expertise Needed: Pharmacy, nursing management and administration

Contact: Mr Frank Krorisky
Director of Human Resources
(201) 261-5151

ROCHESTER GENERAL HOSPITAL
1425 PORTLAND AVENUE
ROCHESTER, NEW YORK 14621-3001

Description: General medical and surgical hospital
Founded: 1847
Annual Sales: $176.0 million

Number of Employees: 2,700
Expertise Needed: Physicians, nursing, laboratory
technology, medical technology
Contact: Ms. Karen Oliver
Manager of Employment
(716) 338-4000

ROCHESTER ST. MARY'S HOSPITAL
89 GENESEE STREET
ROCHESTER, NEW YORK 14611-3201

Description: Private hospital
Founded: 1857
Annual Sales: $71.4 million
Number of Employees: 1,560
Expertise Needed: Nursing, physical therapy, laboratory
technology, medical technology
Contact: Ms Virginia Cassath-Wilson
Manager of Recruitment
(716) 464-3000

ROCKFORD MEMORIAL HOSPITAL
2400 NORTH ROCKTON AVENUE
ROCKFORD, ILLINOIS 61103-3655

Description: General hospital
Founded: 1883
Annual Sales: $156.6 million
Number of Employees: 2,200
Expertise Needed: Cardiology, oncology, physicians,
orthopedics
Contact: Ms Mary Beth Wallace
Human Resources Associate
(815) 961-6115

ROCKY MOUNTAIN HELICOPTERS, INC.
800 SOUTH 3110 WEST
PROVO, UTAH 84601

Description: Provides air ambulance services
Founded: 1970
Expertise Needed: Mechanical engineering, sales,
accounting
Contact: Ms Beverly Ware
Manager of Human Resources
(801) 375-1124

ROCKY MOUNTAIN ORTHODONTICS
650 WEST COLFAX AVENUE
DENVER, COLORADO 80204

Description: Manufactures orthodontic devices
Founded: 1933
Number of Employees: 250
Expertise Needed: Mechanical engineering, industrial
engineering
Contact: Ms Jodi Whitson
Manager of Human Resources
(303) 592-8200

ROGUE VALLEY MEDICAL CENTER
2825 EAST BARNETT ROAD
MEDFORD, OREGON 97504-8332

Description: General hospital
Annual Sales: $104.9 million
Number of Employees: 1,500
Expertise Needed: Registered nursing, licensed practical
nursing
Contact: Ms Lois Shanks
Director of Human Resources
(503) 773-6281

ROPER HOSPITAL
316 CALHOUN STREET
CHARLESTON, SOUTH CAROLINA 29401-1113

Description: General hospital
Founded: 1845
Annual Sales: $129.5 million
Number of Employees: 1,950
Expertise Needed: Cardiac care, physical therapy,
occupational therapy, respiratory therapy, radiology,
nuclear medicine, nursing, licensed practical
nursing
Contact: Ms Elizabeth West
Manager of Human Resources
(803) 724-2000

ROSS-LOOS HEALTHPLAN OF CALIFORNIA
505 NORTH BRAND BOULEVARD
GLENDALE, CALIFORNIA 91203-1925

Description: Provides health-care services
Parent Company: Cigna Healthplans of California
Founded: 1983
Annual Sales: $751.7 million
Number of Employees: 3,200
Expertise Needed: Registered nursing, licensed practical
nursing, data processing, physicians
Contact: Ms Barbara Vosin
Director of Recruiting
(818) 500-6660

ROTECH MEDICAL CORPORATION
4506 L.B. MCLEOD ROAD
ORLANDO, FLORIDA 32811

Description: Provides home infusion therapy and
respiratory care services
Annual Sales: $48.4 million
Number of Employees: 400
Expertise Needed: Pharmacology, accounting, finance,
data processing, nursing
Contact: Ms Rosa Howard
Payroll/Personnel
(407) 841-2115

ROXANE LABORATORIES, INC.
1809 WILSON ROAD
COLUMBUS, OHIO 43228-9579

Description: Manufactures and distributes
pharmaceuticals
Parent Company: Boehringer Ingelheim Corporation
Founded: 1978
Annual Sales: $90.0 million
Number of Employees: 570
Expertise Needed: Laboratory technology
Contact: Ms Judy Orniski
Director of Human Resources
(614) 276-4000

ROYAL DENTAL MANUFACTURING, INC.
12414 HIGHWAY 99
EVERETT, WASHINGTON 98204

Description: Manufactures patient chairs and dentist
stools
Founded: 1969
Number of Employees: 100
Expertise Needed: Accounting, customer service and
support
Contact: Mr Carl Grinold
Controller
(206) 743-0988

ROYAL INTERNATIONAL OPTICAL
2760 IRVING BOULEVARD
DALLAS, TEXAS 75207-2314

Description: Operates retail optical stores
Parent Company: Westinghouse Electric Corporation
Annual Sales: $210.9 million
Number of Employees: 3,355
Expertise Needed: Management, business, sales
Contact: Mr Charles Como
Vice President of Human Resources
(214) 638-1397

RUSH-PRESBYTERIAN SAINT LUKE'S MEDICAL CENTER
1653 WEST CONGRESS PARKWAY
CHICAGO, ILLINOIS 60612

Description: General medical and surgical hospital
Founded: 1837
Annual Sales: $700.4 million
Number of Employees: 9,000
Expertise Needed: Nursing, physical therapy, pharmacy
Contact: Ms Colleen Kelly
Director of Recruitment and Career Services
(212) 942-5000

RYDER INTERNATIONAL CORPORATION
100 CURT FRANCIS ROAD
ARAB, ALABAMA 35016

Description: Manufactures automotive parts and plastic
diagnostic medical products

Founded: 1968
Annual Sales: $22.5 million
Number of Employees: 175
Expertise Needed: Manufacturing engineering, plastics
engineering
Contact: Human Resources Department
(205) 586-1580

S&S X-RAY PRODUCTS, INC.
1101 LINWOOD STREET
BROOKLYN, NEW YORK 11208

Description: Manufactures radiography equipment and
X-ray supplies
Founded: 1959
Annual Sales: $28.0 million
Number of Employees: 300
Expertise Needed: Accounting, finance, data processing,
electrical engineering
Contact: Mr Harold Shoenfeld
President
(718) 649-8500

SAAD ENTERPRISES, INC.
6207 COTTAGE HILL ROAD
MOBILE, ALABAMA 36609

Description: Manufactures medical supplies
Annual Sales: $28.5 million
Number of Employees: 1,000
Expertise Needed: Nursing, licensed practical nursing
Contact: Ms Barbara Mowdy
Nurse Recruiter
(205) 343-9600

SACRED HEART HOSPITAL OF PENSACOLA
5151 NORTH 9TH AVENUE
PENSACOLA, FLORIDA 32504-8721

Description: Nonprofit public hospital
Founded: 1915
Annual Sales: $210.0 million
Number of Employees: 2,300
Expertise Needed: Nursing, physical therapy,
administration, accounting, finance
Contact: Ms Lee Ann Kimbrough
Health Care Recruiter
(904) 474-7000

SAFEGUARD HEALTH PLANS, INC.
505 NORTH EUCLID STREET
ANAHEIM, CALIFORNIA 92801-5537

Description: Provides dental and vision insurance
Founded: 1974
Annual Sales: $60.8 million
Number of Employees: 324

Expertise Needed: Actuarial, finance, accounting, marketing

Contact: Mr Hal Nutter
Human Resources Assistant
(714) 778-1005

SAFESKIN CORPORATION
5100 TOWN CENTER CIRCLE
BOCA RATON, FLORIDA 33486-1008

Description: Manufactures latex examination and surgical gloves
Annual Sales: $33.9 million
Number of Employees: 2,200
Expertise Needed: Manufacturing engineering, chemical engineering, sales, marketing, accounting, finance
Contact: Ms Pat Hayes
Office Manager
(407) 395-9988

SAGE PRODUCTS, INC.
815 TEK DRIVE
CRYSTAL LAKE, ILLINOIS 60014

Description: Manufactures urological infection control, laboratory and general disposable medical products
Founded: 1974
Number of Employees: 360
Expertise Needed: Manufacturing engineering, design engineering, mechanical engineering, marketing
Contact: Director of Human Resources
(815) 455-4700

SAGINAW GENERAL HOSPITAL
1447 NORTH HARRISON STREET
SAGINAW, MICHIGAN 48602-4727

Description: General medical and surgical hospital
Annual Sales: $76.5 million
Number of Employees: 1,300
Expertise Needed: Registered nursing, licensed practical nursing, occupational therapy, physical therapy, radiology, administration, EKG technology, hospital administration, laboratory technology, nursing management and administration
Contact for College Students and Recent Graduates:
Ms Vickie Henige
Nursing Recruiter
(517) 771-4000

Contact for All Other Candidates:
Ms Beverley Daubert
Employment Specialist
(517) 771-4000

S.A.I.C.
6725 ODYSSEY DRIVE
HUNTSVILLE, ALABAMA 35806-3302

Description: Provides research and development services
Founded: 1980
Annual Sales: $20.9 million

Number of Employees: 260
Expertise Needed: Design engineering, chemical engineering, mechanical engineering, electrical engineering
Contact: Ms Joan Arnold
Employment Manager
(205) 971-6400

SAINT AGNES HOSPITAL OF THE CITY OF BALTIMORE
900 SOUTH CATON AVENUE
BALTIMORE, MARYLAND 21229-5201

Description: Church-operated medical and surgical hospital
Founded: 1862
Annual Sales: $140.3 million
Number of Employees: 2,800
Expertise Needed: Registered nursing, licensed practical nursing, physical therapy, radiology
Contact: Human Resources Department
(410) 368-6000

SAINT AGNES MEDICAL CENTER
1303 EAST HERNDON AVENUE
FRESNO, CALIFORNIA 93720

Description: Private hospital
Parent Company: Holy Cross Health System Corporation
Founded: 1978
Annual Sales: $175.9 million
Number of Employees: 2,000
Expertise Needed: Registered nursing
Contact: Ms Julie Wilson
Manager of Employment and Development
(209) 449-3000

SAINT ANTHONY HOSPITAL SYSTEMS
4231 WEST 16TH AVENUE
DENVER, COLORADO 80204

Description: Church-operated medical and surgical hospital
Parent Company: Provenant Health Partners
Founded: 1892
Annual Sales: $123.8 million
Number of Employees: 1,800
Contact: Mr David Black
Vice President of Human Resources
(303) 629-3511

SAINT ANTHONY MEDICAL CENTER, INC.
1201 SOUTH MAIN STREET
CROWN POINT, INDIANA 46307

Description: Private hospital
Founded: 1970
Annual Sales: $91.2 million
Number of Employees: 1,400

Saint Anthony Medical Center, Inc. (continued)

Expertise Needed: Occupational therapy, physical therapy

Contact: Ms Pat Fritch
Employment Specialist
(219) 663-8120

SAINT BARNABAS CORPORATION
94 OLD SHORT HILLS ROAD
LIVINGSTON, NEW JERSEY 07039-5601

Description: Public general hospital
Annual Sales: $179.3 million
Number of Employees: 2,600
Expertise Needed: Nursing, medical technology, licensed practical nursing, physical therapy, occupational therapy, certified nursing and nursing assistance

Contact: Ms Lorraine Marino
Assistant Director of Human Resources
(201) 533-5000

SAINT CATHERINE'S MEDICAL CENTER
4321 FIR STREET
EAST CHICAGO, INDIANA 46312-3049

Description: Nonprofit hospital
Founded: 1963
Annual Sales: $163.5 million
Number of Employees: 2,525
Expertise Needed: Registered nursing, medical technology, respiratory therapy

Contact: Ms Rebecca Anderson
Professional Recruiter

SAINT CHARLES MEDICAL CENTER
2500 NORTHEAST NEFF ROAD
BEND, OREGON 97701-6015

Description: Nonprofit private hospital
Founded: 1971
Annual Sales: $68.1 million
Number of Employees: 1,100
Expertise Needed: Licensed practical nursing, registered nursing

Contact: Ms Laurie Turner
Recruiter
(503) 382-4321

SAINT CLARE'S RIVERSIDE MEDICAL CENTER
25 POCONO ROAD
DENVILLE, NEW JERSEY 07834

Description: Nonprofit medical and surgical hospital
Parent Company: Sisters of the Sorrowful Mother
Annual Sales: $110.5 million
Number of Employees: 2,000

Expertise Needed: Physical therapy, occupational therapy, nursing, registered nursing, X-ray technology, respiratory technology

Contact: Ms Lynette Ubarri-Carr
Senior Recruiter
(201) 625-6629

SAINT DAVID'S HOSPITAL
919 EAST 32ND STREET
AUSTIN, TEXAS 78705-2703

Description: Public hospital specializing in acute care
Founded: 1925
Annual Sales: $98.9 million
Number of Employees: 1,896
Expertise Needed: Occupational therapy, registered nursing

Contact: Ms Dana Dumphy
Employment Manager
(512) 476-7111

SAINT DOMINIC JACKSON MEMORIAL HOSPITAL
969 LAKELAND DRIVE
JACKSON, MISSISSIPPI 39216-4699

Description: General hospital
Parent Company: Saint Dominic Health Services
Founded: 1946
Annual Sales: $88.2 million
Number of Employees: 1,600
Expertise Needed: Cardiac care, pediatric care, registered nursing, licensed practical nursing, occupational therapy

Contact: Ms Dee Craig
Recruitment Coordinator
(601) 982-0124

SAINT EDWARD'S MERCY MEDICAL CENTER
7301 ROGERS AVENUE
FORT SMITH, ARKANSAS 72903-4165

Description: Nonprofit hospital
Founded: 1973
Annual Sales: $94.8 million
Number of Employees: 1,700
Expertise Needed: Nursing, physical therapy, pharmacy, computer science, laboratory assistance

Contact: Human Resources Department
(501) 484-6000

SAINT ELIZABETH HOSPITAL
2830 CALDER STREET
BEAUMONT, TEXAS 77702-1809

Description: Church-operated medical and surgical hospital and nursing home
Founded: 1945
Annual Sales: $221.2 million
Number of Employees: 2,355

Expertise Needed: Radiology, physical therapy, licensed practical nursing, occupational therapy, cardiology, registered nursing

Contact: Ms Ann Haulk
   Human Resource Administrator
   (409) 892-7171

SAINT ELIZABETH HOSPITAL, INC.

225 WILLIAMSON STREET
ELIZABETH, NEW JERSEY 07207-3625

Description: Church-operated hospital
Founded: 1905
Annual Sales: $103.2 million
Number of Employees: 1,325
Expertise Needed: Licensed practical nursing, registered nursing

Contact: Ms Mary Ann Purcell
   Recruitment Manager
   (908) 527-5000

SAINT ELIZABETH MEDICAL CENTER

601 SOUTH EDWIN C. MOSES BOULEVARD
DAYTON, OHIO 45408-1498

Description: Church-operated medical and surgical hospital and nursing home
Parent Company: Franciscan Health Systems of Dayton
Founded: 1878
Annual Sales: $137.4 million
Number of Employees: 2,350
Expertise Needed: Physical therapy, registered nursing, licensed practical nursing, medical technology, medical laboratory technology, respiratory therapy, radiology

Contact: Ms Elizabeth Alexander
   Manager of Employment
   (513) 229-6000

SAINT ELIZABETH MEDICAL CENTER

401 EAST 20TH STREET
COVINGTON, KENTUCKY 41014

Description: Nonprofit hospital
Founded: 1861
Annual Sales: $159.1 million
Number of Employees: 2,800
Expertise Needed: Medical technology, physical therapy, occupational therapy, pathology, respiratory therapy, pharmacy, nuclear medicine, registered nursing

Contact: Human Resources Department
   (606) 292-4000

SAINT ELIZABETH'S HOSPITAL OF BOSTON

736 CAMBRIDGE STREET
BRIGHTON, MASSACHUSETTS 02135-2997

Description: General hospital
Founded: 1872
Annual Sales: $148.8 million
Number of Employees: 2,600

Expertise Needed: Cardiology, medical technology, cardiovascular, nursing, licensed practical nursing, occupational therapy, physical therapy

Contact: Ms Karen Cleaves
   Employment Representative
   (617) 789-3000

SAINT FRANCIS HOSPITAL

100 PORT WASHINGTON BOULEVARD
ROSLYN, NEW YORK 11576-1353

Description: Nonprofit hospital specializing in cardiac care
Founded: 1964
Annual Sales: $121.7 million
Number of Employees: 1,502
Expertise Needed: Nursing, HVAC engineering, radiology, registered nursing

Contact: Ms Dianne Day
   Manager of Recruitment
   (516) 562-6000

SAINT FRANCIS HOSPITAL AND MEDICAL CENTER

1700 SOUTHWEST 7TH STREET
TOPEKA, KANSAS 66606-1674

Description: Nonprofit hospital
Parent Company: Sisters of Charity, Levenworth Health, Inc.
Founded: 1972
Annual Sales: $139.6 million
Number of Employees: 1,724
Expertise Needed: Physical therapy, anesthesiology, registered nursing, radiation therapy

Contact: Ms Janet Kerby-Vitt
   Human Resources Manager
   (913) 295-8000

SAINT FRANCIS HOSPITAL AND MEDICAL CENTER

114 WOODLAND STREET
HARTFORD, CONNECTICUT 06105-1200

Description: Nonprofit private hospital
Founded: 1897
Annual Sales: $217.9 million
Number of Employees: 2,960
Expertise Needed: Physical therapy, registered nursing

Contact: Mr William Walton
   Divisional Director of Human Resources
   (203) 548-4000

SAINT FRANCIS HOSPITAL, INC.

1 SAINT FRANCIS DRIVE
GREENVILLE, SOUTH CAROLINA 29601

Description: General hospital
Founded: 1932
Annual Sales: $83.9 million

Saint Francis Hospital, Inc. (continued)

Number of Employees: 1,500
Expertise Needed: Oncology, rehabilitation, cardiac care, orthopedics, pediatrics
Contact: Ms Sharon Parhell
Director of Human Resources
(803) 255-1000

SAINT FRANCIS MEDICAL CENTER
309 JACKSON STREET
MONROE, LOUISIANA 71210-7407

Description: Medical center specializing in cancer and open heart surgery
Founded: 1913
Annual Sales: $90.8 million
Number of Employees: 1,945
Expertise Needed: Nursing, physical therapy, rehabilitation
Contact: Ms Lea Ann Reynolds
Director of Professional Recruiting
(318) 362-4112

SAINT FRANCIS REGIONAL MEDICAL CENTER
925-29 NORTH SAINT FRANCIS STREET
WICHITA, KANSAS 67214

Description: Nonprofit hospital
Parent Company: St. Francis Ministry Corporation
Founded: 1982
Annual Sales: $269.7 million
Number of Employees: 3,300
Expertise Needed: Registered nursing, occupational therapy, physical therapy, respiratory therapy
Contact: Ms Dee Ann Henning
Nursing Recruiter
(316) 268-5000

SAINT JOHN HEALTH CORPORATION
22101 MOROSS ROAD
DETROIT, MICHIGAN 48236

Description: General medical and surgical hospital
Founded: 1978
Annual Sales: $302.9 million
Number of Employees: 4,412
Expertise Needed: Nursing, medical technology
Contact: Mr Mario Bologna
Human Resources Representative
(313) 343-7491

SAINT JOHN HOSPITAL AND MEDICAL CENTER CORPORATION
22101 MOROSS ROAD
DETROIT, MICHIGAN 48236

Description: Church-operated medical and surgical hospital
Parent Company: Saint John Health Corporation
Founded: 1978

Annual Sales: $260.9 million
Number of Employees: 4,412
Expertise Needed: CAT/MRI technology, physical therapy, occupational therapy, broadcast engineering, nursing, medical technology
Contact: Lisa Straparo
Human Resources Representative

SAINT JOHN'S HOSPITAL
800 EAST CARPENTER STREET
SPRINGFIELD, ILLINOIS 62769-0002

Description: Private general hospital specializing in cardiac care
Founded: 1955
Annual Sales: $175.5 million
Number of Employees: 3,425
Expertise Needed: Physical therapy, occupational therapy, nuclear medicine, technology, registered nursing, respiratory therapy
Contact: Ms Tracie Sayre
Nursing Recruiter
(217) 544-6464

SAINT JOHN'S MERCY MEDICAL CENTER
615 SOUTH NEW BALLAS ROAD
SAINT LOUIS, MISSOURI 63141-8221

Description: Public general hospital
Founded: 1891
Annual Sales: $301.0 million
Number of Employees: 5,741
Expertise Needed: Physical therapy, occupational therapy, respiratory therapy
Contact: Ms Mary Jo Lehman
Nursing Recruiter
(314) 569-6000

SAINT JOHN'S REGIONAL HEALTH CENTER
1235 EAST CHEROKEE STREET
SPRINGFIELD, MISSOURI 65804-2203

Description: General medical and surgical hospital
Annual Sales: $214.8 million
Number of Employees: 4,657
Expertise Needed: Physical therapy, pharmacology, occupational therapy, nursing, respiratory therapy
Contact: Human Resources
(417) 885-2765

SAINT JOSEPH HEALTH CENTER
1000 CARONDELET DRIVE
KANSAS CITY, MISSOURI 64114

Description: General hospital
Parent Company: Carondelet Health Corporation
Annual Sales: $95.5 million
Number of Employees: 1,260
Number of Managerial and Professional Employees Hired 1993: 150

Expertise Needed: Management information systems, radiation technology, medical technology, EKG technology, histology

Contact: Ms Karen Scheunemann
Manager of Employee Relations
(816) 942-4400

SAINT JOSEPH HOSPITAL HEALTH CARE CENTER

1717 SOUTH J STREET
TACOMA, WASHINGTON 98405-4944

Description: Nonprofit hospital
Founded: 1896
Annual Sales: $134.1 million
Number of Employees: 2,182
Expertise Needed: Registered nursing

Contact: Ms Chris Prentice
Nursing Recruiter
(206) 627-4101

SAINT JOSEPH HOSPITAL, INC.

1835 FRANKLIN STREET
DENVER, COLORADO 80218-1126

Description: Nonprofit hospital
Founded: 1972
Annual Sales: $163.0 million
Number of Employees: 2,347
Expertise Needed: Respiratory therapy, laboratory technology, social work, pharmacology, physical therapy, occupational therapy

Contact: Ms Sandy Navarro
Employment Manager
(303) 837-7111

SAINT JOSEPH HOSPITAL, INC.

7620 YORK ROAD
BALTIMORE, MARYLAND 21204-7508

Description: Church-operated medical and surgical hospital
Annual Sales: $137.3 million
Number of Employees: 2,350
Expertise Needed: Nursing, medical technology, physical therapy

Contact: Mr Keith Mariner
Human Resources Recruiting
(301) 337-1285

SAINT JOSEPH'S HOSPITAL OF ATLANTA

5665 PEACHTREE DUNWOODY ROAD
ATLANTA, GEORGIA 30342-1701

Description: General medical and surgical hospital
Parent Company: St. Joseph's Health System, Inc.
Annual Sales: $189.4 million
Number of Employees: 1,950

Expertise Needed: Respiratory therapy, laboratory technology, registered nursing, licensed practical nursing, occupational therapy, physical therapy, radiology, pharmacology

Contact: Human Resources Department
(404) 851-7581

SAINT JOSEPH'S HOSPITAL

428 BILTMORE AVENUE
ASHEVILLE, NORTH CAROLINA 28801

Description: General hospital
Founded: 1901
Annual Sales: $92.8 million
Number of Employees: 1,400
Expertise Needed: Oncology, orthopedics, urology

Contact: Ms Ruby Greene
Employment Manager
(800) 627-8975

SAINT JOSEPH'S HOSPITAL

301 PROSPECT AVENUE
SYRACUSE, NEW YORK 13203-1807

Description: Private hospital
Founded: 1870
Annual Sales: $154.1 million
Number of Employees: 2,700

Contact: Ms Patricia Sesonske
Employment Manager
(315) 448-5111

SAINT JOSEPH'S HOSPITAL OF MARSHFIELD

611 SAINT JOSEPH AVENUE
MARSHFIELD, WISCONSIN 54449-1832

Description: Teaching hospital
Founded: 1890
Annual Sales: $142.0 million
Number of Employees: 2,410
Expertise Needed: Physical therapy, occupational therapy, respiratory therapy

Contact: Personnel Department
(715) 387-1713

SAINT JUDE HOSPITAL

101 EAST VALENCIA MESA DRIVE
FULLERTON, CALIFORNIA 92635-3809

Description: General hospital
Founded: 1942
Annual Sales: $120.7 million
Number of Employees: 1,670
Expertise Needed: Medical technology, radiation technology, physical therapy, occupational therapy, laboratory technology

Contact: Mr Bob O'Neil
Manager of Human Relations
(714) 992-3920

SAINT JUDE MEDICAL, INC.
ONE LILLHEI PLAZA
SAINT PAUL, MINNESOTA 55117

Description: Manufactures surgical devices and supplies and electromedical equipment
Founded: 1976
Annual Sales: $239.5 million
Number of Employees: 700
Expertise Needed: Manufacturing engineering, design engineering, packaging engineering, mechanical engineering, marketing, accounting
Contact: Mr David Vied
Director of Human Resources
(612) 483-2000

SAINT LOUIS CHILDREN'S HOSPITAL
500 SOUTH KINGS HIGHWAY BOULEVARD
SAINT LOUIS, MISSOURI 63110-1014

Description: Nonprofit private pediatric hospital
Founded: 1879
Annual Sales: $142.5 million
Number of Employees: 2,078
Expertise Needed: Physical therapy, occupational therapy
Contact: Ms Carol Sullivan
Employment Manager
(314) 454-6090

SAINT LUKE'S EPISCOPAL HOSPITAL
6720 BERTNER STREET
HOUSTON, TEXAS 77030-2604

Description: Church-operated medical and surgical hospital
Founded: 1947
Annual Sales: $294.0 million
Number of Employees: 3,957
Expertise Needed: Physical therapy, nursing management and administration, cardiovascular nursing, cardiac lab technology, cardiac rehabilitation, cardiology, licensed practical nursing, radiology, veterinary, occupational therapy
Contact: Employment Department
(713) 791-4131

SAINT LUKE'S HEALTH CORPORATION
232 SOUTH WOODS MILL ROAD
CHESTERFIELD, MISSOURI 63017-3417

Description: Private general hospital
Annual Sales: $147.7 million
Number of Employees: 2,847
Expertise Needed: Nursing, physical therapy, occupational therapy, respiratory therapy
Contact: Ms Jane Kerns
Nursing Recruitment
(314) 434-1500

SAINT LUKE'S HOSPITAL
720 4TH STREET NORTH
FARGO, NORTH DAKOTA 58102-4520

Description: Nonprofit hospital specializing in acute care
Annual Sales: $122.1 million
Number of Employees: 2,200
Expertise Needed: Physical therapy, occupational therapy, radiology, registered nursing
Contact: Ms Sharon Carpenter
Employee Relations Manager
(701) 234-5875

SAINT LUKE'S HOSPITAL OF BETHLEHEM, PENNSYLVANIA
801 OSTRUM STREET
BETHLEHEM, PENNSYLVANIA 18015

Description: Nonprofit medical and surgical hospital
Founded: 1872
Annual Sales: $132.6 million
Number of Employees: 2,400
Expertise Needed: Physical therapy, occupational therapy, radiation technology, oncology, medical technology
Contact: Ms Carmen Ferry
Employment Recruiter
(215) 954-4000

SAINT LUKE'S HOSPITAL
700 COOPER AVENUE
SAGINAW, MICHIGAN 48602

Description: Nonprofit medical and surgical hospital
Number of Employees: 1,860
Expertise Needed: Licensed practical nursing, radiation technology, anesthesiology, respiratory therapy, occupational therapy, physical therapy, registered nursing
Contact: Ms Joyce Soderquist
Employment Specialist
(517) 771-6000

SAINT LUKE'S HOSPITAL
101 PAGE STREET
NEW BEDFORD, MASSACHUSETTS 02740-3464

Description: General medical and surgical hospital
Founded: 1884
Annual Sales: $118.2 million
Number of Employees: 2,157
Expertise Needed: Laboratory technology, radiology, registered nursing
Contact: Ms Debra Pickup
Director of Human Resources
(508) 997-1515

SAINT LUKE'S HOSPITAL, INC.
85 NORTH GRAND AVENUE
FORT THOMAS, KENTUCKY 41075-1718

Description: General hospital
Founded: 1954
Annual Sales: $101.6 million
Number of Employees: 1,950
Expertise Needed: Nursing, licensed practical nursing, accounting, physical therapy, occupational therapy, social work, nutrition, pharmacy
Contact: Ms Ronda Schmalzried
Staff Recruiting
(606) 572-3434

SAINT LUKE'S MEDICAL CENTER, INC.
2900 WEST OKLAHOMA AVENUE
MILWAUKEE, WISCONSIN 53215-4330

Description: Public hospital specializing in acute care
Founded: 1928
Annual Sales: $256.3 million
Number of Employees: 2,772
Expertise Needed: Registered nursing, physical therapy, occupational therapy, respiratory therapy
Contact: Ms Karla Bronaugh
Director of Employment
(414) 649-6000

SAINT LUKE'S METHODIST HOSPITAL
1026 A AVENUE NORTHEAST
CEDAR RAPIDS, IOWA 52402-5036

Description: Nonprofit private hospital
Founded: 1884
Annual Sales: $122.8 million
Number of Employees: 2,400
Expertise Needed: Registered nursing, respiratory therapy, occupational therapy, physical therapy
Contact: Mr David Rossate
Manager of Employment
(319) 369-7211

SAINT LUKE'S REGIONAL MEDICAL CENTER
190 EAST BANNOCK STREET
BOISE, IDAHO 83712

Description: General hospital
Founded: 1906
Annual Sales: $129.0 million
Number of Employees: 2,000
Expertise Needed: Pediatric care, maternity care, cardiac care, oncology, orthopedics
Contact: Professional Recruitment
(208) 386-2470

SAINT MARY'S HOSPITAL FOR CHILDREN
2901 216TH STREET
BAYSIDE, NEW YORK 11360-2810

Description: Pediatric hospital
Founded: 1888
Annual Sales: $20.2 million
Number of Employees: 400
Expertise Needed: Physical therapy
Contact: Human Resources Department

SAINT MARY'S HEALTH CARE CORPORATION
235 WEST 6TH STREET
RENO, NEVADA 89520-0112

Description: General medical and surgical hospital
Annual Sales: $47.7 million
Number of Employees: 1,400
Expertise Needed: Nursing, medical technology
Contact: Ms Terri Dibble
Senior Recruitor
(702) 789-3500

SAINT MARY'S HOSPITAL
36475 FIVE MILE ROAD
LIVONIA, MICHIGAN 48154-1971

Description: Church-operated medical and surgical hospital
Founded: 1952
Annual Sales: $60.5 million
Number of Employees: 1,304
Expertise Needed: Cardiac care, licensed practical nursing, medical technology, nuclear medicine, physical therapy, respiratory therapy, pharmacy, phlebotomy, operating room, EKG technology
Contact: Human Resources Department

SAINT MARY'S HOSPITAL
2323 NORTH LAKE DRIVE
MILWAUKEE, WISCONSIN 53211-4508

Description: Non profit private hospital
Founded: 1859
Annual Sales: $189.2 million
Number of Employees: 2,500
Expertise Needed: Registered nursing, physical therapy, respiratory therapy, occupational therapy
Contact: Ms Janice Teuscher
Director of Human Resources
(414) 291-1000

SAINT MARY'S HOSPITAL
LANGHORNE NEWTOWN ROAD
LANGHORNE, PENNSYLVANIA 19047

Description: Public hospital
Founded: 1973
Annual Sales: $94.0 million
Number of Employees: 1,645
Expertise Needed: Cardiac care, oncology, maternity care, physical therapy, occupational therapy
Contact: Mr Thomas Kupinewski
Employment Manager
(215) 750-2000

SAINT MARY'S HOSPITAL CORPORATION

56 FRANKLIN STREET
WATERBURY, CONNECTICUT 06706-1200

Description: Church-operated medical and surgical
    hospital
Annual Sales: $131.7 million
Number of Employees: 2,000
Expertise Needed: Nursing, physical therapy,
    occupational therapy, speech therapy, respiratory
    therapy, radiology, radiation technology, medical
    technology, pharmacy, dietetics
Contact: Ms Katie Bunn
        Human Resources Specialist
        (203) 574-6000

SAINT MARY'S HOSPITAL, INC.

901 45TH STREET
WEST PALM BEACH, FLORIDA 33407-2413

Description: General hospital
Founded: 1938
Annual Sales: $172.8 million
Number of Employees: 2,500
Expertise Needed: Licensed practical nursing, medical
    technology, occupational therapy, accounting,
    respiratory therapy, registered nursing, urology
Contact: Ms Regina Anderson
        Recruitment Director
        (407) 844-6300

SAINT MARY'S MEDICAL CENTER

3700 WASHINGTON AVENUE
EVANSVILLE, INDIANA 47750-0001

Description: Church-operated general hospital and
    nursing home
Founded: 1872
Annual Sales: $142.0 million
Number of Employees: 1,816
Expertise Needed: Registered nursing, licensed practical
    nursing, physical therapy
Contact: Human Resources Department
        (812) 479-4473

SAINT PATRICK HOSPITAL

500 WEST BROADWAY STREET
MISSOULA, MONTANA 59802-4008

Description: General hospital
Founded: 1888
Annual Sales: $109.9 million
Number of Employees: 1,989
Expertise Needed: Cardiac care, cardiology, operating
    room, radiation therapy
Contact: Ms. Jan VanFossen
        Personnel Coordinator
        (406) 721-9666

SAINT PAUL MEDICAL CENTER

5909 HARRY HINES BOULEVARD
DALLAS, TEXAS 75235-6285

Description: General hospital
Founded: 1927
Annual Sales: $137.2 million
Number of Employees: 1,800
Expertise Needed: Nursing, critical care, general surgery,
    maternity care
Contact: Mr Joel Nugent
        Manager of Employment
        (214) 879-1000

SAINT PETER'S HOSPITAL

315 SOUTH MANNING BOULEVARD
ALBANY, NEW YORK 12208

Description: Public hospital
Annual Sales: $130.6 million
Number of Employees: 3,000
Expertise Needed: Registered nursing, occupational
    therapy, physical therapy
Contact: Ms Gaye McCafferty
        Nursing Recruitment
        (518) 792-3151

SAINT RITA'S MEDICAL CENTER

730 WEST MARKET STREET
LIMA, OHIO 45801-4602

Description: Private hospital
Founded: 1918
Annual Sales: $104.6 million
Number of Employees: 1,944
Expertise Needed: Nursing, physical therapy
Contact: Ms Jennifer Vantelberg
        Employment Recruiter
        (419) 227-3361

SAINT THOMAS HOSPITAL

4220 HARDING ROAD
NASHVILLE, TENNESSEE 37205-2005

Description: Church-operated medical and surgical
    hospital
Founded: 1898
Annual Sales: $220.8 million
Number of Employees: 3,000
Expertise Needed: Home health care, registered nursing,
    biomedical engineering, cardiology, cardiac care
Contact: Human Resources Department
        (615) 222-2133

SAINT VINCENT HOSPITAL

835 SOUTH VAN BUREN STREET
GREEN BAY, WISCONSIN 54301-3526

Description: Private hospital specializing in
    rehabilitation, renal dialysis, neonatal intensive care,
    and trauma
Founded: 1890

Annual Sales: $119.1 million
Number of Employees: 2,250
Expertise Needed: Physical therapy, nursing, information services, occupational therapy, respiratory therapy
Contact: Ms Gwen Baumel
Employment Specialist
(414) 433-0111

SAINT VINCENT HOSPITAL & HEALTH CENTER
1233 NORTH 30TH STREET
BILLINGS, MONTANA 59101-0127

Description: Public hospital specializing in maternity and cardiac services
Founded: 1899
Annual Sales: $109.0 million
Number of Employees: 1,600
Expertise Needed: Registered nursing, physical therapy
Contact: Ms Mary Thompson
Nursing Employment Coordinator
(406) 657-0008

SAINT VINCENT HOSPITAL HEALTH CARE CENTER
2001 WEST 86TH STREET
INDIANAPOLIS, INDIANA 46260-1902

Description: Public hospital
Founded: 1881
Annual Sales: $354.6 million
Number of Employees: 4,528
Expertise Needed: Systems analysis, social work, accounting, physical therapy, occupational therapy, dietetics, cardiology, cardiac care, registered nursing, respiratory therapy
Contact: Ms Leazel McDonald
Nursing Recruiter
(317) 871-2345

SAINT VINCENT'S HOSPITAL
2800 UNIVERSITY BOULEVARD
BIRMINGHAM, ALABAMA 35205-1601

Description: General hospital
Founded: 1898
Annual Sales: $121.9 million
Number of Employees: 1,449
Expertise Needed: Radiology, nuclear medicine, information systems, systems analysis, laboratory technology, mechanical engineering, biology
Contact: Ms Terri Brennan
Employment Supervisor
(205) 939-7295

SAINT VINCENT'S HOSPITAL AND MEDICAL CENTER
153 WEST 11TH STREET
NEW YORK, NEW YORK 10011

Description: Hospital
Founded: 1849
Annual Sales: $330.7 million
Number of Employees: 3,852
Expertise Needed: Registered nursing
Contact: Ms Susan Roti
Employment Manager
(212) 790-7000

SAINT VINCENT'S MEDICAL CENTER
355 BARD AVENUE
STATEN ISLAND, NEW YORK 10310-1664

Description: Church-operated medical and surgical hospital
Annual Sales: $139.8 million
Number of Employees: 2,347
Number of Managerial and Professional Employees Hired 1993: 10
Expertise Needed: Physical therapy, registered nursing, radiology, licensed practical nursing, occupational therapy, nursing management and administration, accounting, finance, data processing
Contact: Ms Nancy DeGennarro
Manager of Employment
(718) 876-1234

SAJ DISTRIBUTORS
3017 NORTH MIDLAND DRIVE
PINE BLUFF, ARKANSAS 71603-4828

Description: Distributes health and beauty aids and over-the-counter drugs
Founded: 1968
Annual Sales: $88.3 million
Number of Employees: 303
Expertise Needed: Marketing, accounting, sales
Contact: Ms Sandi Nelling
Manager of Employment
(501) 535-5171

SALEM HOSPITAL
665 WINTER STREET SOUTHEAST
SALEM, OREGON 97301-3919

Description: Nonprofit general hospital
Founded: 1969
Annual Sales: $136.6 million
Number of Employees: 2,600
Expertise Needed: Registered nursing, physical therapy, occupational therapy
Contact: Ms Beverly Spink
Manager of Employment
(503) 370-5227

SALEM HOSPITAL, INC.
81 HIGHLAND AVENUE
SALEM, MASSACHUSETTS 01970-2714

Description: General hospital
Annual Sales: $120.4 million
Number of Employees: 1,848
Expertise Needed: Nursing, licensed practical nursing

Contact: Mr John Lenoti
    Employment Manager
    (508) 741-1200

SALICK HEALTH CARE, INC.
8201 BEVERLY BOULEVARD
LOS ANGELES, CALIFORNIA 90048

Description: Operates cancer diagnostic and treatment
    centers and dialysis centers, and distributes medical
    supplies
Founded: 1972
Annual Sales: $95.1 million
Number of Employees: 840
Expertise Needed: Dialysis, oncology, nursing, laboratory
    technology, medical technology, radiation
    technology, social work, registered nursing

Contact: Ms Barbara Blanchard
    Vice President of Human Resources
    (213) 966-3400

SANDOZ PHARMACEUTICALS CORPORATION
59 STATE HIGHWAY 10
EAST HANOVER, NEW JERSEY 07936

Description: Manufactures and distributes proprietary
    and ethical pharmaceuticals
Parent Company: Sandoz Corporation
Founded: 1919
Annual Sales: $494.0 million
Number of Employees: 3,846
Expertise Needed: Accounting, marketing, finance, law,
    data processing, chemistry, biochemistry, chemical
    engineering, mechanical engineering, management
    information systems

Contact: Ms Bea Sherman
    Associate Director of Staffing
    (201) 503-7500

SANOFI ANIMAL HEALTH, INC.
7101 COLLEGE BOULEVARD
OVERLAND PARK, KANSAS 66210-1891

Description: Manufactures and distributes animal
    pharmaceuticals
Founded: 1979
Annual Sales: $63.3 million
Number of Employees: 350
Expertise Needed: Chemistry, microbiology, animal
    sciences

Contact: Ms Mary Ann Deering
    Director of Human Resources
    (913) 451-3434

SANOFI DIAGNOSTICS PASTEUR, INC.
1000 LAKE HAZELTINE DRIVE
CHASKA, MINNESOTA 55318

Description: Manufactures diagnostic test kits and
    instruments
Annual Sales: $67.3 million
Number of Employees: 704
Expertise Needed: Research and development, sales,
    marketing

Contact: Ms Mary Jo Eayrs
    Recruiting Assistant
    (612) 448-4848

SANTA FE HEALTHCARE, INC.
720 SOUTH WEST 2ND AVENUE
GAINESVILLE, FLORIDA 32601-6260

Description: Provides health-care insurance services
Annual Sales: $437.8 million
Number of Employees: 500
Expertise Needed: Registered nursing, licensed practical
    nursing, physical therapy, respiratory therapy,
    occupational therapy

Contact: Ms Susan Garcia
    Manager of Recruiting
    (904) 372-4321

SANUS CORPORATE HEALTH SYSTEMS
1 PARKER PLAZA
FORT LEE, NEW JERSEY 07024-2937

Description: Provides health-care insurance services
Parent Company: New York Life, Inc.
Annual Sales: $800.0 million
Number of Employees: 2,000
Expertise Needed: Underwriting, health insurance

Contact: Ms Dianne Robertson
    Director of Personnel
    (201) 947-6000

SANUS TEXAS HEALTH PLAN, INC.
4500 FULLER DRIVE
IRVING, TEXAS 75038-6529

Description: Health maintenance organization
Parent Company: Sanus Corporate Health Systems
Annual Sales: $156.3 million
Number of Employees: 178
Expertise Needed: Health insurance, health care, claims
    adjustment/examination, actuarial

Contact: Ms Sandra Foster
    Manager of Personnel
    (214) 791-3900

SARASOTA MEMORIAL HOSPITAL
1700 SOUTH TAMIAMI TRIANGLE
SARASOTA, FLORIDA 34239-3509

Description: General medical and surgical hospital
Founded: 1949
Annual Sales: $195.3 million

Number of Employees: 2,700
Expertise Needed: Registered nursing, licensed practical nursing, occupational therapy, physical therapy, radiology
Contact: Mr Michael Moran
Professional Staffing Recruiter
(813) 953-1410

SCANLAN INTERNATIONAL

1 SCANLAN PLAZA
SAINT PAUL, MINNESOTA 55107

Description: Distributes surgical instruments and supplies
Founded: 1921
Number of Employees: 100
Expertise Needed: Manufacturing engineering, mechanical engineering
Contact: Julie Reilly
Vice President of Operations
(612) 298-0997

SCH HEALTH CARE SYSTEM

2600 NORTH LOOP WEST
HOUSTON, TEXAS 77092-8903

Description: Owns and operates hospitals and medical centers
Founded: 1866
Annual Sales: $1.3 billion
Number of Employees: 20,000
Expertise Needed: Finance, quality control, nursing management and administration, planning
Contact: Ms Kay Saathoff
Personnel Manager
(713) 681-8877

SCHEIN PHARMACEUTICAL

1033 STONELEIGH AVENUE
CARMEL, NEW YORK 10512-2404

Description: Manufactures and distributes pharmaceutical products
Annual Sales: $101.6 million
Number of Employees: 800
Expertise Needed: Chemistry, biochemistry
Contact: Ms. Kim Kinnelley
Recruiter
(914) 225-1700

SCHERING-PLOUGH CORPORATION

ONE GIRALDA FARMS
MADISON, NEW JERSEY 07940-1027

Description: Manufactures pharmaceuticals and consumer health products
Founded: 1864
Annual Sales: $4.1 billion
Number of Employees: 21,100

Expertise Needed: Accounting, finance, data processing, sales, research, human resources
Contact: Human Resources Department
(201) 822-7000

SCHNEIDER (USA), INC.

5905 NATHAN LANE
PLYMOUTH, MINNESOTA 55442

Description: Manufactures surgical and medical instruments
Number of Employees: 925
Expertise Needed: Manufacturing engineering, plastics engineering
Contact: Ms Loraine Pistulka
Senior Human Resources Representative
(612) 550-5500

SCHWARTZ PHARMACEUTICAL USA

5600 WEST COUNTY LINE ROAD
MEQUON, WISCONSIN 53092-4751

Description: Manufactures pharmaceutical products
Annual Sales: $51.1 million
Number of Employees: 350
Expertise Needed: Chemistry, biology
Contact: Ms Ruth Shipp
Employee Relations Manager
(414) 354-4300

SCIENCE APPLICATIONS INTERNATIONAL CORPORATION

10260 CAMPUS POINT DRIVE
SAN DIEGO, CALIFORNIA 92121-1522

Description: Provides high-tech security, health, and environmental products
Founded: 1969
Annual Sales: $1.5 billion
Number of Employees: 14,965
Expertise Needed: Electrical engineering, computer programming, computer science, mechanical engineering, environmental science, data processing, treasury management, finance, accounting
Contact: Ms Mary Lou Dunford
Corporate Staffing Manager
(619) 458-2590

SCIMED LIFE SYSTEMS, INC.

8200 SCIMED PLACE
MAPLE GROVE, MINNESOTA 55311

Description: Manufactures balloon angioplasty equipment
Founded: 1972
Annual Sales: $222.7 million
Number of Employees: 1,300
Number of Managerial and Professional Employees Hired 1993: 300

SCIMED Life Systems, Inc. (continued)

Expertise Needed: Engineering, electrical engineering, chemical engineering, marketing, laboratory technology, mechanical engineering

Contact for College Students and Recent Graduates:
    Mr Lou Gilbert
    Vice President of Human Resources
    (612) 494-2740

Contact for All Other Candidates:
    Ms Sherry Bromley
    Employment Manager
    (612) 494-2846

SCIOS-NOVA, INC.
2450 BAYSHORE PARKWAY
MOUNTAIN VIEW, CALIFORNIA 94043-1173

Description: Researches and develops pharmaceutical products
Founded: 1981
Annual Sales: $25.1 million
Number of Employees: 350
Expertise Needed: Biotechnology, biology, chemistry
Contact: Ms Juniel Butler
    Executive Administrator

SCOTT & WHITE MEMORIAL HOSPITAL
2401 SOUTH 31ST STREET
TEMPLE, TEXAS 76508-0001

Description: General hospital and nursing home
Founded: 1950
Annual Sales: $152.6 million
Number of Employees: 2,650
Expertise Needed: Registered nursing, licensed practical nursing, occupational therapy, physical therapy, radiology, pharmacy, management information systems, medical technology, social work, physician assistant
Contact: Human Resources Department
    (817) 774-2353

SCOTT SPECIALTIES, INC.
512 MAIN STREET
BELLEVILLE, KANSAS 66935

Description: Manufactures and markets orthopedic devices and patient aids
Founded: 1962
Number of Employees: 145
Expertise Needed: Sales
Contact: Mr Tim Wellendorf
    Vice President
    (913) 527-5627

SCRIPPS MEMORIAL HOSPITALS
9888 GENESEE AVENUE
LA JOLLA, CALIFORNIA 92037-1205

Description: General medical and surgical hospitals and nursing homes

Founded: 1924
Annual Sales: $286.6 million
Number of Employees: 3,000
Expertise Needed: Allied health, management, nursing, licensed practical nursing, physician assistant
Contact: Human Resources Department
    (619) 554-8725

SDK HEALTHCARE INFORMATION SYSTEMS
1550 SOLDIERS FIELD ROAD
BOSTON, MASSACHUSETTS 02135

Description: Provides computer systems for hospitals and physicians
Founded: 1961
Number of Employees: 50
Expertise Needed: Computer programming, computer engineering, computer operations, customer service and support, administration, sales, marketing
Contact: Ms Deborah Wishner
    Manager of Human Resources
    (617) 783-7351

SECOMERICA, INC.
100 BAYVIEW CIRCLE
NEWPORT BEACH, CALIFORNIA 92660-2985

Description: Provides home health-care and ambulance services
Annual Sales: $202.0 million
Number of Employees: 4,400
Expertise Needed: Accounting, finance
Contact for College Students and Recent Graduates:
    Ms Judy Bonny
    Executive Secretary to the President
    (714) 725-6600

Contact for All Other Candidates:
    Mr Peter Deiser
    Vice President of Human Resources
    (714) 725-6500

SENTARA ALTERNATIVE DELIVERY SYSTEMS
4417 CORPORATION LANE
VIRGINIA BEACH, VIRGINIA 23462

Description: Provides managed care and health-care insurance services
Number of Employees: 500
Expertise Needed: Health care, registered nursing, accounting, finance, medical records, physical therapy
Contact: Ms Pat Sandeal
    Manager of Human Resources
    (804) 852-7190

SENTARA ENTERPRISES
6015 POPLAR HALL DRIVE
NORFOLK, VIRGINIA 23502-3819

Description: Operates outpatient health-care facilities
Annual Sales: $31.0 million

Number of Employees: 380
Expertise Needed: Nursing, licensed practical nursing, physical therapy, occupational therapy
Contact: Ms Sandy Wheelous
Recruiter
(804) 466-7674

SENTARA HEALTH SYSTEM

6015 POPLAR HALL DRIVE
NORFOLK, VIRGINIA 23502-3819

Description: Owns and operates hospitals and medical centers
Annual Sales: $581.8 million
Number of Employees: 10,000
Expertise Needed: Marketing, print production, printing, accounting, administration, business management, customer service and support
Contact: Human Resources Department
(804) 455-7020

SENTARA HOSPITALS OF NORFOLK

600 GRESHAM DRIVE
NORFOLK, VIRGINIA 23502-3819

Description: Owns and operates general medical and surgical hospitals
Parent Company: Sentara Health System
Annual Sales: $300.7 million
Number of Employees: 5,200
Expertise Needed: Nursing
Contact: Ms Rose Marie Cybart
Nursing Recruiter
(804) 628-3831

SENTARA LIFE CARE CORPORATION

251 SOUTH NEWTOWN ROAD
NORFOLK, VIRGINIA 23502-5718

Description: Operates nursing homes and assisted-care facilities
Annual Sales: $18.9 million
Number of Employees: 950
Expertise Needed: Nursing, licensed practical nursing, accounting, data processing, dietetics, nutrition
Contact: Ms Betty Andrews
Administrator
(804) 461-8500

SENTINEL CONSUMER PRODUCTS

7750 TYLER BOULEVARD
MENTOR, OHIO 44060-4802

Description: Manufactures health and beauty aids
Founded: 1974
Annual Sales: $25.0 million
Number of Employees: 360

Expertise Needed: Accounting, finance, sales, data processing, mechanical engineering, marketing, design engineering
Contact: Ms Trish McGonnell
Director of Human Resources
(216) 974-8144

SEQUANA THERAPEUTICS

11099 NORTH TORREY PINES ROAD
LA JOLLA, CALIFORNIA 92037

Description: Genetic testing laboratory
Number of Employees: 65
Expertise Needed: Genetics engineering, biology
Contact: Ms Anita Wiseth
Human Resources Director
(619) 452-6550

SERA TEC BIOLOGICALS, INC.

223 NORTH CENTER DRIVE
NORTH BRUNSWICK, NEW JERSEY 08902-4247

Description: Operates blood plasma centers
Parent Company: Rite Aid Corporation
Founded: 1969
Annual Sales: $45.0 million
Number of Employees: 500
Expertise Needed: Biochemistry, nursing, laboratory technology, sales
Contact: Employment Department
(908) 422-4200

SERFILCO, LTD.

1777 SHERMER ROAD
NORTHBROOK, ILLINOIS 60062-5360

Description: Manufactures pumps, pumping equipment, and service industry machinery
Founded: 1961
Number of Employees: 165
Expertise Needed: Manufacturing engineering, mechanical engineering
Contact: Ms Lisa Prier
Human Resources Manager
(708) 559-1777

SERONO LABORATORIES, INC.

100 LONGWATER CIRCLE
NORWELL, MASSACHUSETTS 02061

Description: Manufactures pharmaceutical products
Parent Company: Ares Serono, Inc.
Founded: 1971
Annual Sales: $150.0 million
Number of Employees: 300
Expertise Needed: Chemistry, biology, microbiology, laboratory technology, marketing, sales, statistics, research, finance, customer service and support
Contact: Mr Mark Iorio
Human Resources Manager
(617) 982-9000

SERVANTCOR

175 SOUTH WALL STREET
KANKAKEE, ILLINOIS 60901

Description: Health-care services provider
Founded: 1982
Annual Sales: $151.8 million
Number of Employees: 2,600
Expertise Needed: Accounting, administration

Contact: Mr Craig Copper
Vice President of Human Resources
(815) 937-2034

SERVICEMASTER COMPANY

ONE SERVICEMASTER WAY
DOWNERS GROVE, ILLINOIS 60515-1700

Description: Provides building maintenance, sanitation, and industrial services
Annual Sales: $2.5 billion
Number of Employees: 27,700
Expertise Needed: Business management, finance, marketing, chemical engineering, logistics, clinical engineering

Contact: Ms Terry Welch
Manager of Personnel Selection
(708) 964-1300

SETON MEDICAL CENTER

1900 SULLIVAN AVENUE
DALY CITY, CALIFORNIA 94015-2200

Description: Private hospital specializing in cardiac care
Annual Sales: $123.1 million
Number of Employees: 1,211
Expertise Needed: Physical therapy, nursing, networking, licensed practical nursing, criminal investigation

Contact: Ms Kathy Green
Manager of Employment
(415) 991-6829

SHANDS HOSPITAL AT THE UNIVERSITY OF FLORIDA

1600 SOUTHWEST ARCHER ROAD
GAINESVILLE, FLORIDA 32610

Description: Teaching hospital
Founded: 1979
Annual Sales: $317.6 million
Number of Employees: 4,059
Expertise Needed: Nursing, physical therapy, occupational therapy, medical technology, respiratory therapy

Contact: Ms Denise L. Huggins
Director, Employment/Recruitment
(904) 395-0111

SHARED MEDICAL SYSTEMS CORPORATION

51 VALLEY STREAM PARKWAY
MALVERN, PENNSYLVANIA 19355-1406

Description: Develops and distributes computer software for medical applications
Founded: 1969
Annual Sales: $469.6 million
Number of Employees: 3,943
Expertise Needed: Accounting, finance, marketing, sales, software engineering/development

Contact: Ms Christie Robinson
Human Resources
(610) 219-6300

SHARP HEALTH CARE

3131 BERGER AVENUE
SAN DIEGO, CALIFORNIA 92123-4201

Description: General hospital
Founded: 1946
Annual Sales: $614.7 million
Number of Employees: 9,800
Expertise Needed: Quality control, occupational therapy, physical therapy, genetics, radiation technology, oncology, rehabilitation, cardiology

Contact: Ms Jean Graves
Director of Recruiting
(619) 627-5290

SHAWNEE MISSION MEDICAL CENTER

9100 WEST 74TH STREET
SHAWNEE MISSION, KANSAS 66204-4004

Description: Private hospital
Annual Sales: $127.8 million
Number of Employees: 1,700
Expertise Needed: Occupational therapy, physical therapy, medical technology, registered nursing

Contact: Mr Dan Curtis
Employment Interviewer
(913) 676-2000

SHEPHERD SPINAL CENTER, INC.

2020 PEACHTREE ROAD NORTHWEST
ATLANTA, GEORGIA 30309-1402

Description: Not-for-profit rehabilitation hospital
Founded: 1975
Annual Sales: $32.9 million
Number of Employees: 510
Expertise Needed: Registered nursing, critical care, rehabilitation, medical technology, general surgery

Contact: Human Resources
(404) 350-7340

SHEPPARD AND ENOCH PRATT HOSPITAL

6501 NORTH CHARLES STREET
BALTIMORE, MARYLAND 21204

Description: Private nonprofit hospital specializing in mental health

Annual Sales: $59.2 million
Number of Employees: 1,350
Expertise Needed: Nursing, psychiatry, psychology
Contact: Ms Joann Sherrer
　　　　Manager of Recruitment and Selection
　　　　(410) 938-3000

SHERWOOD MEDICAL COMPANY
1915 OLIVE STREET
ST. LOUIS, MISSOURI 63103-1625

Description: Manufactures and distributes disposable
　　medical products
Parent Company: American Home Products
　　Corporation
Annual Sales: $677.0 million
Number of Employees: 6,500
Expertise Needed: Accounting, marketing, finance,
　　chemical engineering, mechanical engineering,
　　electrical engineering
Contact: Mr Herbert Martin
　　　　Vice President of Human Resources
　　　　(314) 241-5700

SHORE MEMORIAL HOSPITAL
1 EAST NEW YORK AVENUE
SOMERS POINT, NEW JERSEY 08244-2300

Description: Public hospital
Parent Company: Shore Memorial Health Foundation
Annual Sales: $96.0 million
Number of Employees: 1,510
Expertise Needed: Nursing, physical therapy,
　　occupational therapy
Contact: Ms Sheila Boyle
　　　　Nursing Recruiter
　　　　(609) 653-3500

SIDMAK LABORATORIES, INC.
17 WEST STREET
EAST HANOVER, NEW JERSEY 07936-2822

Description: Manufactures pharmaceuticals
Founded: 1978
Annual Sales: $85.0 million
Number of Employees: 375
Expertise Needed: Chemistry
Contact: Ms Georgeann Pratt
　　　　Human Resources Manager
　　　　(201) 386-5566

SIEBE NORTH, INC.
4090 AZALEA DRIVE
CHARLESTON, SOUTH CAROLINA 29405-7527

Description: Manufactures medical care and
　　dermatological treatment products
Annual Sales: $114.0 million
Number of Employees: 1,200

Expertise Needed: Manufacturing engineering, research
　　and development, mechanical engineering,
　　industrial engineering, chemical engineering,
　　chemistry
Contact: Ms Jenni Turner
　　　　Personnel Administrator
　　　　(803) 554-0660

SIEMENS HEARING INSTRUMENTS, INC.
10 CONSTITUTION AVENUE
PISCATAWAY, NEW JERSEY 08854-6145

Description: Manufactures and distributes hearing aids
　　and auditory testing equipment
Parent Company: Siemens Medical Corporation
Annual Sales: $50.0 million
Number of Employees: 413
Expertise Needed: Mechanical engineering, production,
　　sales, marketing
Contact: Ms Crystal Ruiz
　　　　Director of Human Resources
　　　　(908) 562-6600

SIEMENS MEDICAL ELECTRONICS
16 ELECTRONICS AVENUE
DANVERS, MASSACHUSETTS 01923-1047

Description: Manufactures patient monitoring systems
Parent Company: Siemens Medical Corporation
Annual Sales: $50.0 million
Number of Employees: 360
Expertise Needed: Electrical engineering, electronics/
　　electronics engineering, design, mechanical
　　engineering, manufacturing engineering,
　　production
Contact: Ms Chris Hall
　　　　Human Resources Administrator
　　　　(508) 750-7500

SIEMENS MEDICAL SYSTEMS, INC.
10950 NORTH TANTAU AVENUE
CUPERTINO, CALIFORNIA 95014-0716

Description: Manufactures and markets medical and
　　diagnostic equipment
Parent Company: Siemens Medical Corporation
Founded: 1847
Annual Sales: $1.8 billion
Number of Employees: 3,200
Expertise Needed: Marketing, sales, accounting, finance,
　　management information systems, medical
　　technology, electrical engineering, electronics/
　　electronics engineering, mechanical engineering,
　　law
Contact: Mr Cort Montross
　　　　Manager of Human Resources
　　　　(908) 321-4300

SIEMENS MEDICAL SYSTEMS, INC., ULTRASOUND GROUP
1040 12TH AVENUE NORTHWEST
ISSAQUAH, WASHINGTON 98027-8929

Description: Manufactures ultrasound equipment
Parent Company: Siemens Medical Corporation
Annual Sales: $69.0 million
Number of Employees: 415
Number of Managerial and Professional Employees Hired 1993: 100
Expertise Needed: Electrical engineering, design engineering
Contact: Ms Barbara Grote
　　　　Employment Manager
　　　　(206) 392-9180

SIERRA HEALTH SERVICES, INC.
333 NORTH RANCHO DRIVE
LAS VEGAS, NEVADA 89106-3797

Description: Provides managed care services
Annual Sales: $235.9 million
Number of Employees: 1,300
Expertise Needed: Laboratory technology
Contact: Ms Carmel Fritz
　　　　Employment Manager
　　　　(702) 646-8170

SIERRA NEVADA LABORATORIES
888 WILLOW STREET
LAS VEGAS, NEVADA 89119-5645

Description: Clinical laboratory
Parent Company: Washoe Professional Center
Annual Sales: $27.5 million
Number of Employees: 419
Expertise Needed: Registered nursing, physical therapy, claims adjustment/examination, actuarial
Contact: Ms Carmel Fritz
　　　　Employment Manager
　　　　(702) 292-7100

SIERRA TUCSON COMPANIES
16500 NORTE LAGO DEL ORO
TUCSON, ARIZONA 85737

Description: Provides hospital and medical clinic management services
Annual Sales: $36.0 million
Number of Employees: 375
Expertise Needed: Activity therapy, behavioral research, casework, chemical dependency, health care, hospital administration, substance abuse treatment and counseling, psychiatric social work, psychotherapy, data processing
Contact: Department of Human Resources
　　　　(602) 624-4000

SIGNET ARMORLITE, INC.
1001 ARMORLITE DRIVE
SAN MARCOS, CALIFORNIA 92069

Description: Manufactures contact lenses
Parent Company: Falcon Manufacturing, Inc.
Annual Sales: $59.3 million
Number of Employees: 936
Expertise Needed: Sales, mechanical engineering
Contact: Ms Donna Peterson
　　　　Director of Human Resources
　　　　(619) 744-4000

SILVER HILL HOSPITAL, INC.
208 VALLEY ROAD
NEW CANAAN, CONNECTICUT 06840-3812

Description: Not-for-profit psychiatric hospital
Founded: 1934
Annual Sales: $15.1 million
Number of Employees: 320
Expertise Needed: Psychiatry, psychology, social work, occupational therapy, counseling
Contact: Ms Merrilyn Payne
　　　　Director of Human Resources
　　　　(203) 966-3567

SINGING RIVER HOSPITAL
2809 DENNY AVENUE
PASCAGOULA, MISSISSIPPI 39581-5301

Description: County medical and surgical hospital
Founded: 1959
Annual Sales: $129.3 million
Number of Employees: 1,800
Expertise Needed: Accounting, data processing, laboratory technology, pediatric care, registered nursing, radiology, licensed practical nursing, occupational therapy, physical therapy, cardiology
Contact: Mr Paul Carter
　　　　Assistant Director of Personnel
　　　　(601) 938-5005

SIOUX VALLEY HOSPITAL ASSOCIATION
1100 SOUTH EUCLID AVENUE
SIOUX FALLS, SOUTH DAKOTA 57105-0411

Description: General hospital
Founded: 1928
Annual Sales: $158.4 million
Number of Employees: 2,900
Expertise Needed: Radiology, CAT/MRI technology, physical therapy, occupational therapy, technical writing
Contact: Mr Donna Dettman
　　　　Nurse Recruiter
　　　　(605) 333-1000

SISTERS OF PROVIDENCE IN OREGON

520 PIKE TOWER
SEATTLE, WASHINGTON 98101-4001

Description: Owns and operates general hospitals and
    health-care centers
Founded: 1876
Annual Sales: $419.1 million
Number of Employees: 4,801
Expertise Needed: Nursing, registered nursing

Contact: Ms Susan Byington
        Employment Manager
        (206) 464-3355

SISTERS OF SAINT JOSEPH OF TEXAS

4000 24TH STREET
LUBBOCK, TEXAS 79410-1894

Description: General hospital
Parent Company: Saint Joseph Health System
Founded: 1939
Annual Sales: $191.1 million
Number of Employees: 1,800
Expertise Needed: Pharmacy, licensed practical nursing,
    nursing, pharmacology, respiratory therapy, medical
    technology, physical therapy

Contact: Ms Ann Bertaia
        Director of Human Resources
        (806) 796-6000

SISTERS OF SAINT JOSEPH'S HOME HEALTH SERVICE

15325 SOUTHEAST 30TH PLACE
BELLEVUE, WASHINGTON 98007

Description: Provides home health-care services
Founded: 1892
Annual Sales: $428.9 million
Number of Employees: 4,565
Expertise Needed: Accounting, finance

Contact: Mr Scott Houston
        Vice President of Human Resources
        (206) 747-1711

SISTERS OF ST. FRANCIS HEALTH SERVICES

1515 WEST DRAGOON TRAIL
MISHAWAKA, INDIANA 46544-4710

Description: Owns and operates hospitals and medical
    centers
Founded: 1974
Annual Sales: $597.1 million
Number of Employees: 6,717
Expertise Needed: Accounting, finance, data processing,
    auditing

Contact: Sister Jane Marte Klein
        President
        (219) 256-3935

SMART PRACTICE

3400 EAST MCDOWELL ROAD
PHOENIX, ARIZONA 85008-3846

Description: Distributes medical and dental equipment
    and supplies
Founded: 1972
Annual Sales: $25.0 million
Number of Employees: 275
Expertise Needed: Business, marketing, sales

Contact: Employment Department
        (602) 225-9090

J. M. SMITH CORPORATION

450 WOFFORD STREET
SPARTANBURG, SOUTH CAROLINA 29301-2242

Description: Wholesale drug distributor
Founded: 1944
Annual Sales: $157.3 million
Number of Employees: 310
Expertise Needed: Data processing, sales, accounting

Contact: Ms Maryanne Hall
        Payroll Manager
        (803) 582-1216

SMITH & NEPHEW DYONICS, INC.

160 DASCOMB ROAD
ANDOVER, MASSACHUSETTS 01810-5885

Description: Manufactures arthroscopic medical
    instruments
Parent Company: SNP, Inc.
Annual Sales: $100.0 million
Number of Employees: 500
Expertise Needed: Design engineering, electrical
    engineering, mechanical engineering

Contact: Ms Rachel Beckmon
        Manager of Compensation and Staffing
        (508) 470-2800

SMITH & NEPHEW RICHARDS, INC.

1450 EAST BROOKS ROAD
MEMPHIS, TENNESSEE 38116

Description: Designs, markets, and manufactures
    implants and medical specialty products
Annual Sales: $326.1 million
Number of Employees: 4,200
Expertise Needed: Sales, biology, mechanical
    engineering, marketing, materials engineering,
    finance, accounting, biomedical engineering, data
    processing

Contact: Mr Steve Ammons
        Manager of Human Resources
        (901) 396-2121

SMITHKLINE BEECHAM CLINICAL LABORATORIES
1201 SOUTH COLLEGEVILLE ROAD
COLLEGEVILLE, PENNSYLVANIA 19426

Description: Provides clinical and medical laboratory services
Parent Company: SmithKline Beecham Corporation
Founded: 1969
Annual Sales: $1.1 billion
Number of Employees: 10,500
Expertise Needed: Marketing, finance, accounting, management information systems, data processing
Contact: Ms Nancy Shapiro
Manager of Human Resources
(610) 454-6000

SMITHKLINE BEECHAM CORPORATION
1 FRANKLIN PLAZA
PHILADELPHIA, PENNSYLVANIA 19102-1225

Description: Manufactures health and personal care products
Founded: 1830
Annual Sales: $9.0 billion
Number of Employees: 53,000
Expertise Needed: Human resources, finance, marketing, management information systems, government affairs/relations, safety engineering, health care
Contact for College Students and Recent Graduates:
Mr Joseph Ambrosino
U.S. College Recruiter
(215) 751-3238

Contact for All Other Candidates:
Ms Diane Doyle
Manager of Employee Development
(215) 751-4000

SOCIETY OF NEW YORK HOSPITAL, INC.
525 EAST 68TH STREET
NEW YORK, NEW YORK 10021-4873

Description: General medical and surgical hospital
Founded: 1771
Annual Sales: $568.9 million
Number of Employees: 6,400
Expertise Needed: Cardiology, oncology, physicians, nursing
Contact: Ms Debra Fuller
Vice President of Human Resources
(212) 746-5454

THE SOCIETY OF THE VALLEY HOSPITAL
223 NORTH VAN DIEN AVENUE
RIDGEWOOD, NEW JERSEY 07450-2736

Description: General medical and surgical hospital
Parent Company: Valley Care Corporation
Founded: 1925
Annual Sales: $144.0 million
Number of Employees: 2,060

Expertise Needed: Nursing, physical therapy, registered nursing, occupational therapy, medical technology, laboratory technology, general surgery, cardiac care
Contact: Human Resources Department

SOFAMOR/DANEK GROUP, INC.
3092 DIRECTORS ROW
MEMPHIS, TENNESSEE 38131-0401

Description: Manufactures and markets spinal implants
Annual Sales: $75.5 million
Number of Employees: 500
Expertise Needed: Accounting, finance, data processing, mechanical engineering
Contact: Mr Jack Young
Director of Human Resources
(901) 396-2695

SOLA BARNES HIND
2420 SANDHILL ROAD
MENLO PARK, CALIFORNIA 94025

Description: Designs and manufactures vision care products
Parent Company: Pilkington Visioncare Holdings
Annual Sales: $435.3 million
Number of Employees: 3,390
Expertise Needed: Management
Contact: Mr Stephen Lee
Vice President of Human Resources
(415) 324-6868

SOMERSET MEDICAL CENTER
110 REHILL AVENUE
SOMERVILLE, NEW JERSEY 08876

Description: Medical center
Parent Company: Somerset Health Care Corporation
Annual Sales: $93.4 million
Number of Employees: 1,600
Expertise Needed: Nursing, physical therapy
Contact: Ms Mary Gibbons
Personnel Interviewer
(908) 685-2200

SONORA LABORATORY SCIENCES
3279 EAST HARBOUR DRIVE
PHOENIX, ARIZONA 85034-7227

Description: Clinical laboratory
Parent Company: Samaritan Health System
Annual Sales: $18.3 million
Number of Employees: 380
Expertise Needed: Phlebotomy, microbiology, medical technology
Contact: Mr Byron Farwell
Director of Human Resources
(602) 470-0000

SOPHA MEDICAL SYSTEMS, INC.

7155 COLUMBIA GATEWAY DRIVE
COLUMBIA, MARYLAND 21046-2138

Description: Manufactures magnetic resonance imaging
  equipment and computer systems
Annual Sales: $38.2 million
Number of Employees: 143
Expertise Needed: Design engineering, electrical
  engineering, software engineering/development,
  manufacturing engineering, sales
Contact: Mr Gary Bethling
        Director of Human Resources
        (410) 290-0100

SORIN BIOMEDICAL, INC.

17600 GILLETTE AVENUE
IRVINE, CALIFORNIA 92714-5702

Description: Manufactures cardiopulmonary and
  respiratory products
Annual Sales: $90.0 million
Number of Employees: 750
Expertise Needed: Mechanical engineering,
  manufacturing engineering, plastics engineering,
  accounting, marketing
Contact: Ms Judy Cable
        Human Resources Representative
        (714) 250-0500

SOUTH CAROLINA BAPTIST HOSPITAL

1330 TAYLOR STREET
COLUMBIA, SOUTH CAROLINA 29220-2910

Description: Private hospital
Founded: 1913
Annual Sales: $210.0 million
Number of Employees: 2,700
Expertise Needed: Nursing, physical therapy,
  occupational therapy, radiology
Contact for College Students and Recent Graduates:
        Ms Val Richardson
        Nursing Employment Coordinator
        (803) 771-5306
Contact for All Other Candidates:
        Ms Rowena Jackson
        Employment Coordinator
        (803) 771-5010

SOUTH SHORE HOSPITAL, INC.

55 FOGG ROAD
SOUTH WEYMOUTH, MASSACHUSETTS 02190-2455

Description: Public hospital
Founded: 1922
Annual Sales: $111.4 million
Number of Employees: 1,775
Contact: Ms Jean Jackson
        Director of Human Resources
        (617) 340-8000

SOUTHEAST ALABAMA MEDICAL CENTER

HIGHWAY 84 EAST
DOTHAN, ALABAMA 36301

Description: Regional hospital
Founded: 1949
Annual Sales: $112.8 million
Number of Employees: 2,000
Expertise Needed: Nursing, occupational therapy,
  physical therapy, radiology, trauma, emergency
  services, cardiac care, anesthesiology, maternity
  care, general surgery
Contact: Department of Personnel
        (205) 793-8111

SOUTHERN BAPTIST HOSPITAL OF FLORIDA

800 PRUDENTIAL DRIVE
JACKSONVILLE, FLORIDA 32207

Description: Private, general hospital
Annual Sales: $188.0 million
Number of Employees: 2,400
Expertise Needed: Physical therapy, occupational therapy,
  speech therapy, social work, medical technology,
  registered nursing
Contact: Ms Susan Rust
        Employment Manager
        (904) 393-2000

SOUTHERN CALIFORNIA PERMANENTE MEDICAL

393 WALNUT STREET
PASADENA, CALIFORNIA 91188

Description: Provides health-care services
Founded: 1952
Annual Sales: $3.7 billion
Number of Employees: 9,500
Expertise Needed: Accounting, auditing, data processing,
  computer programming
Contact: Mr Hugo Aguas
        Regional Director of Personnel
        (818) 405-5757

SOUTHERN HEALTH SYSTEMS, INC.

1785 NONCONNAH BOULEVARD
MEMPHIS, TENNESSEE 38132-2140

Description: Provides health-care services
Annual Sales: $44.7 million
Number of Employees: 400
Expertise Needed: Accounting, finance, data processing,
  licensed practical nursing, pharmacology,
  respiratory therapy, physical therapy, registered
  nursing
Contact: Ms Jill Stem
        Director of Human Resources
        (901) 348-8100

SOUTHERN OPTICAL COMPANY
1909 NORTH CHURCH STREET
GREENSBORO, NORTH CAROLINA 27405-5631

Description: Manufactures optical products
Annual Sales: $36.1 million
Number of Employees: 458
Expertise Needed: Optics, design engineering,
    mechanical engineering
Contact: Mr Jim Price
        Director of Human Resources
        (910) 272-8146

SOUTHWEST LOUISIANA HOSPITAL ASSOCIATION
1701 OAK PARK BOULEVARD
LAKE CHARLES, LOUISIANA 70601-8911

Description: General hospital
Founded: 1950
Annual Sales: $141.9 million
Number of Employees: 1,250
Expertise Needed: Respiratory therapy, management,
    occupational therapy, physical therapy
Contact: Ms Judy Meyer
        Director of Human Resources
        (318) 494-3000

SOUTHWEST TEXAS METHODIST HOSPITAL
7700 FLOYD CURL DRIVE
SAN ANTONIO, TEXAS 78229-3902

Description: General medical and surgical hospital
Founded: 1955
Annual Sales: $163.7 million
Number of Employees: 2,500
Expertise Needed: Cardiac care, allied health, home
    health care, hospital administration, intensive care,
    maternity care, nursing, registered nursing, tax
    accounting
Contact: Human Resources Department
        (210) 692-4000

SOUTHWEST WASHINGTON MEDICAL CENTER
400 NORTHEAST MOTHER JOSEPH PLACE
VANCOUVER, WASHINGTON 98664-3269

Description: General hospital
Annual Sales: $106.3 million
Number of Employees: 2,000
Expertise Needed: Registered nursing, respiratory
    technology
Contact: Ms Ann Nordquist
        Director of Employment
        (206) 256-2097

SPACELABS MEDICAL, INC.
15220 NORTHEAST 40TH STREET
REDMOND, WASHINGTON 98052-5305

Description: Develops and manufactures patient
    monitoring equipment and clinical information
    systems
Founded: 1958
Annual Sales: $252.2 million
Number of Employees: 1,630
Expertise Needed: Quality control, software engineering/
    development
Contact: Vice President of Human Resources
        (206) 882-3700

SPAN-AMERICA MEDICAL SYSTEMS, INC.
70 COMMERCE CENTER
GREENVILLE, SOUTH CAROLINA 29615-5814

Description: Manufactures therapeutic cushions, and
    packaging materials
Founded: 1975
Annual Sales: $30.3 million
Number of Employees: 250
Expertise Needed: Marketing, accounting
Contact: Ms Melinda Gage
        Director of Human Resources
        (803) 288-8877

SPARKS REGIONAL MEDICAL CENTER
1311 SOUTH I STREET
FORT SMITH, ARKANSAS 72917

Description: General medical and surgical hospital
Founded: 1902
Annual Sales: $101.4 million
Number of Employees: 1,900
Expertise Needed: Physical therapy, nursing
Contact: Mr Gary Allen
        Recruiter and Benefits Manager
        (501) 441-4000

EDWARD W. SPARROW HOSPITAL
1215 EAST MICHIGAN AVENUE
LANSING, MICHIGAN 48912-1811

Description: General medical and surgical hospital
Founded: 1910

Annual Sales: $167.5 million
Number of Employees: 3,000
Expertise Needed: HVAC engineering, medical technology, nuclear medicine, occupational therapy, pharmacy, physical therapy, networking, radiation technology
Contact: Ms Maureen Pusateri
Director of Employment
(517) 483-2700

SPARTANBURG REGIONAL MEDICAL CENTER
101 EAST WOOD STREET
SPARTANBURG, SOUTH CAROLINA 29303-3016

Description: Public hospital specializing in trauma and acute care
Founded: 1917
Annual Sales: $153.8 million
Number of Employees: 3,127
Expertise Needed: Registered nursing, occupational therapy, physical therapy, pharmacology, respiratory therapy
Contact: Mr Ed Booknight
Director of Personnel
(803) 560-6387

SPECIAL TOUCH HOME HEALTH CARE SERVICES
1305 EAST 19TH STREET
BROOKLYN, NEW YORK 11230

Description: Provides home health-care services
Annual Sales: $16.0 million
Number of Employees: 985
Expertise Needed: Social service, licensed practical nursing, registered nursing
Contact: Ms Linda Keene
Personnel Director
(718) 258-1197

SPECIALTY SILICONE FABRICATORS
3077 ROLLIE GATES DRIVE
PASO ROBLES, CALIFORNIA 93446

Description: Custom designs and manufactures silicone components for medical devices
Founded: 1982
Number of Employees: 105
Number of Managerial and Professional Employees Hired 1993: 4
Expertise Needed: Mechanical engineering
Contact: Ms Roxanna Taylor
Personnel Manager
(805) 239-4284

SPECTRASCAN IMAGING SERVICES
200 DAY HILL ROAD
WINDSOR, CONNECTICUT 06095

Description: Provides mammography and ultrasound services
Founded: 1981
Number of Employees: 150
Expertise Needed: Computer programming, information systems
Contact: Ms Valerie Standisch
Personnel Director
(203) 285-0545

SPECTRONICS CORPORATION
956 BRUSH HOLLOW ROAD
WESTBURY, NEW YORK 11590

Description: Manufactures lighting and electrical equipment and supplies
Founded: 1955
Number of Employees: 150
Expertise Needed: Electrical engineering, design engineering, mechanical engineering
Contact: Ms Lynn Mauro
Human Resources Manager
(516) 333-4840

SPHINX PHARMACEUTICALS CORPORATION
4 UNIVERSITY PLACE
DURHAM, NORTH CAROLINA 27707

Description: Biopharmaceutical company
Founded: 1987
Number of Employees: 150
Expertise Needed: Research and development, chemistry, biology
Contact: Human Resources Department
(919) 489-0909

SPRING HILL MEMORIAL HOSPITAL
3715 DAUPHIN STREET
MOBILE, ALABAMA 36608-1771

Description: Owns and operates a community hospital, home health-care agency, and claims processing service
Founded: 1975
Annual Sales: $37.6 million
Number of Employees: 1,200
Number of Managerial and Professional Employees Hired 1993: 350
Expertise Needed: Registered nursing, licensed practical nursing, certified nursing and nursing assistance, respiratory therapy, radiological technology
Contact: Ms Linda Compher
Professional/Technical Recruiter
(205) 460-5296

SQUIRE-COGSWELL COMPANY
1111 LAKESIDE DRIVE
GUERNEE, ILLINOIS 60031

Description: Designs, manufactures, and distributes
   suction systems
Founded: 1916
Number of Employees: 130
*Number of Managerial and Professional Employees Hired
   1993:* 10
Expertise Needed: Mechanical engineering, sales,
   computer-aided design, mechanical engineering
Contact: Ms Donna Martin
         Human Resources Manager
         (708) 272-8900

S&S X-RAY PRODUCTS, INC.
1101 LINWOOD STREET
BROOKLYN, NEW YORK 11208

Description: Manufactures radiography and X-ray
   equipment
Founded: 1947
Number of Employees: 220
Expertise Needed: Manufacturing engineering, sales
Contact: Mr Harold Schoenfeld
         President
         (718) 649-8500

THE STAMFORD HOSPITAL
SHELBURNE ROAD
STAMFORD, CONNECTICUT 06902

Description: Nonprofit medical and surgical hospital
Annual Sales: $100.9 million
Number of Employees: 1,166
Expertise Needed: Phlebotomy, EKG technology,
   accounting, emergency medical technology,
   physician assistant
Contact: Personnel Department
         (203) 325-7000

STARKEY LABORATORIES, INC.
6700 WASHINGTON AVENUE SOUTH
EDEN PRAIRIE, MINNESOTA 55344-3405

Description: Manufactures hearing aids and auditory
   testing equipment
Founded: 1970
Annual Sales: $220.3 million
Number of Employees: 2,900
*Number of Managerial and Professional Employees Hired
   1993:* 400
Expertise Needed: Electronics/electronics engineering,
   audio engineering, research and development,
   mechanical engineering, electrical engineering,
   process engineering, design engineering, product
   design and development, quality control
Contact: Mr Larry Miller
         Director of Human Resources
         (612) 941-6401

STERIS LABORATORIES, INC.
620 NORTH 51ST AVENUE
PHOENIX, ARIZONA 85043

Description: Distributes medical, surgical, and hospital
   supplies
Annual Sales: $75.8 million
Number of Employees: 600
Expertise Needed: Chemistry, production, sales,
   marketing, finance, accounting, chemical
   engineering, microbiology
Contact: Mr James Lolli
         Human Resources Manager
         (602) 278-1400

STERLING OPTICAL CORPORATION
10 PENNINSULA BOULEVARD
LYNBROOK, NEW YORK 11563

Description: Owns and operates a chain of optical goods
   stores
Founded: 1914
Number of Employees: 500
Expertise Needed: Sales, marketing
Contact: Ms Mary Ellen Lyons
         Controller
         (516) 887-2100

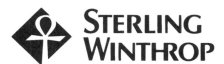

STERLING WINTHROP
90 PARK AVENUE
NEW YORK, NEW YORK 10016

Description: Pharmaceuticals manufacturer
Founded: 1901
Annual Sales: $2.0 billion
Expertise Needed: Manufacturing, research and
   development, marketing, finance, engineering
Contact: Ms Alana M Schuster
         Manager of Employee Relations
         (212) 907-2000

CORPORATE PROFILE

Founded in 1901 in Wheeling, West Virginia, to market
an over-the-counter pain reliever, the Sterling Winthrop
of today is a worldwide developer, manufacturer, and
marketer of pharmaceuticals and consumer health
products. The company has strong brand franchises,
such as Bayer aspirin, Phillips' milk of magnesia, Midol
pain reliever, Neo-Synephrine nasal decongestant, Dairy
Ease natural nutritional supplement, and Stri-Dex acne
medication. The company is structured along two global
lines of business, pharmaceuticals and consumer health
products, each supported by world-class research and
development. Sterling Winthrop markets its products to
customers in more than 100 countries.

The company, a subsidiary of the Eastman Kodak
Company since 1988, entered into a unique and innova-

tive alliance with Elf Sanofi, a France-based health-care company, in January 1991. As a result, the combined operations rank among the top 20 worldwide pharmaceutical groups, with over $2 billion in sales. The alliance is among the world leaders in R&D spending with expenditures of about $500 million.

The administrative arm of the corporation, Sterling Winthrop Inc., includes the Finance, Legal, Information Services, Regulatory and Environmental Affairs, Corporate Relations, and Human Resources departments, as well as many technical support areas. Its goal is to provide direction, stewardship, and support to the two line-of-business groups.

The **Sterling Winthrop Pharmaceuticals Group** is a global manufacturer and marketer of prescription pharmaceuticals, including diagnostic imaging agents, analgesics, anti-infectives, cardiovascular agents, contrast media, and hormonal products. As a result of an innovative pharmaceutical alliance with Elf Sanofi, pharmaceutical products are marketed under the name Sanofi Winthrop in countries around the world, except Japan.

The **Sterling Winthrop Consumer Health Group**, a world leader, manufactures and markets products in four core categories: analgesics, which account for half of the group's sales; gastrointestinal products (antacids and laxatives), comprising the second-largest category; skin care; and cough/cold.

Sterling Winthrop is committed to being a leading company in the global pharmaceuticals and consumer health products industries. It intends to achieve its mission through the research and development of new and effective medicines to cure diseases and by intensifying its efforts to capitalize on the company's well-established brand franchises through marketing excellence.

STEVENS MEMORIAL HOSPITAL
21601 76TH AVENUE WEST
EDMONDS, WASHINGTON 98026-7506

Description: Public hospital
Founded: 1962
Annual Sales: $70.4 million
Number of Employees: 1,250
Expertise Needed: Physical therapy, occupational therapy, registered nursing, licensed practical nursing
Contact: Ms Nancy Borgan
Nurse Recruiter
(206) 744-4190

STORMONT VAIL HEALTH SERVICES CORPORATION
1500 SOUTHWEST 10TH AVENUE
TOPEKA, KANSAS 66604-1301

Description: General hospital
Annual Sales: $83.9 million
Number of Employees: 1,800

Expertise Needed: Cardiology, pediatrics, oncology, maternity care, orthopedics, respiratory therapy, occupational therapy, physical therapy
Contact: Ms Carey Hoit
Personnel Assistant
(913) 354-6000

STORZ INSTRUMENT COMPANY
3365 TREE COURT INDUSTRIAL
SAINT LOUIS, MISSOURI 63122

Description: Manufactures surgical instruments and equipment
Parent Company: American Cyanamid Company
Annual Sales: $241.0 million
Number of Employees: 1,100
Expertise Needed: Sales, mechanical engineering, electrical engineering, marketing, manufacturing engineering, ophthalmological engineering, design engineering
Contact: Mr Web Sant
Manager of Employment
(314) 225-5057

STRATAGENE CLONING SYSTEMS
11099 NORTH TORREY PINES ROAD
LA JOLLA, CALIFORNIA 92037-1029

Description: Biotechnology research company
Annual Sales: $28.9 million
Number of Employees: 250
Expertise Needed: Microbiology, biology, chemistry, molecular biology
Contact: Ms Karen Rahilly
Human Resources Administrator
(619) 535-5400

STRATEGIC HEALTH SERVICES
511 BROOKS STREET
CHARLESTON, WEST VIRGINIA 25301

Description: Home health-care agency
Parent Company: Camcare, Inc.
Annual Sales: $22.1 million
Number of Employees: 400
Expertise Needed: Registered nursing, licensed practical nursing, certified nursing and nursing assistance, physical therapy, occupational therapy, social service, waste management
Contact: Ms Lisa Hackett
Director of Human Resources
(304) 343-8542

STRATO-INFUSAID CORPORATION
123 BRIMBAL AVENUE
BEVERLY, MASSACHUSETTS 01915

Description: Manufactures blood fusion equipment
Parent Company: Pfizer, Inc.
Founded: 1984
Number of Employees: 200

Expertise Needed: Mechanical engineering, manufacturing engineering

Contact: Human Resources Department
(508) 927-9419

STRYKER CORPORATION
2725 FAIRFIELD ROAD
KALAMAZOO, MICHIGAN 49002-1747

Description: Manufactures specialty medical equipment and instruments
Founded: 1938
Annual Sales: $364.8 million
Number of Employees: 2,448
Expertise Needed: Accounting, sales, mechanical engineering, design engineering, electrical engineering
Contact: Ms Vicki Gordon
Benefits Administrator
(616) 385-2600

STYL-RITE OPTICAL
3850 NORTHWEST 35TH AVENUE
MIAMI, FLORIDA 33142

Description: Manufactures and distributes eyeglass frames
Number of Employees: 185
Expertise Needed: Manufacturing engineering, mechanical engineering
Contact: Mr Jose Ramos
Manager of Human Resources
(305) 634-7895

SUBURBAN HOSPITAL
8600 OLD GEORGETOWN ROAD
BETHESDA, MARYLAND 20814

Description: Private hospital
Founded: 1942
Annual Sales: $103.4 million
Number of Employees: 1,550
Expertise Needed: Nursing, radiology, respiratory therapy, physical therapy
Contact: Ms Beth Murphy
Employment Coordinator
(301) 530-3100

SULLIVAN DENTAL PRODUCTS, INC.
10920 WEST LINCOLN AVENUE
MILWAUKEE, WISCONSIN 53227-1130

Description: Distributes dental instruments and equipment
Founded: 1980
Annual Sales: $74.6 million
Number of Employees: 450
Expertise Needed: Sales, marketing
Contact: Department of Human Resources
(424) 321-8881

SULZER BROTHERS, INC.
200 PARK AVENUE
NEW YORK, NEW YORK 10166-0001

Description: Manufactures and distributes heating, air conditioning and refrigeration equipment
Founded: 1940
Annual Sales: $880.7 million
Number of Employees: 4,400
Expertise Needed: Marketing, accounting, finance, sales, mechanical engineering
Contact: Mr John Bird
Corporate Director of Human Resources
(212) 949-0999

BG SULZLE, INC.
1 NEEDLE LANE
SYRACUSE, NEW YORK 13212

Description: Manufactures surgical needles
Annual Sales: $41.9 million
Number of Employees: 500
Expertise Needed: Mechanical engineering, electrical engineering
Contact: Mr Thomas Coleman
Personnel Director
(315) 454-3221

SUMMA HEALTH SYSTEM
525 EAST MARKET STREET
AKRON, OHIO 44304-1619

Description: Public hospital
Parent Company: Summa Health System
Founded: 1890
Annual Sales: $217.2 million
Number of Employees: 3,300
Expertise Needed: Nursing, occupational therapy, physical therapy, radiology, respiratory therapy
Contact: Ms Carol Owen
Nursing Recruiter
(216) 375-3000

SUN COAST HOSPITAL, INC.
2025 INDIAN ROCKS ROAD
LARGO, FLORIDA 34644-1035

Description: Not-for-profit general hospital and nursing home
Founded: 1955
Annual Sales: $46.2 million
Number of Employees: 700
Expertise Needed: Registered nursing, radiology, broadcast engineering, nursing, intensive care, dietetics, certified nursing and nursing assistance, general surgery, medical technology
Contact: Human Resources
(813) 587-7640

SUN HEALTH CORPORATION, WALTER O. BOSWELL MEMORIAL HOSPITAL

13180 NORTH 103RD DRIVE
SUN CITY, ARIZONA 85351-3038

Description: Hospital specializing in geriatric care
Founded: 1981
Annual Sales: $121.7 million
Number of Employees: 1,900
Expertise Needed: Geriatrics, cardiology, dialysis, registered nursing, licensed practical nursing

Contact: Ms Judy Boyd
Manager of Human Resources
(602) 876-5301

SUNHEALTH ALLIANCE, INC.

4501 CHARLOTTE PARK DRIVE
CHARLOTTE, NORTH CAROLINA 28217-1979

Description: Provides data processing services for health-care facilities
Founded: 1983
Annual Sales: $38.1 million
Number of Employees: 515
Expertise Needed: Registered nursing, licensed practical nursing, purchasing, consulting, finance, marketing, occupational therapy, physical therapy, radiology, nursing management and administration

Contact: Ms Ada White
Manager of Human Resources
(704) 529-3300

SUNRISE COMMUNITY, INC.

22300 SOUTHWEST 162ND AVENUE
MIAMI, FLORIDA 33170-3907

Description: Provides health-care for individuals with disabilities
Parent Company: Phineas Corporation
Founded: 1969
Annual Sales: $24.3 million
Number of Employees: 1,000
Expertise Needed: Licensed practical nursing, registered nursing, certified nursing and nursing assistance

Contact: Ms Beatrice Meza
Recruitment
(305) 245-6150

SUNRISE HEALTHCARE CORPORATION

5600 WYOMING BOULEVARD NORTHEAST
ALBUQUERQUE, NEW MEXICO 87109-3149

Description: Owns and operates nursing homes
Annual Sales: $80.0 million
Number of Employees: 3,000
Expertise Needed: Accounting, administration

Contact: Mr Gary Stagner
Director of Human Resources
(505) 821-3355

SUNRISE HOSPITAL & MEDICAL CENTER

3186 SOUTH PARKWAY
LAS VEGAS, NEVADA 89109-2306

Description: General medical and surgical hospital
Parent Company: Humana, Inc.
Founded: 1958
Annual Sales: $219.5 million
Number of Employees: 2,500
Expertise Needed: Registered nursing, occupational therapy, respiratory therapy, physical therapy, radiological technology

Contact: Ms Barbara Reed
Vice President of Human Resources
(702) 731-8000

SUNRISE MEDICAL, INC.

2355 CRENSHAW BOULEVARD
TORRANCE, CALIFORNIA 90501-3329

Description: Manufactures home medical equipment and rehabilitation products
Annual Sales: $319.2 million
Number of Employees: 3,125
Expertise Needed: Electrical engineering, mechanical engineering, test engineering, design engineering

Contact: Ms Deborah Beasley
Director of Human Resources
(310) 328-8018

SUPELCO, INC.

SUPELCO PARK
BELLEFONTE, PENNSYLVANIA 16823

Description: Manufactures and distributes products to research laboratories and hospitals
Founded: 1968
Number of Employees: 430
Expertise Needed: Chemistry, biochemistry, data processing

Contact: Ms Dianne Lidgett
Director of Human Resources
(814) 359-3441

SUPER D DRUGS, INC.

4895 OUTLAND CENTER DRIVE
MEMPHIS, TENNESSEE 38118

Description: Discount drug store chain
Parent Company: Vestar Capital Partners, Inc.
Annual Sales: $185.0 million
Number of Employees: 1,503
Expertise Needed: Pharmaceutical, sales, management

Contact: Human Resources Department
(901) 366-1144

SUPERIOR HEALTHCARE GROUP, INC.

35 INDUSTRIAL ROAD
CUMBERLAND, RHODE ISLAND 02864-7413

Description: Manufactures medical supplies and equipment

Superior Healthcare Group, Inc. (continued)

Founded: 1965
Annual Sales: $30.0 million
Number of Employees: 280
Expertise Needed: Manufacturing engineering, mechanical engineering, accounting
Contact: Ms Kim Hess
Human Resources Representative
(401) 333-6061

SURGICAL APPLIANCE INDUSTRIES, INC.
3960 ROSSLYN DRIVE
CINCINNATI, OHIO 45209-1110

Description: Manufactures orthopedic devices and appliances, prostheses, and convalescent aids
Founded: 1971
Annual Sales: $50.0 million
Number of Employees: 650
Expertise Needed: Accounting, marketing, finance, management information systems, sales
Contact: Ms Gina Faught
Human Resources Department
(513) 271-4594

SURGIMEDICS, INC.
2828 NORTH CRESCENT RIDGE DRIVE
THE WOODLANDS, TEXAS 77381

Description: Manufactures medical and surgical equipment
Founded: 1984
Annual Sales: $30.0 million
Number of Employees: 250
Expertise Needed: Manufacturing engineering, mechanical engineering, research and development, medical technology
Contact: Human Resources Department
(713) 363-4949

SURVIVAL TECHNOLOGY, INC.
2275 RESEARCH BOULEVARD
ROCKVILLE, MARYLAND 20850-3268

Description: Manufactures pharmaceutical products
Founded: 1968
Annual Sales: $30.1 million
Number of Employees: 237
Expertise Needed: Accounting, mechanical engineering, chemical engineering, chemistry, research and development
Contact: Human Resources Department
(301) 926-1800

SUTTER COMMUNITY HOSPITAL
2800 L STREET
SACRAMENTO, CALIFORNIA 95816-5616

Description: Public hospital
Annual Sales: $24.1 million
Number of Employees: 650

Expertise Needed: Registered nursing, nursing management and administration, licensed practical nursing, occupational therapy, physical therapy, radiology, respiratory therapy, finance
Contact: Employment Department
(916) 733-3730

SUTTER CORPORATION
9425 CHESAPEAKE DRIVE
SAN DIEGO, CALIFORNIA 92123-1302

Description: Manufactures and distributes orthopedic products
Founded: 1979
Number of Employees: 250
Expertise Needed: Sales, marketing, research and development, production, customer service and support
Contact: Department of Human Resources
(619) 569-8148

THE SWEDISH HOSPITAL MEDICAL CENTER
747 BROADWAY
SEATTLE, WASHINGTON 98114-0999

Description: Nonprofit general hospital
Founded: 1905
Annual Sales: $282.6 million
Number of Employees: 5,300
Expertise Needed: Registered nursing, licensed practical nursing, physical therapy, occupational therapy, respiratory therapy, medical technology, radiation technology
Contact: Ms Lisa Brock
Human Resources Director
(206) 386-6000

SWEDISH MEDICAL CENTER
501 EAST HAMPDEN AVENUE
ENGLEWOOD, COLORADO 80110-2702

Description: Nonprofit general hospital
Founded: 1909
Annual Sales: $116.5 million
Number of Employees: 2,000
Expertise Needed: Trauma, maternity care, cardiac care, neurology, registered nursing
Contact: Ms Betty Hines
Recruiter
(303) 788-5000

SYNCOR INTERNATIONAL CORPORATION
20001 PRAIRIE STREET
CHATSWORTH, CALIFORNIA 91311

Description: Provides pharmacy services and distributes radiopharmaceuticals used for diagnostic imaging
Founded: 1974
Annual Sales: $230.9 million
Number of Employees: 2,034

Expertise Needed: Accounting, human resources, management information systems, pharmacy

Contact: Ms Deborah Hildebrand
Supervisor of Human Resources
(818) 886-7400

SYNERGEN, INC.
1885 33RD STREET
BOULDER, COLORADO 80301-2505

Description: Researches and develops pharmaceuticals
Founded: 1981
Annual Sales: $51.4 million
Number of Employees: 612
Expertise Needed: Biological engineering, biology, microbiology, chemistry, biochemistry
Contact: Ms Karen Hildebrand
Director of Human Resources
(303) 938-6200

SYNETIC, INC.
100 SUMMIT AVENUE
MONTVALE, NEW JERSEY 07645

Description: Provides pharmaceutical dispensing and management services
Parent Company: Medco Containment Services
Founded: 1989
Annual Sales: $93.7 million
Number of Employees: 1,090
Expertise Needed: Pharmacy
Contact: Ms Doreen Adams
Employment Manager
(201) 358-5300

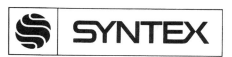

SYNTEX CORPORATION
3401 HILLVIEW AVENUE, M/S A1-160
PALO ALTO, CALIFORNIA 94303

Description: International pharmaceuticals manufacturer
Founded: 1944
Annual Sales: $2.1 billion
Number of Employees: 9,500
Number of Managerial and Professional Employees Hired 1993: 312
Expertise Needed: Chemistry, biology, biochemistry, statistics, clinical research
Contact for College Students and Recent Graduates:
College Relations Coordinator
(415) 354-7201
Contact for All Other Candidates:
Corporate Employment
(415) 354-7201

SYNTEX CHEMICALS, INC.
2075 NORTH 55TH STREET
BOULDER, COLORADO 80301-2803

Description: Manufactures pharmaceutical products
Parent Company: Syntex USA, Inc.
Founded: 1966
Annual Sales: $41.5 million
Number of Employees: 330
Expertise Needed: Chemistry, chemical engineering
Contact: Ms Pat Bassallow
Director of Human Resources
(303) 442-1926

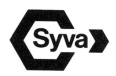

SYVA
3401 HILLVIEW AVENUE
PALO ALTO, CALIFORNIA 94303

Description: Develops and manufactures medical diagnostics
Parent Company: Syntex Corporation
Founded: 1966
Annual Sales: $211.9 million
Number of Employees: 1,250
Number of Managerial and Professional Employees Hired 1993: 82
Expertise Needed: Chemistry, biology, biochemistry, statistics
Contact for College Students and Recent Graduates:
College Relations Coordinator
(415) 354-7281
Contact for All Other Candidates:
Corporate Employment

TAG PHARMACEUTICALS, INC.
1285 AVENUE OF THE AMERICAS
NEW YORK, NEW YORK 10019-6028

Description: Manufactures pharmaceuticals
Annual Sales: $43.6 million
Number of Employees: 350
Expertise Needed: Biochemistry, chemistry, chemical engineering, laboratory technology, pharmaceutical science, pharmacology, pharmaceutical chemistry, manufacturing engineering
Contact: Ms Donna Fikes
Manager of Human Resources
(800) 824-7427

TAKE CARE HEALTH PLAN, INC.
2300 CLAYTON ROAD
CONCORD, CALIFORNIA 94520-2148

Description: Health maintenance organization
Annual Sales: $364.1 million
Number of Employees: 235

Take Care Health Plan, Inc. (continued)

Expertise Needed: Sales, customer service and support, claims adjustment/examination, actuarial, accounting, registered nursing

Contact: Personnel Department
(510) 246-1300

TAMARACK INTERNATIONAL, INC.

625 FOURTH STREET
CHETEK, WISCONSIN 54728

Description: Manufactures medical braces
Founded: 1982
Annual Sales: $34.3 million
Number of Employees: 450
Expertise Needed: Industrial engineering, accounting, business

Contact: Ms Barb Geborec
Assistant Human Resources Manager
(715) 924-4525

TAMPA GENERAL HEALTH CARE

1 COLUMBIA DRIVE
TAMPA, FLORIDA 33601

Description: Public hospital
Annual Sales: $310.7 million
Number of Employees: 3,750
Expertise Needed: Nursing, occupational therapy, physical therapy

Contact: Ms Pam Stone
Professional and Technical Recruiter
(813) 251-7000

TAP PHARMACEUTICALS, INC.

2355 WAUKEGAN ROAD
DEERFIELD, ILLINOIS 60015-5501

Description: Distributes pharmaceutical products
Founded: 1977
Annual Sales: $164.0 million
Number of Employees: 550
Expertise Needed: Sales, marketing, accounting, human resources, management information systems

Contact: Ms Denise Kitchen
Director of Human Resources
(708) 317-5711

TARGET THERAPEUTICS, INC.

47201 LAKEVIEW BOULEVARD
FREMONT, CALIFORNIA 94538-6530

Description: Develops and manufactures disposable medical devices
Parent Company: Collagen Corporation
Annual Sales: $28.1 million
Number of Employees: 249

Expertise Needed: Electrical engineering, manufacturing engineering, medical technology, design engineering, electronics/electronics engineering, instrumentation engineering

Contact: Ms Lisa Schlogeter
Human Resources Administrator
(510) 440-7700

TARRANT COUNTY HOSPITAL DISTRICT

1500 SOUTH MAIN STREET
FORT WORTH, TEXAS 76104-4917

Description: Public hospital specializing in women's services
Founded: 1913
Annual Sales: $142.5 million
Number of Employees: 2,100
Expertise Needed: Nursing

Contact: Ms Ann Henry
Nursing Recruiter
(817) 921-3431

TAYLOR COMPANY

750 NORTH BLACKHAWK BOULEVARD
ROCKTON, ILLINOIS 61072

Description: Manufactures freezing units for reconstructive surgery
Founded: 1926
Number of Employees: 600
Expertise Needed: Manufacturing engineering, mechanical engineering, electrical engineering, electronics/electronics engineering, sales, marketing, accounting

Contact: Ms Jeannie Meichtry
Human Resources Director
(815) 624-8333

TAYLOR-WHARTON CRYOGENICS

4075 HAMILTON BOULEVARD
THEODORE, ALABAMA 36582

Description: Manufactures cryogenic storage tanks
Number of Employees: 278
Expertise Needed: Chemical engineering, mechanical engineering, accounting, marketing, sales

Contact: Ms Paige Walsh
Employee Relations
(205) 443-8680

TECNOL MEDICAL PRODUCTS, INC.

7201 INDUSTRIAL PARK BOULEVARD
FORT WORTH, TEXAS 76180

Description: Designs and manufactures disposal medical and orthopedic products
Founded: 1976
Annual Sales: $71.3 million
Number of Employees: 850
Expertise Needed: Sales, design engineering, plastics engineering, manufacturing engineering,

mechanical engineering, industrial engineering, product design and development, technology research

Contact: Ms Cindy Scruggs
Human Resources Manager
(817) 581-6424

TELECARE CORPORATION
300 PENDLETON WAY
OAKLAND, CALIFORNIA 94621-2102

Description: Owns and operates psychiatric hospitals
Founded: 1966
Annual Sales: $49.0 million
Number of Employees: 1,100
Expertise Needed: Emergency medical technology, cardiology, hospital administration, registered nursing, licensed practical nursing, occupational therapy, physical therapy, radiology, EKG technology, critical care nursing

Contact: Ms Carol Caputo
Director of Human Resources
(510) 632-0133

TELECTRONICS, INC.
7400 SOUTH TUCSON WAY
ENGLEWOOD, COLORADO 80112

Description: Manufactures cardiac pacemakers and electrotherapeutic equipment
Annual Sales: $128.7 million
Number of Employees: 873
Expertise Needed: Electronics/electronics engineering, biomedical engineering

Contact: Ms Sue Eaton
Personnel Administrator
(303) 790-8000

TENNEY ENGINEERING, INC.
1090 SPRINGFIELD ROAD
UNION, NEW JERSEY 07083-8119

Description: Manufactures and markets environmental test and control equipment for laboratories
Founded: 1932
Number of Employees: 185
Expertise Needed: Environmental engineering, mechanical engineering

Contact: Mr Frank Gosztyla
Director of Human Resources
(908) 686-7870

TERUMO MEDICAL CORPORATION
2100 COTTONTAIL LANE
SOMERSET, NEW JERSEY 08873-1271

Description: Manufactures thermometers, medical disposables, and monitors
Founded: 1972
Annual Sales: $140.0 million
Number of Employees: 500

Number of Managerial and Professional Employees Hired 1993: 20
Expertise Needed: Sales, accounting, marketing

Contact: Ms Mary Beth Bubert
Employment Manager
(908) 302-4900

TEX-TENN CORPORATION
HIGHWAY 181 & SUNCREST DRIVE
GRAY, TENNESSEE 37615

Description: Manufactures fabrics for therapy equipment
Annual Sales: $90.0 million
Number of Employees: 100
Expertise Needed: Medical technology, manufacturing engineering, design engineering, chemical engineering

Contact: Human Resources Department
(615) 477-2611

TEXARKANA MEMORIAL HOSPITAL
1000 PINE STREET
TEXARKANA, TEXAS 75501-5100

Description: Public general hospital
Founded: 1959
Annual Sales: $104.6 million
Number of Employees: 1,450
Expertise Needed: Registered nursing

Contact: Ms Lana Matlock
Personnel Department
(903) 793-4511

TEXAS CHILDREN'S HOSPITAL
6621 FANNIN STREET
HOUSTON, TEXAS 77030-2208

Description: Not-for-profit general pediatric hospital
Founded: 1947
Annual Sales: $209.8 million
Number of Employees: 2,121
Expertise Needed: Registered nursing, licensed practical nursing, occupational therapy, physical therapy, radiology, dietetics, dietary services, pharmacy, pharmacology

Contact: Human Resources Department
(713) 770-1000

TFX MEDICAL, INC.
TALL PINES PARK
JAFFREY, NEW HAMPSHIRE 03452

Description: Manufactures and markets medical tubing and related products
Founded: 1982
Number of Employees: 200

TFX Medical, Inc. (continued)

Expertise Needed: Mechanical engineering, industrial engineering, plastics engineering, sales, marketing, design engineering, quality engineering

Contact: Ms Pauline Matthews
Human Resources Manager
(603) 532-7706

THERMEDICS, INC.
470 WILDWOOD STREET
WOBURN, MASSACHUSETTS 01888-1799

Description: Manufactures and markets drug and chemical detection systems
Founded: 1966
Number of Employees: 348
Expertise Needed: Mechanical engineering, design engineering

Contact: Ms Susan Stander
Human Resources Representative
(617) 938-3786

TIMKEN MERCY MEDICAL CENTER
1320-30 TIMKEN MERCY DRIVE
CANTON, OHIO 44708

Description: General hospital
Founded: 1908
Annual Sales: $112.2 million
Number of Employees: 2,100
Expertise Needed: Registered nursing, licensed practical nursing, cardiac care, pediatrics, oncology, diabetes, rehabilitation, maternity care

Contact: Ms Karen Okey
Staffing/Human Resources
(216) 489-1000

TOKOS MEDICAL CORPORATION
1821 EAST DYER ROAD
SANTA ANA, CALIFORNIA 92705-5700

Description: Provides obstetrical home health-care services
Parent Company: Tokos Medical Corporation
Founded: 1985
Annual Sales: $115.2 million
Number of Employees: 1,400
Expertise Needed: Marketing, finance, accounting, gynecology, nursing, obstetrics

Contact: Ms Dana Price
Human Resources Department
(714) 474-1616

TORRANCE MEMORIAL MEDICAL CENTER
3330 LOMITA BOULEVARD
TORRANCE, CALIFORNIA 90505-5002

Description: General hospital
Parent Company: Torrance Health Association
Founded: 1925
Annual Sales: $121.0 million

Number of Employees: 1,700
Expertise Needed: Registered nursing, licensed practical nursing, radiology, medical technology, physical therapy, respiratory therapy, occupational therapy

Contact: Mr Pat Reed
Human Resources Assistant
(310) 325-9110

TOSHIBA AMERICA MEDICAL SYSTEMS, INC.
2441 MICHELLE DRIVE
TUSTIN, CALIFORNIA 92680

Description: Manufactures and markets diagnostic imaging systems
Parent Company: Toshiba America, Inc.
Annual Sales: $119.1 million
Number of Employees: 1,072
Expertise Needed: Marketing, management information systems, accounting, public relations, mechanical engineering, electrical engineering

Contact: Ms Agnes Malloy
Manager of Human Resource Services
(714) 730-5000

TOSHIBA AMERICA MRI, INC.
280 UTAH AVENUE
SOUTH SAN FRANCISCO, CALIFORNIA 94080-6801

Description: Develops and manufactures magnetic resonance imaging systems
Parent Company: Toshiba America Medical Systems
Founded: 1989
Annual Sales: $40.0 million
Number of Employees: 230
Expertise Needed: Research and development, manufacturing engineering, mental health, electrical engineering, software engineering/ development, hardware engineering

Contact: Mr Byron Clendenen
Director of Human Resources
(415) 872-2722

TOURO INFIRMARY
1401 FOUCHER STREET
NEW ORLEANS, LOUISIANA 70115-3515

Description: General hospital
Founded: 1852
Annual Sales: $102.9 million
Number of Employees: 1,850
Expertise Needed: Registered nursing, licensed practical nursing, certified nursing and nursing assistance, cardiology, biology, physical therapy, occupational therapy, respiratory therapy

Contact: Ms Deborah Alexander
Nursing Recruiter
(504) 897-8340

TP ORTHODONTICS, INC.

100 CENTER PLAZA
LAPORTE, INDIANA 46350

Description: Manufactures orthodontic devices
Founded: 1955
Annual Sales: $26.2 million
Number of Employees: 370
Expertise Needed: Accounting, marketing, finance, management information systems
Contact: Ms Elaine Huffman
      Human Resources Director
      (219) 785-2591

TRAVCORPS, INC.

40 EASTERN AVENUE
MALDEN, MASSACHUSETTS 02148

Description: Provides temporary and permanent personnel services to hospitals and health-care facilities
Founded: 1978
Number of Employees: 200
Expertise Needed: Nursing, occupational therapy, physical therapy
Contact: Mr Bruce Cerullo
      President
      (617) 322-2600

TRUE QUALITY PHARMACIES, INC.

222 EAST VIRGINIA STREET
MC KINNEY, TEXAS 75069-4328

Description: Drug store chain
Founded: 1964
Annual Sales: $57.3 million
Number of Employees: 650
Expertise Needed: Biochemistry, chemistry, chemical engineering, laboratory technology, pharmaceutical, manufacturing engineering, pharmaceutical chemistry, pharmacology, pharmaceutical science
Contact: Ms Donna Pultzer
      Director of Human Resources
      (214) 542-0336

TRUSTEES OF MEASE HOSPITAL

601 MAIN STREET
DUNEDIN, FLORIDA 34698-5848

Description: Nonprofit hospital
Founded: 1938
Annual Sales: $107.1 million
Number of Employees: 1,546
Expertise Needed: Nursing, licensed practical nursing, physical therapy, occupational therapy, respiratory therapy
Contact: Ms Sharon Collotta
      Director of Personnel
      (813) 734-6101

TSI MASON RESEARCH INSTITUTE, INC.

57 UNION STREET
WORCESTER, MASSACHUSETTS 01608

Description: Research institute
Founded: 1970
Number of Employees: 175
Expertise Needed: Laboratory technology, chemistry
Contact: Ms Donna Perron
      Human Resources Manager
      (508) 791-0931

T2 MEDICAL, INC.

1121 ALDERMAN DRIVE
ALPHARETTA, GEORGIA 30202-4102

Description: Provides infusion therapy services and operates health-care facilities
Founded: 1984
Annual Sales: $242.1 million
Number of Employees: 1,254
Expertise Needed: Accounting, sales, management, administration
Contact: Mr. Roger Bruce
      Vice President of Human Resources
      (404) 442-2160

TWIN CITY OPTICAL COMPANY

725 HIGHWAY 169 NORTH
MINNEAPOLIS, MINNESOTA 55441-6403

Description: Manufactures eyeglasses
Parent Company: The Churchill Companies
Annual Sales: $45.0 million
Number of Employees: 325
Expertise Needed: Sales, marketing, laboratory technology
Contact: Human Resources Department
      (612) 546-6126

TWIN LABORATORIES, INC.

2120 SMITHTOWN AVENUE
RONKONKOMA, NEW YORK 11779-7327

Description: Manufactures natural and synthetic vitamins
Founded: 1968
Annual Sales: $75.0 million
Number of Employees: 350
Expertise Needed: Food science, nutrition, sales, engineering, marketing, business
Contact: Personnel Department
      (516) 467-3140

UNICARE HEALTH FACILITIES, INC.

105 WEST MICHIGAN STREET
MILWAUKEE, WISCONSIN 53203-2914

Description: Owns and operates nursing homes
Annual Sales: $137.5 million
Number of Employees: 4,457

Expertise Needed: Finance, accounting, hospital administration

Contact: Ms Connie Champnoise
Director of Human Resources
(414) 271-9696

UNIHEALTH AMERICA

4100 WEST ALAMEDA AVENUE
BURBANK, CALIFORNIA 91505-4153

Description: Owns and operates hospitals and insurance companies
Founded: 1970
Assets: $2.8 billion
Number of Employees: 14,000
Expertise Needed: Business management, accounting, finance, auditing, actuarial
Contact: Ms Magaly Juarez
Human Resources Representative
(818) 566-6401

UNIHEALTH AMERICA VENTURES

6300 CANOGA AVENUE
WOODLAND HILLS, CALIFORNIA 91367

Description: Owns and operates not-for-profit general hospitals and medical centers
Founded: 1980
Annual Sales: $24.1 million
Number of Employees: 1,500
Expertise Needed: Health care, health insurance, hospital administration
Contact: Ms Barbara Cook
Vice President of Human Resources
(818) 598-8000

UNION HOSPITAL, INC.

1606 NORTH 7TH STREET
TERRE HAUTE, INDIANA 47804-2706

Description: General hospital
Founded: 1895
Annual Sales: $126.0 million
Number of Employees: 2,000
Expertise Needed: Nursing, licensed practical nursing, occupational therapy, physical therapy, respiratory therapy, radiology, nutrition
Contact: Ms Susan Knapp
Employment Coordinator
(812) 238-7504

UNITED CHURCH HOMES, INC.

170 EAST CENTER STREET
MARION, OHIO 43302-3815

Description: Owns and operates nursing home
Founded: 1916
Annual Sales: $24.1 million
Number of Employees: 900

Expertise Needed: Nursing, licensed practical nursing, physical therapy, occupational therapy
Contact: Mr Tim Hacket
Vice President of Human Resources
(614) 382-4885

UNITED HEALTH, INC.

105 WEST MICHIGAN STREET
MILWAUKEE, WISCONSIN 53203

Description: Provides home health-care and nursing care services
Founded: 1968
Number of Employees: 16,000
Expertise Needed: General nursing, dietetics, occupational therapy
Contact: Ms Nancy Monti
Professional Recruiter
(414) 342-9292

UNITED HEALTHCARE CORPORATION

9900 BREN ROAD EAST
HOPKINS, MINNESOTA 55343-9608

Description: Provides managed care health-care and cost management services
Founded: 1977
Annual Sales: $847.1 million
Number of Employees: 3,500
Expertise Needed: Computer programming, computer science, accounting, credit/credit analysis
Contact: Ms Tracy Heitner
Manager of Recruitment
(612) 936-7395

UNITED INSURANCE COMPANIES

4001 MCEWEN ROAD
DALLAS, TEXAS 75244-5033

Description: Provides life and health insurance
Annual Sales: $371.3 million
Number of Employees: 600
Expertise Needed: Accounting, finance, data processing, law, actuarial, claims adjustment/examination
Contact: Ms Linda Flowers
Personnel Director
(214) 960-8497

UNITED PROFESSIONAL COMPANIES

3724 WEST WISCONSIN AVENUE
MILWAUKEE, WISCONSIN 53208-3153

Description: Operates drug stores and sells medical supplies
Parent Company: United Health, Inc.
Annual Sales: $41.4 million
Number of Employees: 371
Expertise Needed: Pharmacy, nursing, home health care
Contact: Human Resources Department

UNITED STATES SURGICAL CORPORATION

150 GLOVER AVENUE
NORWALK, CONNECTICUT 06850-1308

Description: Manufactures disposable surgical products
Founded: 1964
Annual Sales: $1.2 billion
Number of Employees: 8,100
Expertise Needed: Nutrition, physical therapy,
   mechanical engineering
Contact: Ms Lynnea Prunko
      Vice President of Human Resources
      (203) 845-1000

UNITED WESTERN MEDICAL CENTERS

1301 NORTH TUSTIN AVENUE
SANTA ANA, CALIFORNIA 92701-3530

Description: Public hospital
Founded: 1980
Annual Sales: $174.3 million
Number of Employees: 2,088
Expertise Needed: Registered nursing, physical therapy,
   occupational therapy, respiratory therapy, radiation
   therapy
Contact: Ms Denise Johnson
      Human Resources Associate
      (714) 953-3580

UNIVERSAL CARE, INC.

1600 EAST HILL STREET
LONG BEACH, CALIFORNIA 90806-3612

Description: Provides outpatient medical care services
Founded: 1983
Annual Sales: $39.3 million
Number of Employees: 270
Expertise Needed: Registered nursing, licensed practical
   nursing, physical therapy, occupational therapy
Contact: Ms Sandy Taylor
      Director of Personnel
      (310) 424-6200

UNIVERSAL HEALTH SERVICES

367 SOUTH GULPH ROAD
KING OF PRUSSIA, PENNSYLVANIA 19406-2832

Description: Owns and operates acute-care and
   psychiatric care facilities
Founded: 1978
Annual Sales: $731.2 million
Number of Employees: 9,650
Expertise Needed: Accounting, finance, marketing,
   business, data processing
Contact: Ms Pat White
      Manager of Personnel Administration
      (610) 768-3300

UNIVERSAL HEALTH SERVICES OF NEVADA

620 SHADOW LANE
LAS VEGAS, NEVADA 89106-4119

Description: Owns and operates general medical and
   surgical hospitals
Parent Company: Universal Health Services
Founded: 1979
Annual Sales: $230.9 million
Number of Employees: 1,000
Expertise Needed: Accounting, finance, data processing,
   marketing, business
Contact: Ms Ginger Consigney
      Director of Human Resources
      (702) 388-4000

UNIVERSAL STANDARD MEDICAL LABORATORIES

21705 EVERGREEN ROAD
SOUTHFIELD, MICHIGAN 48075-3968

Description: Owns and operates clinical laboratories
Founded: 1991
Annual Sales: $44.6 million
Number of Employees: 1,000
*Number of Managerial and Professional Employees Hired
   1993:* 12
Expertise Needed: Laboratory technology
Contact: Professional Recruiter

UNIVERSITY COMMUNITY HOSPITAL

3100 EAST FLETCHER AVENUE
TAMPA, FLORIDA 33613-4613

Description: Community general hospital
Founded: 1966
Annual Sales: $104.6 million
Number of Employees: 1,300
Expertise Needed: Registered nursing, physical therapy,
   occupational therapy, respiratory therapy
Contact: Ms Kathy Meloy
      Nursing Recruiter
      (813) 971-6000

UNIVERSITY MEDICAL CENTER, INC.

655 WEST 8TH STREET
JACKSONVILLE, FLORIDA 32209-6511

Description: Private hospital specializing in trauma
Founded: 1971
Annual Sales: $375.0 million
Number of Employees: 2,600
Expertise Needed: Nursing, physical therapy
Contact: Ms Donna Kalkines
      Nurse Recruitment
      (904) 549-5000

UNIVERSITY MEDICAL CENTER OF SOUTHERN NEVADA

1800 WEST CHARLESTON BOULEVARD
LAS VEGAS, NEVADA 89102-2329

Description: County medical and surgical hospital
Founded: 1931
Annual Sales: $184.6 million
Number of Employees: 2,375
Expertise Needed: Respiratory therapy, registered nursing, triage
Contact: Mr. Douglas Pring
　　　Director of Personnel
　　　(702) 383-2000

UNIVERSITY OF MARYLAND MEDICAL SYSTEM

22 SOUTH GREENE STREET
BALTIMORE, MARYLAND 21201

Description: Health-care facility including a hospital, research center, and medical school
Founded: 1984
Annual Sales: $325.0 million
Number of Employees: 5,000
Expertise Needed: Nursing, medical technology, occupational therapy, physical therapy, pharmacology, radiation technology, radiology, research and development
Contact: Mr Rod Flowers
　　　Personnel Manager
　　　(410) 328-2757

UNIVERSITY OF SOUTH ALABAMA MEDICAL CENTER

2451 FILLINGIM STREET
MOBILE, ALABAMA 36617-2238

Description: Public hospital specializing in trauma
Founded: 1963
Annual Sales: $137.8 million
Number of Employees: 2,500
Expertise Needed: Nursing, physical therapy, respiratory therapy, occupational therapy
Contact: Ms Lisa Tanner
　　　Professional Recruiter
　　　(205) 471-7000

THE UPJOHN COMPANY

7000 PORTAGE ROAD
KALAMAZOO, MICHIGAN 49001-0102

Description: Manufactures pharmaceuticals, animal drugs, and consumer health-care products
Founded: 1886
Annual Sales: $3.6 billion
Number of Employees: 18,900
Expertise Needed: Sales, research and development
Contact: Upjohn Applicant Information
　　　(616) 329-5550

UPSHER-SMITH LABORATORIES

14905 23RD AVENUE NORTH
MINNEAPOLIS, MINNESOTA 55447-4708

Description: Manufactures cardiovascular, pharmaceutical, pediatric, vitamin, and hospital products
Founded: 1969
Annual Sales: $26.9 million
Number of Employees: 220
Expertise Needed: Business, chemistry, sales
Contact: Mr Ryan Reisdorfer
　　　Manager of Human Resources Development

U.S. BEHAVIORAL HEALTH

2000 POWELL STREET
EMERYVILLE, CALIFORNIA 94608

Description: Manages health-care benefit and employee assistance programs
Founded: 1979
Number of Employees: 274
Expertise Needed: Behavioral research, casework, chemical dependency, health care, mental health, data processing, psychotherapy, psychiatric social work, substance abuse treatment and counseling
Contact: Ms Suzzane Brennan
　　　Manager of Human Resources
　　　(510) 652-1402

US HEALTHCARE, INC.

1425 UNION MEETING ROAD
BLUE BELL, PENNSYLVANIA 19422-1962

Description: Provides managed care services
Annual Sales: $2.1 billion
Number of Employees: 2,845
Expertise Needed: Management information systems, accounting, sales, applied engineering, imaging technology, claims adjustment/examination, actuarial
Contact: Ms Beth Caulfield
　　　Senior Human Resources Representative
　　　(215) 628-4800

USA NAMIC CORPORATION

PRUYNS ISLAND
GLENS FALLS, NEW YORK 12801-4449

Description: Manufactures disposable medical devices
Founded: 1969
Annual Sales: $54.2 million
Number of Employees: 637
Expertise Needed: Mechanical engineering, project engineering, production
Contact: Mr Kyle Brock
　　　Recruiter
　　　(518) 798-0067

UTAH MEDICAL PRODUCTS, INC.
7043 SOUTH 300 WEST
MIDVALE, UTAH 84047

Description: Develops and manufactures medical
equipment
Founded: 1978
Annual Sales: $36.1 million
Number of Employees: 400
Expertise Needed: Accounting, finance, mechanical
engineering, manufacturing engineering, research
and development, electrical engineering,
production engineering
Contact: Ms Lori Sessions
Manager of Human Resources/Controller
(801) 566-1200

VALLEYLAB, INC.
5920 LONGBOW DRIVE
BOULDER, COLORADO 80301

Description: Manufactures electrosurgical equipment
Parent Company: Pfizer, Inc.
Annual Sales: $160.0 million
Number of Employees: 1,400
Expertise Needed: Electrical engineering, design
engineering, mechanical engineering, plant
engineering, manufacturing engineering, sales,
marketing, chemical engineering
Contact: Ms Jean Arro
Director of Personnel
(303) 530-2300

VALUE BEHAVIORAL HEALTH, INC.
3110 FAIRVIEW PARK DRIVE
FALLS CHURCH, VIRGINIA 22042

Description: Provides health-care insurance services
Parent Company: Value Health, Inc.
Founded: 1983
Annual Sales: $29.9 million
Number of Employees: 500
Expertise Needed: Information systems, case
management, clinical psychology, registered
nursing, licensed practical nursing, automation,
psychiatric social work, claims adjustment/
examination, claims processing/management, and
administration, mar
Contact: Department of Human Resources
(703) 205-7000

VALUE HEALTH, INC.
22 WATERVILLE ROAD
AVON, CONNECTICUT 06001-2066

Description: Provides managed care services
Founded: 1991
Annual Sales: $262.2 million
Number of Employees: 1,400

Expertise Needed: Pharmacy, software engineering/
development, accounting, finance, sales, marketing
Contact: Mr Bob Patricelli
President
(203) 678-3400

VARIAN ASSOCIATES, INC.
3100 HANSEN WAY
PALO ALTO, CALIFORNIA 94304-1030

Description: Manufactures medical, industrial, and
scientific research equipment
Founded: 1948
Annual Sales: $1.3 billion
Number of Employees: 8,000
Expertise Needed: Electrical engineering, mechanical
engineering, software engineering/development,
finance, business administration
Contact: Mr Jack McCarthy
Manager of Human Resources
(415) 493-4000

VECTOR HEALTHSYSTEMS
405 PROMENADE STREET
PROVIDENCE, RHODE ISLAND 02940

Description: Provides software systems for hospitals and
health-care facilities
Founded: 1968
Number of Employees: 400
Expertise Needed: Data processing, software
engineering/development, medical records
Contact: Ms Anna Cote
Administrative Assistant of Employee Services
(401) 453-8360

VENCOR, INC.
BROWN AND WILLIAMSON TOWER
LOUISVILLE, KENTUCKY 40202

Description: Owns and operates long-term, acute-care
hospitals
Annual Sales: $214.7 million
Number of Employees: 1,912
Expertise Needed: Registered nursing, licensed practical
nursing, certified nursing and nursing assistance,
accounting, finance, data processing, law
Contact: Ms Susan Solley
Recruiting Services
(502) 569-7386

VENTRITEX, INC.
709 EAST EVELYN AVENUE
SUNNYVALE, CALIFORNIA 94086-6527

Description: Develops and manufactures defibrilators
and related products
Annual Sales: $25.1 million
Number of Employees: 263

VENTRITEX, INC.

Ventritex, Inc. (continued)

Expertise Needed: Accounting, finance, data processing, electrical engineering, biology, physics, chemistry
Contact: Mr Mark Sobolik
Employment Recruiter
(408) 738-4883

VETERANS MEMORIAL MEDICAL CENTER

1 KING PLACE
MERIDEN, CONNECTICUT 06451-5415

Description: Public general hospital
Annual Sales: $101.3 million
Number of Employees: 1,600
Expertise Needed: Registered nursing, physical therapy, occupational therapy, respiratory therapy
Contact: Ms Cheryl Hopper
Employment Manager
(203) 238-8200

VISTA HILL FOUNDATION

2355 NORTHSIDE DRIVE
SAN DIEGO, CALIFORNIA 92108-2705

Description: Nonprofit psychiatric hospital
Founded: 1957
Annual Sales: $41.6 million
Number of Employees: 1,200
Expertise Needed: Psychology, psychotherapy, licensed practical nursing, registered nursing, clinical psychology, social work, physical therapy, occupational therapy, respiratory therapy
Contact: Mr Scott Nishida
Employment Coordinator
(619) 563-1770

VISITING NURSE ASSOCIATION OF GREATER PHILADELPHIA

1 WINDING ROAD
PHILADELPHIA, PENNSYLVANIA 19131-2903

Description: Provides home health-care services
Parent Company: Philadelphia Home Care
Founded: 1979
Annual Sales: $22.0 million
Number of Employees: 300
Expertise Needed: Physical therapy, occupational therapy, licensed practical nursing, networking, criminal investigation, social work, home health care
Contact: Mr Robert Simon
Director of Human Resources
(215) 581-2010

VISITING NURSE SERVICE OF NEW YORK

107 EAST 70TH STREET
NEW YORK, NEW YORK 10021-5006

Description: Provides home health-care services
Founded: 1893
Annual Sales: $334.7 million
Number of Employees: 2,200

Expertise Needed: Nursing, business, accounting
Contact: Ms Alice Hanks
Director of Recruiting
(212) 560-3370

VITAL SIGNS, INC.

20 CAMPUS ROAD
TOTOWA, NEW JERSEY 07512-1210

Description: Manufactures disposable medical products for anesthesia and respiratory uses
Founded: 1972
Annual Sales: $65.7 million
Number of Employees: 520
Expertise Needed: Mechanical engineering, manufacturing engineering
Contact: Ms Robin Kaminski
Employment Specialist
(201) 790-1300

VITALINK PHARMACY SERVICES, INC.

1250 EAST DIEHL ROAD
NAPERVILLE, ILLINOIS 60563-9367

Description: Provides pharmacy management services
Parent Company: Manor Healthcare Corporation
Founded: 1981
Annual Sales: $65.7 million
Number of Employees: 300
Expertise Needed: Business management, pharmacy, sales
Contact: Human Resources Department
(708) 505-1320

VIVA OPTIQUE, INC.

11 STEWART PLACE
FAIRFIELD, NEW JERSEY 07004-2203

Description: Manufactures eyewear
Founded: 1978
Annual Sales: $50.0 million
Number of Employees: 300
Expertise Needed: Optometry, optics, accounting, marketing
Contact: Ms Leslie Allain
Human Resources Department
(201) 882-3400

VNS HOME CARE, INC.

107 EAST 70TH STREET
NEW YORK, NEW YORK 10021-5006

Description: Provides home health-care services
Annual Sales: $276.7 million
Number of Employees: 1,432
Expertise Needed: Accounting, licensed practical nursing, nursing
Contact: Ms Beth Petersel
Recruitment Assistant
(212) 560-3370

VOLUNTARY HOSPITALS OF AMERICA
220 EAST LAS COLINNAS BOULEVARD
IRVING, TEXAS 75039-3713

Description: Not-for-profit alliance of health-care
    organizations
Founded: 1977
Annual Sales: $110.4 million
Number of Employees: 1,006
Expertise Needed: Radiology, registered nursing, physical
    therapy, licensed practical nursing, occupational
    therapy, health care, accounting, data processing,
    nursing management and administration
Contact: Department of Human Resources
    (214) 830-0000

WAKE COUNTY HOSPITAL SYSTEM
3000 NEW BERN AVENUE
RALEIGH, NORTH CAROLINA 27610-1215

Description: Public hospital
Founded: 1961
Annual Sales: $232.4 million
Number of Employees: 3,800
Expertise Needed: Registered nursing, physical therapy,
    occupational therapy, respiratory therapy
Contact: Ms Jane Grisson
    Recruitment
    (919) 250-8000

WALGREEN COMPANY
300 WILMOT ROAD
DEERFIELD, ILLINOIS 60015

Description: Nationwide retail drug store chain
Founded: 1901
Annual Sales: $7.4 billion
Number of Employees: 55,000
Expertise Needed: Retail, management, business
    management
Contact: Manager of Recruiting
    (708) 940-2500

WARM SPRING REHABILITATION FOUNDATION
FM 1586 AND PARK ROAD 11
OTTINE, TEXAS 78658

Description: Rehabilitation center
Founded: 1937
Annual Sales: $19.3 million
Number of Employees: 480
Expertise Needed: Nursing, respiratory therapy,
    occupational therapy, physical therapy, speech
    therapy, social service, psychology
Contact: Ms Vlasat Perkle
    Employment Manager
    (210) 672-6592

WARNER-LAMBERT COMPANY
201 TABOR ROAD
MORRIS PLAINS, NEW JERSEY 07950

Description: Manufactures and markets
    pharmaceuticals, consumer health-care products,
    and other consumer products
Founded: 1955
Annual Sales: $5.6 billion
Number of Employees: 34,000
Expertise Needed: Pharmaceutical, health care
Contact: Human Resources Department
    (201) 540-2000

WASHINGTON ADVENTIST HOSPITAL
7600 CARROLL AVENUE
TAKOMA PARK, MARYLAND 20912-6392

Description: Church-operated medical and surgical
    hospital
Parent Company: Adventist Healthcare Mid Atlantic
Annual Sales: $107.9 million
Number of Employees: 1,800
Expertise Needed: Cancer care, respiratory therapy,
    occupational therapy, physical therapy, registered
    nursing
Contact: Ms. Janet Hunter
    Associate Director of Human Resources
    (301) 891-5222

MARY WASHINGTON HOSPITAL
1001 SAM PERRY BOULEVARD
FREDERICKSBURG, VIRGINIA 22401

Description: General medical and surgical hospital
Annual Sales: $92.7 million
Number of Employees: 1,371
Expertise Needed: Registered nursing, licensed practical
    nursing, physical therapy
Contact: Ms. JoAnn Abarno
    Manager of Employment
    (703) 899-1400

WASHINGTON TOWNSHIP HOSPITAL DISTRICT
2000 MOWRY AVENUE
FREMONT, CALIFORNIA 94538-1716

Description: General hospital
Founded: 1948
Annual Sales: $121.4 million
Number of Employees: 1,400
Expertise Needed: Registered nursing, licensed practical
    nursing, occupational therapy, physical therapy,
    radiation technology, respiratory therapy
Contact: Personnel Department
    (510) 791-1111

WASHOE MEDICAL CENTER, INC.
77 PRINGLE WAY
RENO, NEVADA 89520

Description: General medical and surgical hospital
Parent Company: Washoe Health System, Inc.
Annual Sales: $199.9 million
Number of Employees: 2,357
Expertise Needed: Registered nursing, occupational therapy, nursing, respiratory therapy, physical therapy
Contact: Mr. Bernard Parks
Manager of Employment
(702) 328-4100

WATERLOO INDUSTRIES, INC.
300 ANSBOROUGH AVENUE
WATERLOO, IOWA 50704

Description: Manufactures hospital furniture and storage equipment
Founded: 1918
Annual Sales: $30.0 million
Number of Employees: 500
Expertise Needed: Manufacturing engineering, design engineering, mechanical engineering, industrial engineering, marketing, management
Contact: Human Resources Department
(319) 235-7131

WATSON PHARMACEUTICALS, INC.
311 BONNIE CIRCLE
CORONA, CALIFORNIA 91720-2882

Description: Manufactures pharmaceutical products and provides commercial research laboratory services
Annual Sales: $34.7 million
Number of Employees: 250
Expertise Needed: Pharmaceutical, laboratory technology, research
Contact: Ms Mary Everetsen
Personnel Manager
(909) 270-1400

WAUKESHA MEMORIAL HOSPITAL
725 AMERICAN AVENUE
WAUKESHA, WISCONSIN 53188-5031

Description: General hospital
Founded: 1956
Annual Sales: $95.5 million
Number of Employees: 1,764
Expertise Needed: Nursing, licensed practical nursing, cardiac care, respiratory therapy, laboratory technology, chemical dependency, management information systems
Contact: Ms Judith Gunkel
Employment Coordinator
(414) 544-2011

WELCH-ALLYN, INC.
4341 STATE STREET ROAD
SKANEATELES FALLS, NEW YORK 13153

Description: Manufactures medical diagnostic instruments
Founded: 1915
Annual Sales: $100.0 million
Number of Employees: 1,600
Expertise Needed: Management, manufacturing, accounting, design engineering, mechanical engineering, computer programming
Contact: Mr Pat Reynolds
Recruiter
(315) 685-4273

WESLEY-JESSEN, INC.
400 WEST SUPERIOR STREET
CHICAGO, ILLINOIS 60610

Description: Manufactures contact lenses, pharmaceuticals, and ophthalmic supplies
Founded: 1946
Number of Employees: 800
Expertise Needed: Accounting, manufacturing engineering, optics
Contact: Mr Michael Southard
Human Resources Director
(312) 751-6200

WEST JERSEY HEALTH SYSTEM CAMDEN
1000 ATLANTIC AVENUE
CAMDEN, NEW JERSEY 08104

Description: Public hospital specializing in substance abuse treatment
Founded: 1884
Annual Sales: $224.0 million
Number of Employees: 4,100
Expertise Needed: Physical therapy, occupational therapy, accounting, management information systems, registered nursing
Contact: Ms Karen Harnish
Director of Human Resources
(609) 342-4055

WESTERN DENTAL SERVICES, INC.
300 PLAZA ALICANTE
GARDEN GROVE, CALIFORNIA 92640-2736

Description: Dental offices
Founded: 1984
Annual Sales: $48.6 million
Number of Employees: 1,600
Expertise Needed: X-ray technology, laboratory technology, dentistry/dental hygiene, office management
Contact: Ms Nia Rojas
Human Resources Associate
(714) 938-1600

WESTERN OPTICAL CORPORATION
1200 MERCER STREET
SEATTLE, WASHINGTON 98109-5511

Description: Owns and operates retail optical stores
Founded: 1967
Annual Sales: $24.7 million
Number of Employees: 249
Expertise Needed: Optics

Contact: Mr Brian Burgher
　　　　Personnel Manager
　　　　(206) 622-7627

WESTERN PENNSYLVANIA HOSPITAL
4800 FRIENDSHIP AVENUE
PITTSBURGH, PENNSYLVANIA 15224-1722

Description: Public hospital
Founded: 1848
Annual Sales: $221.1 million
Number of Employees: 2,800
Expertise Needed: Nursing

Contact: Ms Deborah Stockles
　　　　Nursing Recruiter
　　　　(412) 578-5134

WESTHAVEN SERVICES COMPANY
7643 PONDEROSA ROAD
PERRYSBURG, OHIO 43551-4862

Description: Distributes medical equipment and supplies
Annual Sales: $25.0 million
Number of Employees: 200
Expertise Needed: Accounting, marketing, finance, sales, information systems

Contact: Mr Michael Crabtree
　　　　Chief Financial Officer
　　　　(419) 661-2200

WHITBY PHARMACEUTICALS, INC.
1211 SHERWOOD AVENUE
RICHMOND, VIRGINIA 23220-1212

Description: Manufactures and distributes pharmaceutical products
Annual Sales: $65.0 million
Number of Employees: 100
Expertise Needed: Business administration, diagnostic research, clinical research, pharmacy, biochemistry, chemistry

Contact: Ms Joan Isaac
　　　　Employment Manager
　　　　(804) 254-4400

WHITE OAK MANOR, INC.
2407 SOUTH PINE STREET
SPARTANBURG, SOUTH CAROLINA 29302-4335

Description: Owns and operates retirement centers and nursing homes
Founded: 1968
Annual Sales: $51.4 million

Number of Employees: 2,100
Expertise Needed: Registered nursing, licensed practical nursing, dietetics, social service

Contact: Ms Heidi Edwards
　　　　Human Resources
　　　　(803) 582-7503

WILMAC CORPORATION
209 NORTH BEAVER STREET
YORK, PENNSYLVANIA 17403-5321

Description: Owns and operates a nursing home and retirement center
Founded: 1965
Annual Sales: $20.0 million
Number of Employees: 1,000
Expertise Needed: Registered nursing, licensed practical nursing, health insurance, accounting, data processing

Contact: Mr Tom Shugars
　　　　Director of Human Resources
　　　　(717) 854-7857

WILMAD GLASS COMPANY, INC.
U.S. ROUTE 40 & OAK ROAD
BUENA, NEW JERSEY 08310

Description: Manufactures and markets laboratory glassware
Founded: 1951
Expertise Needed: Mechanical engineering, ceramic engineering

Contact: Ms Eileen Gannon
　　　　Director of Human Resources
　　　　(609) 697-3000

WINCHESTER MEDICAL CENTER, INC.
1840 AMHERST STREET
WINCHESTER, VIRGINIA 22601-2808

Description: Nonprofit private hospital offering acute care services
Annual Sales: $119.3 million
Number of Employees: 1,852
Expertise Needed: Occupational therapy, physical therapy, pharmacology, neurology, intensive care, psychiatry, management information systems, accounting

Contact: Ms Leslie Kelly
　　　　Employment Coordinator
　　　　(703) 722-8800

WINTHROP UNIVERSITY HOSPITAL
259 1ST STREET
MINEOLA, NEW YORK 11501-3957

Description: General hospital
Founded: 1896
Annual Sales: $225.2 million
Number of Employees: 2,850

Winthrop University Hospital (continued)

Expertise Needed: Cardiology, oncology, physicians, chemical dependency, nursing, accounting, management information systems

Contact: Ms Robin Salsberg
Employment Specialist
(516) 663-2351

WISCONSIN PHYSICIANS SERVICE INSURANCE

1717 WEST BROADWAY
MADISON, WISCONSIN 53713-1834

Description: Provides health-care insurance services
Founded: 1977
Annual Sales: $409.6 million
Number of Employees: 3,800
Expertise Needed: Accounting, finance, data processing, law, registered nursing, licensed practical nursing

Contact: Ms Kathy Bennett
Senior Recruiter
(608) 221-4711

WK NURSING HOME CORPORATION

100 WEST KINGSBRIDGE ROAD
BRONX, NEW YORK 10468-4066

Description: Nursing home
Founded: 1966
Annual Sales: $58.7 million
Number of Employees: 1,200
Expertise Needed: Data processing, home health care, nursing, licensed practical nursing

Contact: Personnel
(718) 579-0500

WOMEN & INFANTS HOSPITAL OF RHODE ISLAND

101 DUDLEY STREET
PROVIDENCE, RHODE ISLAND 02905-2401

Description: Hospital specializing in obstetrics, gynecology, and pediatrics
Annual Sales: $97.9 million
Number of Employees: 1,560
Expertise Needed: Gynecology, oncology, registered nursing, licensed practical nursing, computer programming, computer analysis

Contact: Ms Krista Sauvageau
Director of Employment
(401) 274-1100

WOMEN'S HOSPITAL FOUNDATION

9050 AIRLINE HIGHWAY
BATON ROUGE, LOUISIANA 70815-4103

Description: Hospital providing medical and educational services to women and children
Founded: 1968
Annual Sales: $62.8 million
Number of Employees: 1,250

Expertise Needed: Respiratory therapy, nursing, physical therapy, medical technology, accounting, finance, management information systems

Contact: Ms Linda Lee
Recruiting Coordinator
(504) 927-1300

WRIGHT MEDICAL TECHNOLOGY

5677 AIRLINE ROAD
ARLINGTON, TENNESSEE 38002-9501

Description: Manufactures orthopedic implants and instrumentation
Parent Company: Dow Corning Corporation
Founded: 1977
Annual Sales: $45.7 million
Number of Employees: 600
Expertise Needed: Design engineering, marketing

Contact: Mr Jerry Yates
Employment Manager
(901) 867-9971

WUESTHOFF MEMORIAL HOSPITAL

110 LONGWOOD AVENUE
ROCKLEDGE, FLORIDA 32955-2828

Description: Nonprofit hospital specializing in cardiac care
Annual Sales: $92.0 million
Number of Employees: 1,644
Expertise Needed: Nursing, technology, physical therapy, occupational therapy, accounting, management information systems

Contact: Ms Cheryl Miller
Nursing Recruiter
(407) 636-2211

WYCKOFF HEIGHTS MEDICAL CENTER

374 STOCKHOLM STREET
BROOKLYN, NEW YORK 11237-4006

Description: Private hospital
Founded: 1889
Annual Sales: $112.3 million
Number of Employees: 1,600
Expertise Needed: Nursing, licensed practical nursing, physical therapy, occupational therapy, accounting, management information systems

Contact: Ms Fran Heney
Nursing Recruiter
(718) 963-7272

WYETH-AYERST INTERNATIONAL, LTD.

SAINT DAVID'S CENTER
WAYNE, PENNSYLVANIA 19087

Description: Pharmaceuticals manufacturer
Parent Company: American Home Products Corporation
Founded: 1944
Annual Sales: $1.0 billion

Number of Employees: 13,269
Contact: Ms Susan Ford
Supervisor of Employment
(215) 254-4100

XOMA CORPORATION
2910 7TH STREET
BERKELEY, CALIFORNIA 94710-2700

Description: Researches and develops biopharmaceutical products
Founded: 1981
Annual Sales: $5.1 million
Number of Employees: 235
Expertise Needed: Biochemistry, biology, chemistry, microbiology, technical
Contact: Ms Pamela Bailey
Senior Technical Recruiter
(510) 644-1170

XOMED
6743 SOUTHPOINT DRIVE NORTH
JACKSONVILLE, FLORIDA 32216-6218

Description: Manufactures medical equipment
Parent Company: Bristol-Myers Squibb Company
Founded: 1979
Annual Sales: $37.0 million
Number of Employees: 500
Expertise Needed: Electrical engineering, mechanical engineering, industrial engineering, accounting, data processing, marketing, sales, research and development, information services
Contact: Ms Elaine Stallings
Associate Manager of Human Resources
(904) 296-9600

YAKIMA VALLEY MEMORIAL HOSPITAL ASSOCIATION
2811 TIETON DRIVE
YAKIMA, WASHINGTON 98902-3761

Description: Public hospital specializing in trauma care
Founded: 1950
Annual Sales: $62.0 million
Number of Employees: 1,174
Expertise Needed: Registered nursing, licensed practical nursing, physical therapy, respiratory therapy, occupational therapy
Contact: Ms Kathy Franz
Director of Personnel
(509) 575-8000

YALE-NEW HAVEN HOSPITAL, INC.
20 YORK STREET
NEW HAVEN, CONNECTICUT 06510-3220

Description: Teaching hospital
Annual Sales: $356.0 million
Number of Employees: 5,800
Expertise Needed: Nursing, hospital administration, physical therapy, occupational therapy, respiratory therapy
Contact: Ms Maureen Egan
Manager of Personnel
(203) 785-5083

YOUVILLE HOSPITAL REHABILITATION CENTER
1575 CAMBRIDGE STREET
CAMBRIDGE, MASSACHUSETTS 02138-4398

Description: Nonprofit public hospital
Founded: 1894
Annual Sales: $44.4 million
Number of Employees: 902
Expertise Needed: Laboratory technology, medical technology, physical therapy, occupational therapy, speech therapy, respiratory therapy, social service, registered nursing, licensed practical nursing, occupational therapy
Contact: Ms Joann Parsons
Employment Manager
(617) 876-4344

ZANDEX, INC.
1122 TAYLOR STREET
ZANESVILLE, OHIO 43701-2658

Description: Nursing home
Founded: 1968
Annual Sales: $20.7 million
Number of Employees: 800
Expertise Needed: Data processing, finance, registered nursing, licensed practical nursing, accounting
Contact: Ms Rebecca Butts
Controller
(614) 454-1400

CARL ZEISS, INC.
1 ZEISS DRIVE
THORNWOOD, NEW YORK 10594-1939

Description: Manufactures medical and surgical equipment, microscopes, and measuring devices
Founded: 1925

Zandex, Inc. (continued)
Annual Sales: $300.0 million
Number of Employees: 1,700
Expertise Needed: Electronics/electronics engineering, software engineering/development, design engineering, physics, biology, chemistry
Contact: Mr Lawrence Hart
        Vice President of Human Resources
        (914) 747-1800

ZENITH LABORATORIES, INC.
140 LEGRAND AVENUE
NORTHVALE, NEW JERSEY 07647-2403

Description: Manufactures pharmaceuticals
Annual Sales: $59.4 million
Number of Employees: 411
Expertise Needed: Laboratory technology, medical technology
Contact: Ms Winnie Stavras
        Employment Manager
        (201) 767-1700

ZIMMER, INC.
727 NORTH DETROIT STREET
WARSAW, INDIANA 46580-2746

Description: Manufactures orthopedic products
Parent Company: Bristol-Myers Squibb Company
Founded: 1972
Annual Sales: $1.0 billion
Number of Employees: 4,450
Number of Managerial and Professional Employees Hired 1993: 20
Expertise Needed: Design engineering, sales, computer programming, marketing, finance
Contact: Director of Staffing
        (219) 267-6131

GOVERNMENT EMPLOYERS

DEPARTMENT OF CONSUMER & REGULATORY AFFAIRS

614 H STREET NORTHWEST
WASHINGTON, DC 20001

Description: U.S. agency that monitors, investigates, and evaluates consumer product issues

Expertise Needed: Engineering, maintenance, mental health, physicians, nursing, registered nursing, business

Contact: Office of the Director
(202) 727-1000

DEPARTMENT OF HEALTH & HUMAN SERVICES

200 INDEPENDENCE AVENUE SOUTHWEST
WASHINGTON, DC 20201

Description: U.S. agency that establishes and administers policies regarding health-care and social services

Expertise Needed: Social work, finance, business management, accounting

Contact: Ms Theresa Smith
Director of Personnel
(202) 619-0146

DEPARTMENT OF STATE, BUREAU OF MEDICAL SERVICES

2201 C STREET NORTHWEST
WASHINGTON, DC 20520

Description: Provides medical-related services to the Department of State

Expertise Needed: Laboratory technology, nursing, physicians

Contact: Ms Rita Marinucci
Personnel Officer
(202) 647-3617

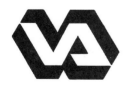

DEPARTMENT OF VETERANS AFFAIRS

810 VERMONT AVENUE NORTHWEST
WASHINGTON, DC 20420

Description: Provides health care for veterans
Founded: 1930
Annual Budget: $33.0 billion
Number of Employees: 259,000
Expertise Needed: Dentistry/dental hygiene, registered nursing, chemistry, health care
Contact: Human Resources Department
(202) 535-8859

For more information, see full organization profile, pg. 212.

FEDERAL EMERGENCY MANAGEMENT AGENCY

500 C STREET SOUTHWEST, FEDERAL CENTER PLAZA
WASHINGTON, DC 20472

Description: U.S. agency that provides emergency and disaster relief services
Founded: 1979
Number of Employees: 10,000
Expertise Needed: Accounting, actuarial, business administration, computer science, criminal justice, civil engineering, electrical engineering, finance, law, military/defense
Contact: Ms Dianne Boha
Chief, Headquarters Personnel Operations Division
(202) 646-4040

FEDERAL TRADE COMMISSION

6TH STREET & PENNSYLVANIA AVENUE NORTHWEST
WASHINGTON, DC 20580

Description: U.S. agency that enforces laws against unfair trade practices
Number of Employees: 950
Number of Managerial and Professional Employees Hired 1993: 15
Expertise Needed: Marketing, advertising, law, business administration, credit/credit analysis
Contact: Mr Elliot Davis
Director of Personnel
(202) 326-2000

FOOD & DRUG ADMINISTRATION, CENTER FOR DEVICES AND RADIOLOGICAL HEALTH

9200 CORPORATE BOULEVARD
ROCKVILLE, MARYLAND 20850

Description: Ensures the safety and effectiveness of medical devices
Founded: 1982
Annual Budget: $88.0 million
Number of Employees: 1,200
Expertise Needed: Health care, chemistry, food chemistry, pharmacology
Contact: CDRH Recruitment Officer (HFZ-405)

GENERAL ACCOUNTING OFFICE

441 G STREET NORTHWEST
WASHINGTON, DC 20548

Description: Provides financial investigation services
Expertise Needed: Economics, accounting, law, finance, auditing
Contact: Ms Francis Garcia
Director of Recruiting
(202) 512-3000

INTERSTATE COMMERCE COMMISSION

12TH STREET & CONSTITUTION AVENUE
NORTHWEST
WASHINGTON, DC 20423

Description: Monitors and regulates interstate trade and business policies and practices
Founded: 1887
Number of Employees: 600
Expertise Needed: Criminal justice, transportation, law
Contact: Ms Mary Sylvester
Acting Chief of Personnel Management
(202) 927-7288

NATIONAL ACADEMY OF SCIENCE

2101 CONSTITUTION AVENUE NORTHWEST
WASHINGTON, DC 20148

Description: Private, nonprofit scientific research organization
Expertise Needed: Biology, physics, environmental engineering, chemistry, environment/forestry
Contact: Mr Richard Lawrence
Manager of Employment and Compensation
(202) 334-2000

NATIONAL INSTITUTE OF STANDARDS & TECHNOLOGY

ADMINISTRATION BUILDING
GAITHERSBURG, MARYLAND 20899

Description: Promotes public health, public safety, and environmental issues
Expertise Needed: Biology, physics, mechanical engineering, civil engineering
Contact: Human Resources Department
(301) 975-2000

NATIONAL INSTITUTES OF HEALTH

9000 ROCKVILLE PIKE
BETHESDA, MARYLAND 20892

Description: Conducts studies for the purpose of preventing, detecting, diagnosing, and treating diseases and disabilities
Expertise Needed: Biology, behavioral research, biotechnology, physics, chemistry
Contact: Mr Herb Carey
Branch Chief- Recruitment
(301) 496-4000

NATIONAL SCIENCE FOUNDATION

4201 WILSON BOULEVARD
ARLINGTON, VIRGINIA 22230

Description: Promotes science, engineering, and technical programs
Expertise Needed: Social work, economics, engineering, behavioral sciences, clinical education, biology, computer science, geology, physical science, mathematics
Contact: Ms Janet Silva
Chief of Employment
(703) 306-1185

OCCUPATIONAL SAFETY & HEALTH ADMINISTRATION

200 CONSTITUTION AVENUE NORTHWEST
WASHINGTON, DC 20210

Description: U.S. agency that ensures the provision and maintenance of safe work places
Number of Employees: 2,300
Number of Managerial and Professional Employees Hired 1993: 10
Expertise Needed: Industrial hygiene, health care, safety engineering, accounting, finance
Contact: Ms Floria Jones
Supervisor of Staffing
(202) 219-8013

OFFICE OF MANAGEMENT & BUDGET

17TH STREET & PENNSYLVANIA AVENUE
WASHINGTON, DC 20503

Description: Branch of the Executive Office in charge of preparing the national budget
Expertise Needed: Public affairs, public policy and planning, economics, law, business administration
Contact: Mr Steve Weigler
Human Resources Manager
(202) 395-7250

PEACE CORPS

1990 K STREET NORTHWEST
WASHINGTON, DC 20526

Description: Provides volunteer services to foreign nations in need
Founded: 1961
Number of Employees: 1,200
Number of Managerial and Professional Employees Hired 1993: 300
Expertise Needed: Medical technology, occupational therapy, health science, education, training and development, computer programming, business development, administration, agriculture
Contact: Ms Sharon Barbe Fletcher
Director of Personnel
(202) 606-3886

SMALL BUSINESS ADMINISTRATION

409 THIRD STREET SOUTHWEST
WASHINGTON, DC 20416

Description: Provides assistance and loans to small businesses
Founded: 1953
Number of Employees: 3,000
Number of Managerial and Professional Employees Hired 1993: 20
Expertise Needed: Business development, criminal justice, law, accounting, credit/credit analysis, computer analysis, project management, investment
Contact: Mr Jose Mendez
Personnel Staffing Specialist
(202) 205-6790

EMPLOYER DESCRIPTIONS

In-depth information on the business activities and employment opportunities at some profiled companies and government organizations

Memorial Sloan-Kettering Cancer Center

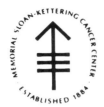

Description of Organization: A nonprofit, comprehensive cancer center that provides medical and hospital services for cancer patients and conducts basic and applied biomedical research

Number of Employees: 6,200

Headquarters Location: New York, New York

Academic Fields of Recruitment Interest: The life sciences, computer science, electrical engineering, physical therapy, pharmacy science, medical technology, statistics, accounting, finance, nursing, health-care administration, management

Major Entry-Level Opportunities for New Graduates: Biomedical research, clinical research, medical technology, computer-based programming, patient finance, engineering, general management, hospital administration

BACKGROUND AND OPERATIONS

For more than a century, the people at Memorial Sloan-Kettering Cancer Center (MSKCC) have been at the forefront in the fight against cancer, leading the way in patient care, biomedical research, and business administration. They have made a real difference and, in so doing, have achieved personal success and the rewards that it brings.

MSKCC offers its employees the opportunity to do a world of good and realize important goals of far-reaching significance.

The Center's varied activities and wide range of career opportunities offer each person a chance to make history.

In 1884, the cornerstone was laid for the New York Cancer Hospital. That hospital would become Memorial Sloan-Kettering Cancer Center; its mission, as stated by the first president, John E. Parsons, was "the exclusive treatment and care of cancer patients."

Success has strengthened that purpose. Today, in its expanding complex of buildings on Manhattan's East Side, MSKCC integrates patient care, research, and educational activities in a multidimensional pursuit of that single goal: to eliminate cancer as a threat to human life.

Since the Center's founding, research has been recognized as vital to the accomplishment of its mission to progressively control and cure cancer. The research programs of the Sloan-Kettering Institute are dedicated to the advancement of the understanding of fundamental biological processes.

The work at MSKCC is interesting and inherently important and represents a dynamic, evolving process. A research career at MSKCC offers the opportunity for growth as a scientist and for mobility within the health-care field. Research technicians work in a scientifically stimulating environment of experimentation and study. Because of the rapid evolution of current initiatives, in both the basic and applied sciences, research personnel consistently find themselves working on the frontiers of science. The Center's laboratories are state-of-the-art; the atmosphere is collegial.

The management and administration story of the nineties is being written in the health-care field. Advances in medicine, changing systems of delivery, and renewed attention—in both the private and public spheres—to medical costs and medical financing make the health services industry a dynamic area in which to apply management skills. MSKCC has been an innovator in this respect, enlisting the aid of management science to realize productivity gains and new levels of efficiency in health-care administration.

In every department, administrative activities receive the same high level of management scrutiny: recordkeeping, patient scheduling, budgeting, communications, the use of systems, project control, and task control. The Center strives to make these functions more efficient, productive, and supportive of MSKCC's overall aim of serving the patient and conducting research.

Information systems play a key role in this dynamic environment. The Center has made a significant commitment to an enhanced role for information systems and has backed it with the essential resources.

The Strategic Plan for Automation calls for a fully automated medical center, integrating systems for clinical and research laboratories, patient-care units, the pharmacy, and an on-line patient registration system. The Center is creating a network of communications links that reflect the multilevel interaction of each component of the organization.

This is development work on a vast scale, which encourages employees to function as team members on a complete project. At MSKCC, this development takes place in a highly professional environment that provides all the needed tools and training for the right people. There is the chance to learn many new technologies as MSKCC maintains its edge in information systems knowledge. There are opportunities for career growth as the Center charts new directions for the application of information systems in the health care field.

EMPLOYMENT OPPORTUNITIES

ENTRY-LEVEL AND EXPERIENCED PERSONNEL

Biomedical Research. Biomedical research personnel are recruited on a needs basis to fill technical support staff positions in the institute. Candidates for employment are exposed to an extraordinary diversity of opportunities over a wide range of basic and/or applied sciences. Five scientific programs have been established that cover the principal areas of research at the institute. They are Molecular Biology, Cell Biology and Genetics, Immunology, Molecular Pharmacology and Therapeutics, and Cellular Biochemistry and Biophysics. A candidate for a technical support position should combine solid theoretical understanding of the contemporary life sciences with practical hands-on experience. To work as a research technician with a project team at Memorial Sloan-Kettering Cancer Center is to embark upon a career in the biomedical sciences that will yield tremendous personal and professional satisfaction.

Clinical Research. Opportunities are available for candidates interested in participating in the acquisition and analysis of data related to therapeutic and/or diagnostic patient protocols. A successful candidate for a research study assistant position must have an interest in automated systems, possess solid analytical skills, and be comfortable working with technical, medical, and scientific terminology.

Medical Technology. The Clinical Laboratories activities at MSKCC rank among the foremost medical technology programs in the country. Work within an academic research environment, combined with the most contemporary technologies, results in a unique professional experience for the medical technologist. The range of clinical laboratories at Memorial Hospital comprise all aspects of the field. A candidate for a medical technologist position should possess an approved New York City license or be license-eligible. The MSKCC Clinical Laboratories staff is committed to high quality patient care through high-quality lab support.

Information Systems. The information systems specialist at MSKCC works with the latest hardware, software, and telecommunications technologies to provide systems support to meet the medical, scientific, and operational needs of the Center. With a long-range strategy that calls for increased automation of functions and full integration of systems, the data processing specialist may look forward to significant opportunities for career growth in operations, project development, and management. Whether employees' interests are in mainframe programming, PC computing, telecommunications, scientific programming, or local area networking, they have the opportunity to become leaders in the application of information systems to a broad range of activities within health care.

Health-Care Administration. A candidate for a management position at MSKCC must possess a special set of talents and abilities combining analytical skills with interpersonal skills. The management support person works closely with the administration and professional staffs to develop, implement, and manage a variety of programs. The Center endeavors to make these functions more efficient, more productive, and more supportive of MSKCC's ultimate aim of serving the patient. A candidate for a position in health-care administration should combine solid theoretical training in health-care or business management with practical experience, preferably in budgeting, automated systems, line supervision, and knowledge of the regulatory environment.

THE ORGANIZATION AS EMPLOYER

Memorial Sloan-Kettering Cancer Center is a world-class institution, known for the exceptional care it provides to patients, for its research initiatives, for the unsurpassed caliber of its staff and facilities, and for the administrative support that ensures optimal functioning. The very purpose for which MSKCC exists makes it a place where creativity and individual initiative are prized and where new ideas are encouraged. This makes for a dynamic environment in which each person has an exceptional opportunity to further his or her personal goals.

At the same time, MSKCC is a place where people from varied backgrounds and with diverse skills work together as a team toward a single goal. Whether it is through the teamwork of care providers, or the efforts of a management team that creates more effective business systems, or a team of researchers who define new answers and new questions—all are part of the effort to control and cure cancer. In this environment, each person's success contributes to the institution's success. The rewards that come from individual achievement are increased by the sense of accomplishment that comes from contributing to the greater goal.

MSKCC's policy is to offer salaries that are current and competitive. To ensure that this policy is carried out effectively, annual compensation reviews keep MSKCC's compensation packages in line with the best in the marketplace. MSKCC offers a comprehensive health-care plan as well as disability, life, dental, and other forms of insurance. In addition, as befits an institution where research and education are of paramount importance, MSKCC offers a 100% tuition reimbursement program for approved courses taken at any accredited educational institution.

APPLICATION AND INFORMATION

Memorial Sloan-Kettering Cancer Center encourages the submission of résumés on a year-round basis from both interested students and experienced personnel. Candidates who match current or anticipated needs will be contacted for a personal interview. MSKCC also conducts an extensive College Relations Program. Students are encouraged to contact their college or university placement office for additional information.

MSKCC is an equal opportunity employer, m/f/d/v.

Direct inquiries to:

Administrator, College Relations
Employment Section CRE:P
Human Resources Division
Memorial Sloan-Kettering Cancer Center
1275 York Avenue
New York, New York 10021

Oxford Health Plans

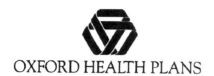

OXFORD HEALTH PLANS

Description of Organization: A regional corporation that provides a full range of innovative and managed health-care services to members in New York, New Jersey, Connecticut, Philadelphia, and New Hampshire

Number of Employees: Approximately 1,000

Headquarters Location: Norwalk, Connecticut

Academic Fields of Recruitment Interest: Business, marketing, management, liberal arts, communications

Major Entry-Level Opportunities for New Graduates: Operations, finance, customer service, claims, provider relations, sales and marketing, management information systems

BACKGROUND AND OPERATIONS

Oxford Health Plans is currently one of the fastest-growing managed health insurance companies in the New York metropolitan area. The company offers one of the most diversified product portfolios in the Metropolitan New York market, from traditional HMOs to flexible, point-of-service HMO/indemnity plans. Oxford currently insures over 3,300 employer groups in the metropolitan area through one of the largest and highest-quality health-care provider networks. In addition, it has recently entered government-sponsored programs, including Medicare and Medicaid, through the development of a tightly controlled, full-capitated subset of this network.

A strong management team, a flat management style, and a corporate willingness to see change as an opportunity and not a threat have enabled Oxford to become a leader in delivering innovative, successful managed-care products to the New York metropolitan area. Oxford's "firsts" include the first true point-of-service program offered in the New York tristate area, the first self-insured HMO-type and POS-type programs available to employers in the New York metropolitan area, and the first managed-care organization in the tristate area to demand that 9,000 participating physicians be board-certified or board-eligible and within five years of having completed residency training.

Since its inception, Oxford's staffing, information systems, and management practices have focused on creating an environment of learning, innovation, and change. One of the company's sustainable competitive advantages is the ability to change quickly in the face of new information and new realities. Oxford's enrollment has increased in sixteen consecutive quarters, off of an ever-expanding membership base. Enrollment growth has exceeded 80 percent for the past two years and now exceeds 300,000 (217,000 at year-end 1993). Revenues for the year ended December 31, 1993, grew to $311 million, a 100 percent increase over 1992. Stockholders' equity increased to approximately $91 million, or $5.84 per share, and the company has no long-term debt.

FUTURE DIRECTIONS

With an exceptionally strong financial position, a large and efficient provider network, and an entire organization designed to accommodate rapid change in the health-care environment, Oxford is extremely well positioned. It is aggressively expanding product offerings, honing marketing skills, refining management information technologies, and upgrading quality control efforts. Some of these efforts include creating subsets of the provider network to meet the specific needs of market segments, developing targeted marketing efforts that use Oxford's extensive database, expanding the company's wellness programs, increasing penetration in New Jersey and Connecticut, and adding new physician Quality Assurance Review protocols and extending the Service Spotlight program, which is designed to monitor Oxford's performance in all service areas through direct, thorough evaluations by its customers. Oxford is committed to its original mission of providing complete, flexible, high-quality medical coverage to all its members and to doing so at a responsible, predictable cost.

EMPLOYMENT OPPORTUNITIES

ENTRY-LEVEL AND EXPERIENCED PERSONNEL

As Oxford expands into various new health-care frontiers, there are diverse opportunities for individuals seeking a rewarding and satisfying career. Positions in all areas are available. These areas include, but are not limited to, finance, operations, customer service, provider relations, claims, sales and marketing, and management information systems.

TRAINING

Informal and formal orientation processes, which include interacting with various members of the Oxford professional team, are offered. These processes help to continually reinforce the importance of new hires to the company's future.

THE ORGANIZATION AS EMPLOYER

Oxford Health Plans offers full medical coverage, tuition reimbursement, and internal education seminars. Employees are also offered a wellness program to help them maintain a more healthy lifestyle and to promote both physical and mental well-being. The three primary components of the wellness program are a personal health risk appraisal, health fairs, and "lunch and learn" seminars.

APPLICATION AND INFORMATION

Oxford Health Plans recruits nationwide for entry-level and experienced professionals who are highly motivated and detail-oriented and have a professional demeanor, entrepreneurial spirit, and excellent interpersonal and communication skills. Applicants are encouraged to send a résumé to the following address.

Direct inquiries to:

Oxford Health Plans
Human Resources Department-PG
800 Connecticut Avenue
Norwalk, Connecticut 06854

Veterans Health Administration

Department of Veterans Affairs

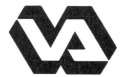

Description of Organization: The largest component of the Department of Veterans Affairs (VA); provides medical, surgical, psychiatric, nursing, and specialty care and also conducts research studies

Number of Employees: Approximately 200,000

Headquarters Location: Washington, D.C.

Academic Fields of Recruitment Interest: Audiology, nutrition, occupational therapy, pharmacy, physical therapy, radiology, rehabilitation, respiratory therapy, speech pathology, social work

BACKGROUND AND OPERATIONS

With almost 200,000 employees, the Veterans Health Administration (VHA) is the largest component of the Department of Veterans Affairs (VA).

Treating more than one million patients on an inpatient basis annually, the VHA provides medical, surgical, psychiatric, and nursing care as well as specialty care, such as hemodialysis, organ transplant, spinal cord injury, substance abuse treatment, ambulatory care, critical care, and long-term care. It also conducts research studies on AIDS, diabetes, drug addiction, epilepsy, nerve regeneration, Alzheimer's disease, and other problems associated with aging.

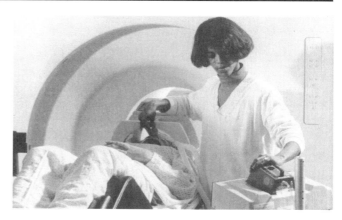

EMPLOYMENT OPPORTUNITIES

ENTRY-LEVEL AND EXPERIENCED PERSONNEL

For allied health professionals, VA offers unparalleled opportunities for career growth.

Under a unique federal personnel system, VA facilities may directly appoint physical therapists, occupational therapists, physician assistants, registered or certified respiratory therapists, and expanded-function dental auxiliaries to positions for which no civil service examination is required. For several other allied health occupations, the VA Delegated Examining Unit (DEU) has national civil service examining authority. To name but a few, the DEU covers audiologists/speech pathologists, dietitians, diagnostic radiologic technicians/technologists, medical record administrators, social workers, and vocational rehabilitation specialists.

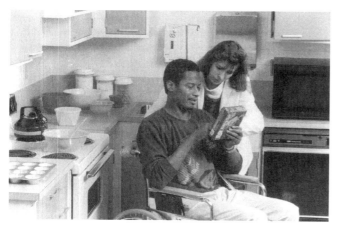

THE ORGANIZATION AS EMPLOYER

VA's mission is to provide the best possible care for the nation's veterans. In recognition of the contributions made by allied health professionals in achieving this goal, VA offers extensive and competitive employment benefits and educational opportunities. Allied health professionals at VA earn thirteen to twenty-six days of paid vacation and personal leave each year. They also earn thirteen days of sick leave annually, with no limit on accumulation. Military leave is authorized up to fifteen days per year for active reservists and members of the National Guard. There are also ten paid federal holidays.

VA offers a variety of group health insurance plans, with premiums partially paid by the federal government. Term life insurance, with coverage based on salary, is available, with the cost shared by the federal government. Family and additional coverage options are available.

Newly hired allied health professionals are covered by the Federal Employees' Retirement System (FERS). FERS is a three-tier retirement plan composed of Social Security benefits, FERS basic benefits, and the Thrift Savings Plan, which is a tax-deferred savings plan similar to 401(k) plans offered in the private sector.

Numerous other benefits are offered by VA, including mobility between facilities, liability protection, cash awards for adopted suggestions, smoke-free and drug-free workplaces, employee wellness programs, credit unions, dining facilities, free parking at most facilities, and child care at some facilities.

In general, starting salaries for allied health professionals are based on education and experience and can vary by location. Therefore, applicants should directly contact the facility where they would like to work for specific information about salaries currently being offered.

212

VA recognizes the importance of ongoing education and the benefit it provides to both veteran patients and VA employees. Opportunities are available through programs such as the Health Professional Scholarship Program for qualifying staff and students, tuition support for job-related and continuing education courses, university- and college-affiliated clinical education programs, VA national and regional education programs, and paid time off for approved continuing education programs.

APPLICATION AND INFORMATION

VA health-care facilities have specialized medical care programs and range in size from 110 to more than 1,400 beds. As such, a variety of opportunities are available for allied health professionals. To gain a firsthand view of VA health care, interested individuals are encouraged to arrange to visit VA facilities in their area by calling or writing for an appointment. Telephone numbers are listed in local directories under "U.S. Government." Those interested may also address correspondence to the Human Resources Management Service at any VA Medical Center.

Pharmacists, physician assistants, physical therapists, and occupational therapists are invited to call 800-949-0002.

For more information about occupations covered by the DEU and for application materials, interested individuals should write or call:

Veterans Affairs Delegated Examining Unit
P.O. Box 24269
Richmond, Virginia 23224-0269
800-368-6008 (toll-free)
800-552-3045 (toll-free in Virginia)

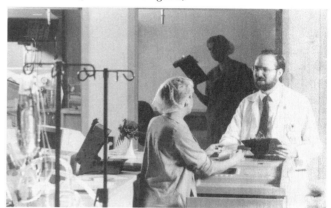

INDEX BY INDUSTRY

Companies are indexed under the following categories in this section.

Biotechnology
Business Services
Chemicals
Clinics and Health Centers
Computer Programming and Consulting
Computer Software
Computer Systems and Peripherals
Consumer and Household Products
Cost Management Services
Data Processing Services
Dental Products and Services
Educational Services
Electronics and Electrical Equipment
Environmental Products and Equipment
Finance and Investments
Foundations and Nonprofits
Furniture and Fixtures
Government Organizations
Health Care Services
Health Maintenance and Preferred
    Provider Organizations
Heating and Air Conditioning
Home Health-Care Services
Hospice Care
Hospitals and Medical Centers
Hospital Management Services

Industrial Machinery and Equipment
Information Services
Instruments
Insurance
Laboratories
Medical Equipment and Services
Medical Practices
Nursing Homes/Convalescent Care
Office Equipment
Optical Products
Outpatient, Rehabilitation, and
    Therapy Services
Paper and Related Products
Personnel and Placement Services
Pharmaceuticals
Pharmacy Management Services
Psychiatric and Mental Health Treatment
Real Estate
Research Organizations
Retail Trade
Rubber and Plastics
Substance Abuse Treatment
Textiles and Clothing
Transportation and Shipping
Wholesale Trade and Distribution

INDEX BY INDUSTRY

This index classifies companies according to the primary industries in which they operate.

Finance and Investments
American Physicians Services
Group, 23

Foundations and Nonprofits
National Academy of Science, 206
Nemours Foundation, 135
Voluntary Hospitals of America, 199

Furniture and Fixtures
Midmark Corporation, 129
National Service Industries, Inc., 134

Government Organizations
Department of Consumer &
Regulatory Affairs, 205
Department of Health & Human
Services, 205
Department of State, Bureau of
Medical Services, 205
Department of Veterans Affairs, 205
Federal Emergency Management
Agency, 205
Federal Trade Commission, 205
Food & Drug Administration,
Center for Devices and
Radiological Health, 205
General Accounting Office, 205
Interstate Commerce
Commission, 206
National Institutes of Health, 206
National Institute of Standards &
Technology, 206
National Science Foundation, 206
Occupational Safety & Health
Administration, 206
Office of Management &
Budget, 206
Peace Corps, 206
Small Business Administration, 206

Health Care Services
ARA Environmental Services,
Inc., 25
Caremark International, Inc., 46
Employee Benefit Plans, Inc., 68
EMSI, 68
Ethix Healthcare Corporation, 69
First Hospital Wyoming Valley, 71
Healthcare Services Group, Inc., 86
Home X-Ray Services of America, 91
Humana, Inc., 94
Isomedix, Inc., 101
I-Stat, 95
Johnson & Johnson Health
Management, 103
Johns Hopkins Health System
Corporation, 103
JSA Healthcare Corporation, 104
Kaiser Foundation Health Plan of
Colorado, Inc., 104
Kaiser Permanente, 105

Kaiser Permanente, Northeast
Division Headquarters, 105
Kaiser Permanente, Southeast
Division Headquarters, 105
Lifesource Blood Services, 110
Medical America Health Systems
Corporation, 117
Mediq, Inc., 120
OSF Healthcare System, 142
Permanente Medical Group,
Inc., 146
PHP Healthcare Corporation, 148
Physicians Health Plan
Corporation, 148
Rocky Mountain Helicopters,
Inc., 161
Ross-Loos Healthplan of
California, 161
Sentara Alternative Delivery
Systems, 174
Servantcor, 176
Sierra Health Services, Inc., 178
Southern California Permanente
Medical, 181
Southern Health Systems, Inc., 181
Sunrise Community, Inc., 187
Universal Care, Inc., 195
U.S. Behavioral Health, 196
Vector Healthsystems, 197

**Health Maintenance and Preferred
Provider Organizations**
Aetna Health Plans of Southern
California, 19
Blue Care Network, East
Michigan, 37
Blue Care Network, Health
Central, 37
Capital Area Community Health
Plan, 45
Central Massachusetts Health
Care, 48
Chicago HMO, Ltd., 50
Community Health Care Plan, 56
Complete Health Services, Inc., 57
Comprecare Health Care
Services, 57
Continental Health Affiliates,
Inc., 58
Corvel Corporation, 60
Corvel Healthcare Corporation, 60
Dean Health Plan, Inc., 63
Fallon Health Care System, 70
FHP Takecare, 71
Foundation Health, 73
Greater Atlantic Health Service, 79
Group Health Cooperative, 80
Group Health Cooperative of Puget
Sound, 80
Group Health Northwest, 80
Healthplus of Michigan, Inc., 87
Healthsource, Inc., 87

Health Plan of Nevada, Inc., 85
Health Plus of New Mexico, Inc., 85
HMO America, Inc., 89
HMO Colorado, Inc., 89
HMO Missouri, Inc., 89
Independent Health Association, 97
Intergroup Healthcare
Corporation, 99
Medcenters Healthcare, Inc., 117
MVP Health Plan, 131
National HMO (New York),
Inc., 133
Ochsner Health Plan, 139
Pacificare of California, 143
Pacificare of Texas, Inc., 143
Pilgrim Health Care, Inc., 149
Preferred Care, 151
Primecare Health Plan, Inc., 153
Principal Health Care, Inc., 153
Private Healthcare Systems, Ltd., 153
Qual-Med, Inc., 155
Qual-Med Plans for Health, 155
Sanus Texas Health Plan, Inc., 172
Sierra Health Services, Inc., 178
Take Care Health Plan, Inc., 189
United Healthcare Corporation, 194
US Healthcare, Inc., 196
Value Health, Inc., 197

Heating and Air Conditioning
Neslab Instruments, Inc., 135

Home Health Care Services
Advantage Health Corporation, 18
Alacare Home Health Service, 19
Allen Healthcare Services, Inc., 20
Baton Rouge Health Care, 30
Bestcare, Inc., 33
Care Group, Inc., 46
Community Hospice Care, Inc., 56
Family Aides, Inc., 70
Family Home Care, 70
Fidelity, 71
Girling Health Care, Inc., 77
Helping Care, Inc., 88
HHC, Inc., 88
HMSS, Inc., 89
Homecare Management, Inc., 91
Homedco Group, Inc., 91
Home Care Affiliates, Inc., 91
Home Health Corporation of
America, 91
Home Nursing Services, Inc., 91
Hospital Staffing Services, 93
Housecall, Inc., 93
In Home Health, Inc., 97
Jordan Health Services, Inc., 104
Kelly Assisted Living Services, 105
Lincare, Inc., 110
National Homecare Systems,
Inc., 133

Hospice Care

Hospitals and Medical Centers

Medical Equipment and Services

Medical Practices

Nursing Homes/Convalescent Care

FoxMeyer Corporation, 73
Fujisawa USA, Inc., 74
Genentech, Inc., 75
General Injectibles & Vaccines, 75
Geneva Pharmaceuticals, Inc., 76
Genica Pharmaceuticals, 76
Gensia Pharmaceuticals, Inc., 76
Glaxo Americas, Inc., 77
Glaxo, Inc., 77
G. C. Hanford Manufacturing
    Company, 81
Halsey Drug Company, Inc., 81
Hazelton Washington, 83
Herbalife International, Inc., 88
Hoechst-Roussel Pharmaceuticals,
    Inc., 90
Hoffmann-La Roche, Inc., 90
HyClone Laboratories, Inc., 94
ICN Pharmaceuticals, Inc., 95
IDEC Pharmaceuticals
    Corporation, 95
IGI, Inc., 96
Immucor, Inc., 96
ImmuLogic Pharmaceutical
    Corporation, 97
ImmunoGen, Inc., 97
Isis Pharmaceuticals, 100
Ivax Corporation, 101
Johnson & Johnson, 103
J. M. Smith Corporation, 179
Knoll Pharmaceuticals, 107
KV Pharmaceutical Company, 107
Lemmon Company, 108
Marion Merrell Dow, Inc., 114
Marion Merrell Dow
    Pharmaceuticals, 114
Marsam Pharmaceuticals, Inc., 114
McGaw, Inc., 116
McNeil Consumer Products, 116
Mead Johnson & Company, 116
Melaleuca, Inc., 121
Millennium Pharmaceuticals, 129
Mylan Laboratories, Inc., 132
Nature's Bounty, Inc., 134
Nature's Sunshine Products,
    Inc., 134
Neuman Distributors, Inc., 135
Nu Skin International, 139
Oncogene Science, Inc., 140
Organon, Inc., 141
Ortho Biotech, 141
Ortho Pharmaceutical
    Corporation, 141
Paco Pharmaceutical Services,
    Inc., 143
Parexel International
    Corporation, 144
Parke-Davis, Division of
    Warner-Lambert Company, 144
Par-Pharmaceutical, 144
Perdue Frederick Company, 146
Perrigo Company, 146

Pfizer, Inc., 147
PharmaKinetics Laboratories,
    Inc., 148
Plantation Botanicals, Inc., 150
Private Formulations, Inc., 153
Procter & Gamble
    Pharmaceuticals, 153
Purepac, Inc., 154
Rhone-Poulenc Rorer, Inc., 158
Rhone-Poulenc Rorer
    Pharmaceuticals, 158
Rhone Merieux, Inc., 158
Roberts Pharmaceutical
    Corporation, 160
Roxane Laboratories, Inc., 162
Sandoz Pharmaceuticals
    Corporation, 172
Schein Pharmaceutical, 173
Schwartz Pharmaceutical USA, 173
SCIOS-Nova, Inc., 174
Sera Tec Biologicals, Inc., 175
Serono Laboratories, Inc., 175
Sidmak Laboratories, Inc., 177
SmithKline Beecham
    Corporation, 180
Sphinx Pharmaceuticals
    Corporation, 183
Sterling Winthrop, 184
Survival Technology, Inc., 188
Synergen, Inc., 189
Syntex Chemicals, Inc., 189
Syntex Corporation, 189
Tag Pharmaceuticals, Inc., 189
Tap Pharmaceuticals, Inc., 190
Twin Laboratories, Inc., 193
Upsher-Smith Laboratories, 196
Watson Pharmaceuticals, Inc., 200
Wesley-Jessen, Inc., 200
Whitby Pharmaceuticals, Inc., 201
Xoma Corporation, 203
Zenith Laboratories, Inc., 204

Pharmacy Management Services
HPI Health Care Services, Inc., 93
Insta-Care Pharmacy Services
    Corporation, 98
National Institutional
    Pharmaceutical Services, 133
Omnicare, Inc., 140
Pharmacy Management Services,
    147
Syncor International
    Corporation, 188
Vitalink Pharmacy Services, Inc., 198

Psychiatric and Mental Health Treatment
Carrier Foundation, Inc., 47
Center for Health Care Service, 48
Charter Fairmount Institute, 49
Charter Hospital of Corpus
    Christi, 49

Charter Lakeside Hospital, Inc., 49
Charter Lakeside Hospital, Inc., 49
Charter Real, Inc., 49
Charter Westbrook Hospital, 49
Christian Health Care Center, 53
First Hospital Corporation, 71
First Hospital Corporation of
    Portsmouth, 71
First Hospital Wyoming Valley, 71
Innovative Healthcare Systems, 98
Introspect Healthcare
    Corporation, 100
Menninger Foundation, Inc., 122
Mental Health Management,
    Inc., 123
North Central Health Care
    Facility, 137
Park HealthCare Company, 144
Preferred Health Care, Ltd., 151
Telecare Corporation, 191
Universal Health Services, 195

Real Estate
NME Properties, Inc., 136

Research Organizations
Aldrich Chemical Company, Inc., 20
Enzo Biochem, Inc., 69
Hazelton Washington, 83
Hycor Biomedical, Inc., 94
Immunex Corporation, 97
Life Technologies, Inc., 109
Lovelace Medical Foundation, 111
Methodist Hospital Foundation, 125
National Academy of Science, 206
National Institutes of Health, 206
National Science Foundation, 206
Panlabs, Inc., 144
Pharmaco LSR International,
    Inc., 147
Promega Corporation, 154
Research Triangle Institute, 157
S.A.I.C., 163
TSI Mason Research Institute,
    Inc., 193

Retail Trade
Allied Pharmacy Management, 21
American Drug Stores, Inc., 22
America's Best Contacts &
    Eyeglasses, 22
Big B, Inc., 34
Buckeye Discount, Inc., 43
ChemD, Inc., 50
Drug Emporium, Inc., 65
Eye Care Centers of America, 70
Family Vision Centers, Inc., 71
Hannaford Brothers, 82
Hook-SupeRx, Inc., 91
Kinney Drugs, Inc., 107

Rubber and Plastics

Substance Abuse Treatment

Textiles and Clothing

Transportation and Shipping

Wholesale Trade and Distribution

GEOGRAPHIC INDEX

An index of profiled companies in alphabetical order by state.

Massachusetts

Michigan

INDEX BY HIRING NEEDS

An index of profiled companies by areas of expertise sought.

Accounting

Acufex Microsurgical, Inc., 17
Acuson Corporation, 17
Advanced Technology Laboratories, 18
Advantage Health Corporation, 18
Adventist Healthcare/Middle Atlantic, 19
Adventist Health Systems/Sunbelt, 18
Adventist Health Systems/West, 18
A.H. Robins Company, Inc., 160
Aladan Corporation, 19
Alcon Laboratories, Inc., 20
Alco Health Services Corporation, 20
Allergan Medical Optics, Inc., 21
Alliance Health, Inc., 21
Allied Healthcare Products, 21
Allied Pharmacy Management, 21
The Altoona Hospital, 21
Amalgamated Life Insurance Company, Inc., 22
American Baptist Homes of the West, 22
American Brands, Inc., 22
American Family Assurance Collective, 23
American Health Services Corporation, 23
American Medical Electronics, 23
American Medical International, 23
American Shared-Cure Care, 24
America's Best Contacts & Eyeglasses, 22
Amerihealth, Inc., 24
Amersham Medi-Physics, Inc., 24
Amity Care Corporation, 25
AMSCO International, Inc., 25
Angelica Corporation, 25
ARA Environmental Services, Inc., 25
Arbor Health Care Company, 25
Asklepios Hospital Corporation, 26
Associated Group, 27
Baker Cummins Pharmaceuticals, Inc., 28
Bally Manufacturing Corporation, 29
Barco of California, 29
Bard Urological Division, 30
Baystate Medical Center, Inc., 31
Beckman Instruments, Inc., 32
Becton Dickinson, Consumer Products Division, 32

Becton Dickinson & Company, 32
Bennett X-Ray Corporation, 32
Benson Optical Company, Inc., 33
Bergen Brunswig Corporation, 33
Beverly California Corporation, 34
Beverly Enterprises, Inc., 34
Big B, Inc., 34
Bindley Western Industries, 34
BioMedical Applications Management, 35
Biomet, Inc., 35
Bio-Reference Laboratories, Inc., 35
Block Drug Company, Inc., 36
Blue Care Network, East Michigan, 37
Blue Care Network, Health Central, 37
Blue Cross of Idaho Health Service, 40
Blue Cross & Blue Shield Mutual of Ohio, 37
Blue Cross & Blue Shield of Alabama, 37
Blue Cross & Blue Shield of Arkansas, 37
Blue Cross & Blue Shield of Colorado, 37
Blue Cross & Blue Shield of Florida, 37
Blue Cross & Blue Shield of Kansas, 38
Blue Cross & Blue Shield of Maryland, 38
Blue Cross & Blue Shield of Massachusetts, 38
Blue Cross & Blue Shield of Michigan, 38
Blue Cross & Blue Shield of National Capitol Area, 38
Blue Cross & Blue Shield of New Jersey, 39
Blue Cross & Blue Shield of North Carolina, 39
Blue Cross & Blue Shield of Oregon, 39
Blue Cross & Blue Shield of Tennessee, 39
Blue Cross & Blue Shield of Texas, Inc., 39
Blue Cross & Blue Shield of Utica/Watertown, Inc., 40
Blue Cross & Blue Shield of Vermont, 40

Blue Cross & Blue Shield of Western New York, 40
Blue Cross & Blue Shield United of Wisconsin, 40
BMC Industries, Inc., 40
Bon Secours Health Systems, 41
Boston Metal Products Corporation, 41
Boston Scientific Corporation, 41
The Brian Center Corporation, 41
Briggs Corporation, 42
Britthaven, Inc., 42
The Burrows Company, 44
Cabot Medical Corporation, 44
California Pacific Medical Center, 44
California Physicians Service, 44
Cambridge Biotech Corporation, 45
Capital Area Community Health Plan, 45
Capital Blue Cross, Inc., 46
Cardinal Health, Inc., 46
Caremark International, Inc., 46
Caremet, Inc., 46
The Carle Foundation, 47
Carrier Foundation, Inc., 47
Carter-Wallace, Inc., 47
Catholic Healthcare West, 47
Center for Health Care Service, 48
Central Pharmaceuticals, Inc., 48
Charter Hospital of Corpus Christi, 49
Charter Lakeside Hospital, Inc., 49
Charter Medical Corporation, 49
Chase Pharmaceutical Company, 50
Chase Scientific Glass, 50
Chattanooga Group, Inc., 50
Chicago HMO, Ltd., 50
Children's Hospital of Wisconsin, 52
Choice Drug Systems, Inc., 53
Christian Homes, Inc., 53
Cigna Corporation, 54
Cigna Healthplan of Texas, Inc., North Texas Division, 54
Cigna Health Plans of California, 54
Cigna Health Plans of California, 54
CIS Technologies, Inc., 54
Cleveland Clinic Foundation, 55
Coastal Healthcare Group, Inc., 55
Cole Vision Corporation, 55
Columbia HCA Health Care Corporation, 56
Common Brothers, Inc., 56
Community Health Care Plan, 56
Community Hospice, Inc., 57

Chemistry

Pharmavite Corporation, 148
Private Formulations, Inc., 153
Purepac, Inc., 154
Radiometer America, Inc., 156
Research Triangle Institute, 157
Rhone-Poulenc Rorer
    Pharmaceuticals, 158
Rhone Merieux, Inc., 158
Roche Biomedical Laboratories,
    Inc., 160
Sandoz Pharmaceuticals
    Corporation, 172
Sanofi Animal Health, Inc., 172
Schein Pharmaceutical, 173
Schwartz Pharmaceutical USA, 173
SCIOS-Nova, Inc., 174
Serono Laboratories, Inc., 175
Sidmak Laboratories, Inc., 177
Siebe North, Inc., 177
Sphinx Pharmaceuticals
    Corporation, 183
Steris Laboratories, Inc., 184
Stratagene Cloning Systems, 185
Supelco, Inc., 187
Survival Technology, Inc., 188
Synergen, Inc., 189
Syntex Chemicals, Inc., 189
Syntex Corporation, 189
Syva, 189
Tag Pharmaceuticals, Inc., 189
True Quality Pharmacies, Inc., 193
TSI Mason Research Institute,
    Inc., 193
Upsher-Smith Laboratories, 196
Ventritex, Inc., 197
Whitby Pharmaceuticals, Inc., 201
Xoma Corporation, 203

Chemotherapy
Lubbock County Hospital, University
    Medical Center, 111
Mercy Hospital, Inc., 124

Child Therapy
Arkansas Children's Hospital, 26
Minneapolis Children's Medical
    Center, 129

Civil Engineering
Cobe Laboratories, Inc., 55
Continental Medical Systems, 58
Federal Emergency Management
    Agency, 205
Humana, Inc., 94
National Institute of Standards &
    Technology, 206
Research Triangle Institute, 157

Claims Adjustment/Examination
Arizona Physicians IPA, Inc., 26
Blue Cross of Western
    Pennsylvania, 40

Blue Cross & Blue Shield of
    Colorado, 37
Blue Cross & Blue Shield of
    Georgia, 38
Blue Cross & Blue Shield of
    Minnesota, 38
Blue Cross & Blue Shield of
    Oregon, 39
Blue Cross & Blue Shield of
    Rochester Area, 39
Blue Cross & Blue Shield of
    Utica/Watertown, Inc., 40
Blue Cross & Blue Shield of
    Virginia, 40
Capital Blue Cross, Inc., 46
Central Massachusetts Health
    Care, 48
Cigna Healthplan of Texas, Inc.,
    North Texas Division, 54
Comprecare Health Care
    Services, 57
Dean Health Plan, Inc., 63
Employee Benefit Plans, Inc., 68
Ethix Healthcare Corporation, 69
Foundation Health, 73
Healthplus of Michigan, Inc., 87
Health Plan of Nevada, Inc., 85
HMO America, Inc., 89
Independence Blue Cross, 98
Intergroup Healthcare
    Corporation, 99
Johnson & Johnson Health
    Management, 103
Kaiser Permanente, Northeast
    Division Headquarters, 105
Keystone Health Plan East, Inc., 106
King County Medical Blue Shield
    Combined Services
    Northwest, 106
Living Center of America, Inc., 110
Midwest Foundation, 129
MVP Health Plan, 131
Ochsner Health Plan, 139
Pacificare of California, 143
Pierce County Medical Bureau, 149
Qual-Med Plans for Health, 155
Sanus Texas Health Plan, Inc., 172
Sierra Nevada Laboratories, 178
Take Care Health Plan, Inc., 189
United Insurance Companies, 194
US Healthcare, Inc., 196
Value Behavioral Health, Inc., 197

**Claims Processing/Management,
and Administration**
Blue Cross & Blue Shield Mutual of
    Ohio, 37
Central Massachusetts Health
    Care, 48
Focus Healthcare Management, 72
Medical Service Bureau of
    Idaho, 119

Ochsner Health Plan, 139
Oxford Health Plans, Inc., 142
Value Behavioral Health, Inc., 197

Clinical Accounting
HealthPro, 87
Pacificare of Texas, Inc., 143

Clinical Education
National Science Foundation, 206

Clinical Engineering
Evangelical Health Systems, 69
Marquette Electronics, Inc., 114
Servicemaster Company, 176

Clinical Nursing
Continental Health Affiliates,
    Inc., 58
Diabetes Treatment Centers of
    America, 64
Pacificare of California, 143

Clinical Psychology
Carrier Foundation, Inc., 47
C. R. Bard, Inc., 29
Mental Health Management,
    Inc., 123
Value Behavioral Health, Inc., 197
Vista Hill Foundation, 198

Clinical Research
Fisons Corporation, 72
HealthPro, 87
Syntex Corporation, 189
Whitby Pharmaceuticals, Inc., 201

Clinical Services
Blue Cross & Blue Shield of
    Maryland, 38
Electromedics, Inc., 67
Great Lakes Rehabilitation
    Hospital, 79
Kaiser Foundation Health Plan of
    Colorado, Inc., 104
Mental Health Management,
    Inc., 123
Monmouth Medical Center, 130
Occupational Health Services, 139

Clinical Technology
Boston Scientific Corporation, 41
Durham Regional Hospital, 65

Codependency Counseling
Occupational Health Services, 139

Communications
Blue Cross & Blue Shield of New
    Jersey, 39
Ciba-Geigy Corporation, 54

Electronics/Electronics Engineering

Emergency Medical Technology

Emergency Nursing

Emergency Services

Engineering

Manufacturing

Manufacturing Engineering

Richardson Electronics, Ltd., 159
Road Rescue, Inc., 160
Ryder International Corporation, 162
Safeskin Corporation, 163
Sage Products, Inc., 163
Saint Jude Medical, Inc., 168
Scanlan International, 173
Schneider (USA), Inc., 173
SERFILCO, Ltd., 175
Siebe North, Inc., 177
Siemens Medical Electronics, 177
Sopha Medical Systems, Inc., 181
Sorin Biomedical, Inc., 181
S&S X-Ray Products, Inc., 184
Storz Instrument Company, 185
Strato-Infusaid Corporation, 185
Styl-Rite Optical, 186
Superior Healthcare Group, Inc., 188
Surgimedics, Inc., 188
Tag Pharmaceuticals, Inc., 189
Target Therapeutics, Inc., 190
Taylor Company, 190
Tecnol Medical Products, Inc., 190
Tex-Tenn Corporation, 191
Toshiba America MRI, Inc., 192
True Quality Pharmacies, Inc., 193
Utah Medical Products, Inc., 197
Valleylab, Inc., 197
Vital Signs, Inc., 198
Waterloo Industries, Inc., 200
Wesley-Jessen, Inc., 200

Marketing

Abbott Laboratories, 17
Access Health Marketing, 17
Acufex Microsurgical, Inc., 17
Acuson Corporation, 17
Adventist Health Systems/ Sunbelt, 18
Allergan Medical Optics, Inc., 21
American Cyanamid Company, 22
American Family Assurance Collective, 23
American Health Services Corporation, 23
American Home Products, 23
American Medical Electronics, 23
American Medical International, 23
Amerihealth, Inc., 24
Amersham Medi-Physics, Inc., 24
AMRESCO, Inc., 25
Angelica Corporation, 25
Apothecare Products, Inc., 25
ARA Environmental Services, Inc., 25
Bard Access Systems, 29
Bard Patient Care Division, 30
Bausch & Lomb, Inc., 30
Baxter Diagnostics, 31
Baxter International, Inc., 31

Beckman Instruments, Inc., 32
Becton Dickinson, Acutecare Division, 32
Becton Dickinson, Consumer Products Division, 32
Becton Dickinson & Company, 32
Bennett X-Ray Corporation, 32
Berlex Laboratories, Inc., 33
Beverly Enterprises, Inc., 34
Big B, Inc., 34
Biomet, Inc., 35
Bissell Healthcare Corporation, 36
Block Drug Company, Inc., 36
Blue Care Network, Health Central, 37
Blue Cross of Western Pennsylvania, 40
Blue Cross & Blue Shield of Alabama, 37
Blue Cross & Blue Shield of Maryland, 38
Blue Cross & Blue Shield of Michigan, 38
Blue Cross & Blue Shield of Minnesota, 38
Blue Cross & Blue Shield of National Capitol Area, 38
Blue Cross & Blue Shield of New Jersey, 39
Blue Cross & Blue Shield of Texas, Inc., 39
Blue Cross & Blue Shield of Western New York, 40
Bon Secours Health Systems, 41
Boston Metal Products Corporation, 41
Boston Scientific Corporation, 41
Briggs Corporation, 42
Buckeye Discount, Inc., 43
California Physicians Service, 44
Camp International, Inc., 45
Capital Area Community Health Plan, 45
Caremark International, Inc., 46
Caremet, Inc., 46
Carrier Foundation, Inc., 47
Carrington Laboratories, Inc., 47
Central Pharmaceuticals, Inc., 48
Charter Hospital of Corpus Christi, 49
Charter Medical Corporation, 49
Chase Pharmaceutical Company, 50
Chicago HMO, Ltd., 50
Cigna Corporation, 54
CIS Technologies, Inc., 54
Clintec International, Inc., 55
Coastal Healthcare Group, Inc., 55
Cole Vision Corporation, 55
Colonial Life Accident Insurance, 56
Common Brothers, Inc., 56
Community Health Care Plan, 56

Comprehensive Addiction Programs, 57
Compuchem Laboratories, Inc., 57
CONMED Corporation, 58
Connaught Laboratories, Inc., 58
Cooper Development Company, 59
Corometrics Medical Systems, 60
Corvel Corporation, 60
CVS, Inc., 61
Cybex Division, 61
Dahlberg, Inc., 62
Denticare, 63
Depuy, Inc., 63
The Detroit Medical Center, 64
Devon Industries, Inc., 64
Diversicare Corporation America, 64
DLP/INRAD, Inc., 65
Durr Drug Company, 65
Eckerd Drugs of Texas, Inc., 66
E.G. Baldwin & Associates, Inc., 28
Electro-Biology, Inc., 66
Eli Lilly and Company, 67
Elkins-Sinn, Inc., 67
Empi, Inc., 68
EPI Corporation, 69
Ethix Healthcare Corporation, 69
Family Vision Centers, Inc., 71
Federal Trade Commission, 205
Ferno-Washington, Inc., 71
FHP Takecare, 71
First Hospital Corporation, 71
Fisher Hamilton Scientific, Inc., 72
Fisons Corporation, 72
Forest Pharmaceuticals, Inc., 72
Foster Medical Supply, Inc., 73
Franciscan Health System, Inc., 73
Fresenius USA, Inc., 74
Fujisawa USA, Inc., 74
Fuji Medical Systems USA, 74
Gaymar Industries, Inc., 75
GC America Company, 75
General Injectibles & Vaccines, 75
Genesis Health Ventures, Inc., 76
Gensia Pharmaceuticals, Inc., 76
Goldline Laboratories, Inc., 78
Graduate Hospital, 78
Graham Field, Inc., 78
Greenery Rehabilitation Group, 79
Group Health Northwest, 80
Guardian Life Insurance Company of America, 80
Hanger J.E., Inc. of Georgia, 101
Hannaford Brothers, 82
Harmac Medical Products, Inc., 82
Harris Labs, 82
Harvard Community Health Plan, 83
Hausmann Industries, Inc., 83
HCF, Inc., 84
Health-Chem Corporation, 84
Health-O-Meter Products, Inc., 85
Healthplus of Michigan, Inc., 87
HealthPro, 87

Medical Laboratory Technology

Medical Records

Veterans Memorial Medical Center, 198
Visiting Nurse Association of Greater Philadelphia, 198
Vista Hill Foundation, 198
Voluntary Hospitals of America, 199
Wake County Hospital System, 199
Warm Spring Rehabilitation Foundation, 199
Washington Adventist Hospital, 199
Washington Township Hospital District, 199
Washoe Medical Center, Inc., 200
West Jersey Health System Camden, 200
William Beaumont Hospital, 32
Winchester Medical Center, Inc., 201
Wuesthoff Memorial Hospital, 202
Wyckoff Heights Medical Center, 202
Yakima Valley Memorial Hospital Association, 203
Yale-New Haven Hospital, Inc., 203
Youville Hospital Rehabilitation Center, 203
Youville Hospital Rehabilitation Center, 203

Office Management
Western Dental Services, Inc., 200

Oncology
American Oncologic Hospital, 23
Carilion Health System, 46
Charleston Area Medical Center, 48
Charlotte Mecklenburg Hospital Authority, 49
Christ Hospital, 53
Grossmont Hospital Corporation, 79
Gundersen Clinic, Ltd., 80
Kimball Medical Center, 106
Manatee Memorial Hospital, 113
Mercy Health Services, Inc., 123
Monmouth Medical Center, 130
Montefiore Medical Center, 130
NEDH Corporation, 134
Oakwood Hospital Corporation, 139
Ochsner Alton Medical Foundation, 139
Richland Memorial Hospital, 159
Rockford Memorial Hospital, 161
Saint Francis Hospital, Inc., 166
Saint Joseph's Hospital, 167
Saint Luke's Hospital of Bethlehem, Pennsylvania, 168
Saint Luke's Regional Medical Center, 169
Saint Mary's Hospital, 169
Salick Health Care, Inc., 172
Sharp Health Care, 176
Society of New York Hospital, Inc., 180

Stormont Vail Health Services Corporation, 185
Timken Mercy Medical Center, 192
Winthrop University Hospital, 201
Women & Infants Hospital of Rhode Island, 202

Operating Room
Brooklyn Hospital Center, Inc., 43
Children's Memorial Hospital, 51
Detroit-Macomb Hospital Corporation, 64
Maine Medical Center, 113
Mercy Hospital, Inc., 124
Middlesex Hospital, 128
Saint Mary's Hospital, 169
Saint Patrick Hospital, 170

Operations
Bindley Western Industries, 34
Blue Cross & Blue Shield of New Jersey, 39
Diabetes Treatment Centers of America, 64
Harlan Sprague Dawley, Inc., 82
Homedco Group, Inc., 91
Innovative Healthcare Systems, 98
Kimberly-Clark Corporation, 106
KV Pharmaceutical Company, 107
Marion Merrell Dow Pharmaceuticals, 114
McNeil Consumer Products, 116
Mercy Children's Hospital, 123
Oxford Health Plans, Inc., 142

Ophthalmological Engineering
Alcon Surgical, Inc., 20
America's Best Contacts & Eyeglasses, 22
Benson Optical Company, Inc., 33
Chiron Corporation, 53
Kaiser Foundation Health Plan of Colorado, Inc., 104
Storz Instrument Company, 185

Ophthalmology
Empire Vision Center, 68
Health Care Plan, Inc., 84
Optical Radiation Corporation, 140
Optical Radiation Corporation, 141

Optics
Allergan Medical Optics, Inc., 21
America's Best Contacts & Eyeglasses, 22
Benson Eyecare Corporation, 33
Benson Optical Company, Inc., 33
Chiron Vision, Inc., 53
Circon Corporation, 54
Family Vision Centers, Inc., 71
Newport Corporation, 136
NuVision, Inc., 139

Omega Optical Company, Inc., 140
Optical Radiation Corporation, 141
Optometric Eyecare Centers, 141
Polymer Technology Corporation, 150
Southern Optical Company, 182
Viva Optique, Inc., 198
Wesley-Jessen, Inc., 200
Western Optical Corporation, 201

Optometry
America's Best Contacts & Eyeglasses, 22
Benson Eyecare Corporation, 33
Benson Optical Company, Inc., 33
Family Vision Centers, Inc., 71
Group Health Northwest, 80
Kaiser Foundation Health Plan of Colorado, Inc., 104
Meyrowitz Opticians, 127
NuVision, Inc., 139
Optometric Eyecare Centers, 141
Renaissance Eyewear, Inc., 157
Viva Optique, Inc., 198

Orthopedics
Charleston Area Medical Center, 48
Gaston Memorial Hospital, Inc., 74
Hanger Orthopedic Group, Inc., 81
Hospital for Joint Diseases, 92
Orthopaedic Hospital, 141
Osteonics Corporation, 142
Rockford Memorial Hospital, 161
Saint Francis Hospital, Inc., 166
Saint Joseph's Hospital, 167
Saint Luke's Regional Medical Center, 169
Stormont Vail Health Services Corporation, 185

Packaging Engineering
BioWhittaker, Inc., 36
Fujisawa USA, Inc., 74
L & F Products, Inc., 107
Marion Merrell Dow, Inc., 114
Medco Containment Services, Inc., 117
Phoenix Products Company, Inc., 148
Rhone-Poulenc Rorer Pharmaceuticals, 158
Saint Jude Medical, Inc., 168

Pathology
Associated Regional University Pathologists, 27
Kaiser Foundation Health Plan, 104
Mercy Hospital, Inc., 124
Saint Elizabeth Medical Center, 165

Hu-Friedy Manufacturing Company, Inc., 93
I Care Industries, Inc., 95
The Jackson Laboratory, 101
Neuromed, Inc., 135
Perrigo Company, 146
Siemens Hearing Instruments, Inc., 177
Siemens Medical Electronics, 177
Steris Laboratories, Inc., 184
Sutter Corporation, 188
USA Namic Corporation, 196

Production Control
Bausch & Lomb Pharmaceutical Division, 30

Production Engineering
Boston Metal Products Corporation, 41
Cordis Corporation, 59
Nature's Sunshine Products, Inc., 134
Promega Corporation, 154
Utah Medical Products, Inc., 197

Production Management
Microtek Medical, Inc., 128

Product Design and Development
American Medical Electronics, 23
Bear Medical Systems, Inc., 32
Colonial Life Accident Insurance, 56
DLP/INRAD, Inc., 65
Helena Plastics, 88
Hybritech, Inc., 94
Mark Clark Products, 114
Nellcor, Inc., 134
Nordictrack, Inc., 137
Osteonics Corporation, 142
Paco Pharmaceutical Services, Inc., 143
Promega Corporation, 154
Puritan-Bennett Corporation, 154
Starkey Laboratories, Inc., 184
Tecnol Medical Products, Inc., 190

Product Design Engineering
AMSCO International, Inc., 25
Helena Plastics, 88

Product Engineering
Bissell Healthcare Corporation, 36
Cordis Corporation, 59
Medical Data Electronics, Inc., 119
Micropump Corporation, 128
Promega Corporation, 154

Product Management
Nalge Company, 132

Program Analysis
Biosym Technologies, Inc., 35
Blue Cross & Blue Shield of Western New York, 40
Capital Blue Cross, Inc., 46
CSC Healthcare Systems, Inc., 61
Elliot Hospital, 67
Encore Associates, Inc., 68
Foundation Health, 73
IDX Corporation, 95
Living Center of America, Inc., 110
Owen Healthcare, Inc., 142
Phamis, Inc., 147
Primecare Health Plan, Inc., 153

Project Engineering
Ciba Vision Corporation, 54
Diabetes Treatment Centers of America, 64
Harmac Medical Products, Inc., 82
Johnson & Johnson Medical, Inc., 103
McGaw, Inc., 116
Medtronic, Inc., 121
Micropump Corporation, 128
National Medical Care, Inc., 133
USA Namic Corporation, 196

Project Management
Healthdyne Technologies, Inc., 87
National Healthtech Corporation, 133
Paco Pharmaceutical Services, Inc., 143
Rhone-Poulenc Rorer Pharmaceuticals, 158
Small Business Administration, 206

Prosthetics
Hanger Orthopedic Group, Inc., 81

Psychiatric Nursing
Newton Wellesley Hospital, 136

Psychiatric Social Work
Carrier Foundation, Inc., 47
Charter Hospital of Corpus Christi, 49
Sierra Tucson Companies, 178
U.S. Behavioral Health, 196
Value Behavioral Health, Inc., 197

Psychiatry
Carrier Foundation, Inc., 47
Charter Fairmount Institute, 49
Charter Real, Inc., 49
Charter Westbrook Hospital, 49
Christian Health Care Center, 53
Greenleaf Health Systems, Inc., 79
Innovative Healthcare Systems, 98
Introspect Healthcare Corporation, 100

Menninger Foundation, Inc., 122
Mental Health Management, Inc., 123
North Central Health Care Facility, 137
Sheppard and Enoch Pratt Hospital, 177
Silver Hill Hospital, Inc., 178
Winchester Medical Center, Inc., 201

Psychology
Charter Fairmount Institute, 49
Charter Real, Inc., 49
Charter Westbrook Hospital, 49
Christian Health Care Center, 53
Gaston Memorial Hospital, Inc., 74
Glens Falls Hospital, 77
Group Health Northwest, 80
HealthCare Rehabilitation Center, 86
Introspect Healthcare Corporation, 100
Maimonides Medical Center, Inc., 113
Menninger Foundation, Inc., 122
North Central Health Care Facility, 137
NovaCare, Inc., 138
Palomar Pomerado Health System, 144
Preferred Health Care, Ltd., 151
Rivendell of America, Inc., 159
Sheppard and Enoch Pratt Hospital, 177
Silver Hill Hospital, Inc., 178
Vista Hill Foundation, 198
Warm Spring Rehabilitation Foundation, 199

Psychotherapy
Carrier Foundation, Inc., 47
Mercy Hospital, Inc., 124
Sierra Tucson Companies, 178
U.S. Behavioral Health, 196
Vista Hill Foundation, 198

Public Administration
American Medical Systems, Inc., 23

Public Affairs
Office of Management & Budget, 206

Public Policy and Planning
Office of Management & Budget, 206

Public Relations
American Home Products, 23
Toshiba America Medical Systems, Inc., 192

Radio Frequency Engineering

Real Estate

Registered Nursing

Respiratory Care

Respiratory Technology

Respiratory Therapy

Retail

Risk Management

Safety Engineering

Sales

Peterson's Job Opportunities in Health Care 1995

Buy this copy of *Job Opps '95*. Then—
Send For Your <u>FREE</u> Book!

Just complete and return one of these cards to receive your FREE book.

Choose

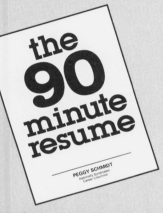

Fresh, Innovative Approach To A Troublesome Task

Or

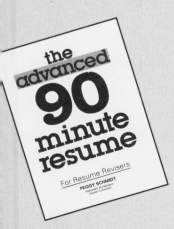

Transforms That Resume From Adequate To Dynamite

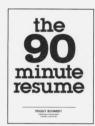

The 90-Minute Resume
by Peggy Schmidt

Turns resume writing into an enjoyable project that can truly show results! This updated best-seller helps test resume expertise, presents resume "makeovers," and offers suggestions for getting your resume to decision makers.

ISBN 1-56079-150-0, 127 pages, 6 x 9, $7.95 value, pb, **2nd edition**

Yes! I have purchased *Job Opps '95*.

Please send me my FREE copy of
The 90-Minute Resume *

I am enclosing my receipt for *Job Opps '95*.

I understand that I must pay shipping/handling of $2.50.

Date_____ Tel. (_____)_____

Ship to: _____

Address:_____

City:_____

State:_____ Zip:_____

Method of payment: Payable to "Peterson's"

___Check or money order for $2.50 enclosed.

* Offer good while supplies last. Not to be combined with any other discount offer.

Please return this completed order form to:
Peterson's, Dept. MM9408, P.O. Box 2123, Princeton, NJ 08543-2123
Call toll-free: 1-800-338-3282

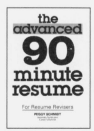

The Advanced 90-Minute Resume
by Peggy Schmidt

Warm, personal advice helps you analyze your current resume for maximum impact. For both business professionals changing careers and those with non-traditional career paths.

ISBN 1-56079-151-9, 126 pages, 6 x 9, $7.95 value, pb

Yes! I have purchased *Job Opps '95*.

Please send me my FREE copy of
The Advanced 90-Minute Resume *

I am enclosing my receipt for *Job Opps '95*.

I understand that I must pay shipping/handling of $2.50.

Date_____ Tel. (_____)_____

Ship to: _____

Address:_____

City:_____

State:_____ Zip:_____

Method of payment: Payable to "Peterson's"

___Check or money order for $2.50 enclosed.

* Offer good while supplies last. Not to be combined with any other discount offer.

Please return this completed order form to:
Peterson's, Dept. MM9408, P.O. Box 2123, Princeton, NJ 08543-2123
Call toll-free: 1-800-338-3282

*Please enclose in an envelope along
with your sales receipt for* **Job Opps '95**
*and your payment of $2.50 for shipping
and handling, and mail to:*

Peterson's
P.O. Box 2123
Princeton, NJ 08543-2123

*Please enclose in an envelope along
with your sales receipt for* **Job Opps '95**
*and your payment of $2.50 for shipping
and handling, and mail to:*

Peterson's
P.O. Box 2123
Princeton, NJ 08543-2123